Notice to the Reader

The opinions and conclusions expressed in this book are mine, and unless indicated otherwise, mine alone. They are based on my scientific research and on specific case studies involving my patients. Be advised that every person is unique and may respond differently to the treatments described in this book. On occasion I have provided dosage recommendations. Again, remember that we are all different and any new treatment should be applied in a cautious, common sense way.

The treatments outlined herein are not intended to be a substitute for other forms of conventional medical treatment. In fact, they are completely compatible. Please feel free to consult with your physician or other health care provider.

I have indicated throughout this book the existence of pollutants in food and other products. These pollutants were identified using a testing device of my invention known as the Syncrometer®. Complete instructions for building and using this device are contained in the *Syncrometer® Science Laboratory Manual*. Therefore anyone can repeat the tests described and verify the data.

The Syncrometer® is more accurate and versatile than the best existing testing methods. A method for determining the degree of precision is also presented (in the *Manual*). However at this point it only yields **Positive** or **Negative** results, it does not quantify. The chance of a false **Positive** or a false **Negative** is about 5%, which can be lessened by test repetition.

It is in the public interest to know when a single bottle of a product tests **Positive** to a serious pollutant. If one does, the safest course is to avoid all bottles of that product entirely, which is what I repeatedly advise. These recommendations should be interpreted as intent to warn and protect the public, not to provide a statistically significant analysis. It is my fervent hope that manufacturers use the new electronic techniques in this book to make purer products than they ever have before.

The Prevention Of All Cancers

Published in the United States by:
New Century Press
1055 Bay Blvd., Ste. C
Chula Vista, CA 91911
www.newcenturypress.com

ISBN 1-890035-34-3
Other books by Dr. Clark available from New Century Press:
- *The Cure For All Cancers*
      (English, German, Italian, Japanese)
- *The Cure For All Diseases*
      (English, Dutch, Finnish, German, Italian, Polish, Russian, Spanish)
- *The Cure For All Advanced Cancers*
      (English, German, Italian)
- *Syncrometer® Science Laboratory Manual*

Your Invitation

This book is about a completely self-sufficient cancer curing therapy that can be carried out by the patient at home at fairly low cost. It seldom requires medical care before it is diagnosed.

Scurvy was once a dreaded disease, as much as cancer is today. Even the CA-word strikes terror in many of us. Now we know that scurvy is a simple vitamin C deficiency disease. It doesn't even require medical care as it always did in the past. It is noteworthy that all the medical care given at that time did not save the scurvy patient. It was palliative. But the women of a Native American Indian tribe, the Iroquois, knew how to cure, not just treat this disease. And to do it quickly, in days.

This is an excerpt from the personal journal of Jacques Cartier, the early French explorer.

> *Thus it was that we lost 25 of our best men to the dreaded sickness. There were another forty who were at the point of death and the remainder, except two or three, were all gravely ill...People from Stadacone... among whom was Agaya...responded that...the liquid and residue from the leaves of a tree...was the sole cure for the illness...Two women...gathered nine or ten branches...to boil them in water...Drink the water every other day...It...turned out to be a miracle... they were cured and restored to health after having drunk the brew only two or three times...After all that, the crew was ready to kill to get to the medicine. This wonderful tree has done in less than a week what all the physicians of Louvain and Montpellier, using all the drugs of Alexandria, would not be able to accomplish in a year...Winter–1535.*

It took 400 years from the discovery of its cure (1535) to the use of the cure by the public in the early 1900's. Yet it had even been published in <u>medical journals</u> many times[1]. Today, we all know how to prevent, not just cure this dreadful disease: eat fresh fruit and vegetables. It is not <u>medical</u> advice. It is nutritional. It took the unrelated <u>orange juice industry</u>, not the medical profession, to bring it to the public's attention in the early 1900's.

Why did it take so long to put into practice a simple cure, the eating of fresh fruit and vegetables? The medical profession was waiting for absolute "proof" on its own "scientific" terms. The cure was called "controversial" by medical professionals, giving it a bad reputation. Sick persons and their families would not have waited to resolve professional or commercial conflicts. Their priorities hold life dearer than financial interests, or analytical reasoning. And ordinary people, not able

[1] Davies, M.B., Austin, J., Partridge, D.A., *Vitamin C, Its Chemistry and Biochemistry,* Royal Society of Chemistry, 1991, chapter 2

to read the medical journals, had no way to even learn about the controversy.

If they had, they would have tried the controversial cure, since that could do no harm and in a few months would have resolved the controversy. Why didn't the doctors do this, just try it? Success would have meant an instant reduction in the number of doctors per ship, from a minimum of two, to one.

It was in the professionals' interest to keep the cure and even the controversy over it <u>out</u> of the hands of the public, "lest they injure themselves with an unproven treatment". The public was held hostage by its medical professionals.

Unless the public has access to the great truths uncovered by scientists, they cannot learn them even now. Books and computers are making it possible for the first time in history.

In this book the true beginning of cancer will be described. From this the first true prevention program can arise.

Cancer as an epidemic is now 100 years old. Some of its true causes were already known 100 years ago, like parasites (in several animals)[2], coal tar,[3] synthetic dyes,[4] and improperly prepared foods.[5] But these discoveries have been ignored rather than treasured, as befell the scurvy cure.

Scientific research pursued a course of finding <u>carcinogens</u> for animal and bacterial models instead of in its real victims, the human race. This was in spite of a warning by Jesse Greenstein, a widely respected cancer researcher, and others in the 1940s <u>not</u> to pursue carcinogens because it would be endless and useless. It certainly did lead to an explosion of research data, altogether overwhelming with promise, but none of it really relevant. By implanting or injecting tumor cells or

---

[2] A good discussion of this topic (more than just dogs) is by Bailey, W.S., *Parasites and Cancer: Sarcoma in Dogs Associated with Spirocerca lupi,* Annals Of the New York Academy of Sciences, v. 108, 1963, pp. 890-923

[3] Greenstein, Jesse P., *Biochemistry of Cancer,* 2nd ed., Academic Press Inc., 1954, pp. 44-56

[4] Ibid., pp. 88-96

[5] Lane, A., Blickenstaff, D., and A.C. Ivy, *The Carcinogenicity of Fat "Browned" by Heating,* Cancer, v. 3, 1950, pp. 1044-51

by working with special transformed culture lines, the beginnings of cancer were already lost. This is not how we get our cancers. Hopelessness then gave birth to the current new direction in research, supplying corrective genes. This in itself is a huge, population-wide human experiment. This time it misses not only the true cause of cancer, but also the mutagens that damage the genes. It seems unwise as an overall strategy.

Hopefully the age of computers will now set free the bird of truth as was never before possible. Patients and their families have easy access to information just like doctors and researchers do.

Only when each layperson and common laborer possess the knowledge about cancer prevention, as they already do for scurvy prevention, will the medical profession stop claiming an exclusive right to cancer treatment. It will no longer be lucrative. Till then its power to restrict and hold hostage the patient will continue. At present this power seems quite misplaced, since medical professionals know neither how cancer begins nor how it progresses. In the future, preventing cancer, like preventing scurvy will not generate high incomes for anybody. Nor will herbal and natural treatments. These therapies will fall to lay health advisers and lay nutritionists. It will be a huge step of progress for humanity.

But making practical use of this new knowledge still depends on wisdom, something that we all have and all lack to some degree.

An example of wisdom for an individual might be changing daily habits before cancer strikes and certainly after, such as improving diet, stopping addictions, and being especially protective of the immune system.

An example of wisdom for the medical profession would be analyzing tumors for the immunity destroyers they contain. Then searching for the same items in the patient's environment, the water, food, cookware and dentalware. Such tests were prohibitively expensive even 10 years ago. Now they are not. A test for PCBs in the drinking water can cost less than $200.00.

The dye, DAB (butter yellow), is known to cause much too high alkaline phosphatase levels in animals. Many cancer patients show high alkaline phosphatase levels. An example of wisdom would be to search for this dye in the white blood cells of these cancer patients. The LDH enzyme can reach sky-high levels in cancer patients, too. This is due to Sudan Black B dye accumulated in the red blood cells. When cobalt has accumulated in these cell types, the enzyme levels are too low instead of too high. With so many dyed foods in the market place and so many heavy metals in our drinking water, cancer patients should be studied for their dye and metal exposure.

To my knowledge such studies have not been done, nor do I see evidence of these rational approaches. Here is another example. Scientists know that broken chromosomes are characteristic of nearly every cancer.[6,7] This means there is extreme genetic damage. They also know that heavy metals, like copper, cadmium, and the lanthanides ("rare earths") cause chromosomes to break.[8] Yet doctors do not send biopsy specimens to a lab for heavy metal analysis! If they did, they would be in a position to search for the patient's source of these mutagenic metals and to advise chelation therapy. EDTA (ethylenediaminetetraacetate) chelation removes heavy metals from the body. Patients should remove heavy metals from dentalware, cookware, plastic ware used for food, eyeglass frames, wristwatches and jewelry, water pipes, and the water itself. The cost of metal analysis is now so low and the test itself so sensitive, no biopsy specimen or drinking water sample should be untested.

---

[6] Weiss, L.M., Warnke, R.A., Sklar, J., Cleary, M.L., *Molecular Analysis of the Chromosomal Translocation in Malignant Lymphomas, (14;18)* N. Eng. Jour. Med., v. 317, no. 19, 1987, pp. 1185-89

[7] Warrell, R.P., et al., *Differentiation Therapy of Acute Promyelocytic Leukemia with Tretinoin (All-Trans-Retinoic Acid),* N. Eng. Jour. Med., v. 324, no. 20, 1991, pp. 1385-93

[8] Komiyama, Makoto, *Sequence-Specific and Hydrolytic Scission of DNA and RNA by Lanthanide Complex-Oligo DNA Hybrids,* J. Biochem, v. 118, no. 4, 1995, pp. 665-70

Ordinary laypersons have a great deal of wisdom. This book will help you to practice and express your own wisdom. Your instincts and questions are well worth pursuing. You can build the same investigative tool that I have used: instructions are in *Cure for all Cancers* and in the *Syncrometer® Science Laboratory Manual*. Your discoveries and experience, together with others', are valuable and very much needed. When wisdom is accumulated, it can contribute to a <u>new</u> bank of information for persons in the future that face the same dilemma that you may have faced. Solutions can be found by communicating and listening to others in similar predicaments. It is my cherished belief that in this way you and others can solve human health problems that lie languishing as orphans as well as our most common ones.

I invite you to do so.

And a special invitation goes out to younger readers. Building the electronic device and searching for cause and effect in all the health problems your family suffers from could stir the heart of any of us who are detectives in spirit. It is much more important than finding a name for an illness. Finding a name is diagnosis. That can be left to doctors. It does not contribute to the study of health. We will be analysts: nutritionists, chiropractors, homeopaths, massage therapists, engineers, biologists, naturopaths, cell physiologists, veterinarians, medical doctors, physicists, dentists, and plain hobbyists, all with a common goal: to analyze our problems, find causes that can be removed, and to improve the health of others and ourselves. That is the essence of <u>curing</u>.

Challenge to Students

This whole book is just one chapter of a very long detective story that began over 100 years ago. Nobody knows why we suddenly develop a lump, then more lumps, all of them growing and spreading like mold on a loaf of bread. This book is about detecting parasite eggs and stages in these lumps, of the most unexpected varieties. Imagine finding a coiled up dog heartworm in every abdominal mass and Hodgkin's lymphoma mass! Imagine finding aluminum holding it all together!

We can detect parasites, bacteria and viruses in many places inside our own bodies, which we always thought was nearly sterile! Some of these cause cancers. Some cause other health problems.

But can't this be done everyday by any doctor or scientist in a laboratory? Yes! But for them it is laborious, costly, and takes years. Their results are unreliable and must wait to be repeated for about another 10 years! They are based on chemistry, immunology, and microbiology, all very difficult and expensive. The electronic method we will use for the studies in this book takes minutes and is highly reliable. But you must train yourself, just as you once did to use a computer or to ride a bike.

Present day medical science does not approach cancer or other disease in the rational way described here. Partly because of the difficulty, and partly because of the cost.

So, instead, chemicals are snatched off the shelves, and tried one after another, to see "what they can do" for some disease! This is inefficient to the extreme and ultimately much more costly. There is almost nothing to show for 100 years of such random research when true detective work could have yielded much more.

My detective device is a new invention. It is an electronic circuit that detects resonance in much the same way a radio does. In your radio a distant frequency produced in a studio is matched to a frequency you produce in your set. The new device used for these experiments matches a frequency produced in your body with one you place on a capacitor plate. Although the new device is simple to build it is much more advanced in principle than a voltmeter. A voltmeter is almost the only device that has ever been used to make electrical measurements in the body. Electrical studies of the human body have lagged far behind other fields. Measuring the voltages of the heart gives us the EKG. Voltages of the brain give us the EEG. There is also a magnetometer that can make magnetic measurements of the body. The newly invented device described here scans for anything in the body—be it an object, an organ, a chemical or virus because everything has a characteristic frequency or set of frequencies. And the capacitance of any body part is easily influenced. The device is so simple to build that even girls and boys can build it. And I hope you do.

Girls and boys have often become radio amateur operators in their teen years. It is not beyond your skill level. Nor beyond your level to learn its uses. With this new technology you will be led into the secret world of the inner body. Not it's outside appearances but the strange inner workings. These have never been seen, heard or measured before. A whole inner world is waiting to be explored. Whether it's the brain or heart or skin, you can go on a detective hunt for what is really going on there. You can search for answers to profound questions. Why did your brother or sister develop a "bad gene"? Why did you develop a little brown spot on your face—or a little red blister on your leg? What is a freckle? Why is your dad beginning to go bald? Why is your grandmother getting pain in her fingers? These are all detective stories waiting to be told, waiting for the detective in you to feel the urge to find the villains.

I call my new device a Syncrometer®. You can build it or buy it. Building it is by far the best. Then you know how it works and can troubleshoot it in minutes at no cost.

You put yourself into the circuit and hear your resistance change as you tune the circuit to different frequency patterns. When you find a pattern that matches yours, a huge current flows that you can hear on a loudspeaker. Any two places you touch on the body can be eavesdropped. A resistance change between them can be heard. It does this by amplifying a signal through an ordinary, inexpensive PNP transistor.

You can tune your Syncrometer® to any organ by placing it on the open capacitor plate, even the genes themselves. You can hear a Herpes virus coming out of the chromosomes. You can hear an enzyme coming out of a gene. You can hear DNA going about its business of transcription. You can hear a CD4 type of white blood cell capture an HIV virus. Will the virus get killed or the cell? Or will it be a standoff? There are telltale signs you can use to eavesdrop on this battle. Simply detecting what is there at any given moment and watching this change with time, gives data beyond anyone's imagination.

You can learn the new Syncrometer® mathematics and find that frequencies rule your body in some yet mysterious way. Maybe you will find the energy sources of these frequencies. Maybe you will find the perfect antidote against any intruder in your body by using this arithmetic. Why does your body add, subtract, multiply and divide these frequencies like regular radio signals? Why does all life come from life? Is the secret in these frequencies? Can they only be handed on (transmitted), not created? Or are they created in the recesses of our mitochondria? Could they have come from outer space? Could they be replaced or duplicated, or at least patched up when the body is sick? Could you find the antidotes to new diseases appearing in our population by searching for missing frequencies?

The world of life is full of too many mysteries to even ask the right questions. But those who <u>think</u> and explore will be rewarded. Applying chemistry was once very rewarding to biologists when it first began. But now it is a slow and costly pathway to find truths. The electronic method gets a whole host of research results in an hour. Best of all, you can make all the research plans yourself.

You are invited to become a Syncrometer® detective. Learn basic electronics from a beginner's amateur radio manual. Scout out this hobby at a Radio Shack store. See how easy it is. Get an amateur radio license while you're at it, though it is not

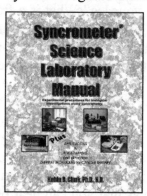

ISBN 1-890035-17-3

*Fig. 1 The underlying science for my "**curing**" books*

essential. Start building electronic kits, and build from scratch. This is a hobby that reaches ages 18 to 80! Use my *Syncrometer® Science Laboratory Manual* to launch your new detective profession. Maybe you can move this beginning science forward to automation or to a whole new application.

Just be sure to write your detective story in a notebook as you unravel mysteries, the way I have done. If 10 students with 10 home-built Syncrometers® wrote 10 such detective stories, and contacted the other nine to form a special Syncrometer® club for students, you could <u>REALLY</u> begin to rescue this planet!

RSVP
The author

Keep in mind a quote from the discoverer of vitamin C:
"Research means going out into the unknown with the hope of finding something new to bring home. If you know in advance what you are going to do, or even to find there, then it is not research at all: then it is only a kind of honorable occupation."

—*Albert Szent-Gyorgyi*
(1893-1986)

To the Cancer Patient

This book is meant for the complete novice.

Even though you have never taken an herb, never used an electrical device, never taken supplements, and know nothing about homeography, you can protect yourself and even get yourself well from this dreadful disease.

All you need is a determination to get well and keep well. You need the intelligence to follow instructions carefully, and the good fortune to have a friend or family who loves you and will help.

It is not incompatible with any other method, clinical or non-clinical. In fact, it would be profoundly helpful.

This book does not have detailed explanations for the advice given, only general explanations. For the details go to *The Cure For All Cancers* book and *The Cure For All Advanced Cancers* book, as well as the *Syncrometer® Science Laboratory Manual*[9], all by this author

Although this book is non-technical, details can be important, especially if you have scientific-minded friends and doctors, who would like to understand why you are advised to make certain changes or take certain things. The underlying science has been recorded in the *Syncrometer® Science Laboratory Manual* so others can repeat it. The essence of science is repeatability. They, as well as you, may wish to analyze and compare my interpretations with others'.

---

[9] New Century Press, www.newcenturypress.com

It is important, too, to have some perspective on the last 100 years of cancer treatment. Reading books like *The Cancer Cure That Worked* and others[10] will give you this perspective.

In reading these books you might feel frustration, and wonder how so many alternative therapies could exist, with such widely different approaches, and yet seeming to claim they had found the one cause and solution for cancer. They saw <u>their</u> patients recover by removing this one cause. Of course they had also <u>changed</u> the diet, water, and residence of their patients. The concept was certainly flawed, that for every single disease there is a single cause, but it seemed so to them. When a chain of causes is responsible for a disease, removing a single <u>one</u> can seem to be the only one. Their findings were nevertheless valid, being science and experience based. Today, we can fit their findings into this chain. Many of us still suffer from the same wrong concepts. When you read this cancer book you will be in awe of cancers' great complexity. I could easily see how very important each early therapist's work was. It contributed to my ideas and others'. They gave a lifetime of dedication and service to American society and science. They did it without a research budget, without a Syncrometer®, and often harassed and scorned. Their writings should be gathered up to be commemorated for their true worth. Their contributions are priceless.

---

[10] Lynes, Barry and Crane, John, *The Cancer Cure That Worked!* Marcus Books, 1987; Livingston-Wheeler, MD, Virginia and Addeo, Edmond G., *The Conquest of Cancer, Vaccines and Diet,* New York, F. Watts, 1984, Chicago, Advanced Century Pub. Co. 1978; Manner, Harold W., DiSanti, Steven and Michalsen, Thomas, *The Death of Cancer*, Cancer Book House, June 1979; Koch, William F., *Natural Immunity, www.williamfkoch.com;* Gerson, MD, Max, *A Cancer Therapy, Results of Fifty Cases,* New York, Whittier Books 1958; Bradford, R., Culbert, M.L., Allen, H.W., *International Protocols For Individualized, Integrated Metabolic Programs In Cancer Management,* 2nd ed., The Robert W. Bradford Foundation, 1983; Krebs Jr, Ernst T. *A collection of papers bearing on the Unitarian or Trophoblastic Fact of Cancer and related works on Metabolic Therapy,* http://www.navi.net/~rsc/krebsall.htm

Using a natural method like mine, and those of earlier therapists, is vastly more important than simply using a clinical method, even though the clinical method is quicker and does not interfere with your lifestyle. A natural method puts you in control of your own health. It reaches into your lifestyle to show you causes of your diseases, causes that you could abolish. It reaches into the environmental causes that need change. It gives you the confidence that you are not just relying on a doctor's promise that "he got it all" in surgery or his or her implication that you could not be struck again.

You may wish to combine this natural method with other natural methods or with a clinical method. There is no conflict between natural and clinical methods. In fact, a natural method added to a standard clinical method should raise the success percentages of clinical treatments astronomically. But your clinician may prefer that you do not take vitamins or herbs or other alternative treatments. This is usually advised from a position of ignorance. We must never lump "vitamins" or "alternative treatments" together as if they did the same thing. Each has individual action and should be individually evaluated for your situation. You could copy the page from the earlier *Cure For All Advanced Cancers* book, with the reference cited that discusses the issue of vitamin taking, and even provide a copy of the research article.[11] Your oncologist may appreciate this gesture. He or she will have a better standing with their peers with this new knowledge, especially after you recover.

One of the main objectives in this book is to reach as many persons as possible with the new knowledge about preventing cancer. And reaching those without access to natural health care, without access to the accumulation of health-related knowledge that already exists. It stretches back over thousands of years! They need to hear the good news that the true causes of cancer have been found, although not published in the

---

[11] Jaakkola, K., et al., *Treatment with Antioxidant and other Nutrients in Combination with Chemotherapy and Irradiation in Patients with Small-Cell Lung Cancer,* Anticancer Research, v. 12, 1992, pp. 599-606

standard scientific journals. Publishing here must wait till the subject is depoliticized. People need to hear that a recipe for prevention as well as cure has been developed that is within their reach, their capability and their finances. These recipes invite innovation; they are open to change as experience is gathered.

The discoveries described in this book create a scientific basis for a cure, in fact, more than one cure. There are always more ways than one to accomplish a task.

Now that health has a scientific path to follow and a device to monitor it, health could become a reality for all of society. We could put cancer "to rest", beside scurvy. Only reaching the afflicted, far and wide, will accomplish this.

Choosing your Program

For Beginning Cancers

If you <u>now have</u> a beginning cancer, with just a small tumor, less than the size of a marble, you may be able to clear it up with the simple program given in the first book, *The Cure For All Cancers*. Many patients reported that they did. But in that program we stopped only the <u>malignancy</u> part of the tumor. Then we went on a major clean up program for your lifestyle. Your teeth, your diet, your home and your body products were all cleared thoroughly from those things that burden your immune system. After this your own immune power returned to remove the tumor without clinical help. You were advised to stay on a *Maintenance Program* of killing parasites regularly and keeping a clean environment. That was ten years ago.

If you <u>once had</u> a beginning cancer and tumors went away without help from a more drastic, clinical method, you know you did the right things then. Nevertheless, you should remember that you WERE TARGETED. You were targeted by a specific parasite, specific bacteria and a specific virus. Your immune system rescued you even while you neglected many important things. That is the magic (not yet understood) power of the immune system. But once targeted, you can never be "untargeted". To live safely past the five-year mark and have a NORMAL lifespan you will <u>always</u> need to kill these former invaders regularly and protect your immune system. You may have done nothing about your dentalware or water supply. But luck does not last. It is an insecure way to live. You should add the new prevention path described in this book.

If you did require the help of clinical doctors at one time, you are even less secure. Your cancer is bound to find a new organ to grow in. Use all the advice in this book to prevent a recurrence.

Cancer recurs because it is a <u>systemic</u> disease based on immunodepression. It can be compared to mold developing in a loaf of bread or termites entering a house. Once you see these, it is already far past the beginning and almost too late. The whole loaf and the whole house are at risk, not just where the trouble was spotted. Organ and body destruction, which happen in cancer, may <u>appear</u> to be stopped. But they may have merely moved to another location or be having their ups and downs. The disease can never be trusted even if you were told by the surgeon "they got it all". The recurrence will not be noticed until it has become advanced. Hurry, to put your prevention program in place before cancer surfaces again.

If you choose the beginners' program from *The Cure For All Cancers*, be sure to add the prevention program described in this book. It is newly discovered. Never before has there been a way to prevent cancer with certainty.

Also be sure to give yourself time limits and objective tests, such as cancer markers and scans, so you know with certainty how effective your chosen program is for you. Avoid x-rays if possible, they are too damaging. Substitute ultrasounds where possible. If x-rays are necessary, use as few exposures as possible, not dozens. If scans are used avoid being injected with dyes, lanthanides (like gadolinium), or radio-activity (like technetium) to make you "glow" on the *Negative*. It makes no sense to inject more immunodepressants, the very cause of the whole disease! The scanning industry has taken on a life of its own, with less regard for yours. Certainly, it is easier to see a detail, but details in minutiae seldom count. Find a cooperative doctor with conservative, least invasive methods, but with realism. In other countries (Europe) you can request these tests yourself. Society's health is better served with such freedoms, without paying extra "middlemen" for referrals when not needed (see *Sources*).

For Advanced Cancers

If you have a cancer recurrence, or a tumor has started in a second organ, you should consider yourself advanced. Compare yourself to the loaf of bread with its second visible green mold spot. You must snatch this loaf and clean it up immediately, this very minute if you treasure it, and then freeze it, which changes its environment. You have no time to lose. You are entered in a race, not of your choosing. The race is between your cancer and your immune system. Can the tumors invade the rest of your body faster than you can get rid of them?

If you decide to get started with the beginners' program, taken from *Cure For All Cancers*, you may get an immediate halt for the disease. But only the malignancy will be gone. That is not enough. Even adding the prevention program is not enough. You need to see the tumors shrink and disappear. Cancer is very deceptive. It is seldom visible or painful or diagnosable until it is very late. Of course, it can be found with a Syncrometer® long before that. To stamp out an advanced cancer completely, you need to add either the *21-Day Program* from *The Cure For All Advanced Cancers* or choose the *3-Week Program* from this book. The difference between these two is that the earlier *21-Day Program* uses mainly supplements plus regular zapping, while the *3-Week Program* given here reduces supplements to a minimum. They are replaced with "plate-zapping" and "drop-taking" (called homeography). We will discuss these later. If you are very hardy and determined, you can do both programs together!

Again, put up time limits for yourself, when you will do tests and scans. You may be able to find a cooperative therapist to schedule these for you and give interpretations. You may be able to find a Syncrometer® tester who can tell you your status. Best of all, do it yourself.

In more progressive countries you can schedule tests and scans for yourself. You may need to go there to save your life. Be fair but critical with your results. If they do not give you proof of progress, you need to change something. Improving your compliance is the easiest option you could choose before it is too late. Don't neglect clinical and other alternative options. Review them to choose the wisest path.

With all this realism in one hand and optimism in your other hand you have the best chance to join the ranks of cured advanced cancer cases.

Speed is important. You can jump into action but you must do each program completely. If parts of any program are left out you are taking the risk of failing.

Both the earlier *21-Day Program* and this new *3-Week Program*, succeed in over 95% of cases when you do it all. Left out in the tragical 5% are only those who are so clinically ill they need a transfusion every week, or need drainage of effusate every week, and those already in jaundice or kidney failure. Even these can often be salvaged with the help of Syncrometer® testing and homeography treatment. It is well suited to emergency care.

Even if you choose to do the present *3-Week Program*, the advanced cancer patient can get extra helpful advice from the earlier *Cure For All Advanced Cancers* book. Where to get items you may want is given there in the *Sources* section. You are free to copy pages from it for yourself or friends (not for commercial purposes). A therapist, too, will find the technical explanations in the earlier book useful. Remember, they were discovered by Syncrometer® and can be verified by yourself, using the *Syncrometer® Science Laboratory Manual*.

Table of Contents

Table of Figures

CHAPTER 1

THE TRUE CAUSE OF CANCER...

...has never been known! In this book I will show you the true beginnings of all cancers.

Whether the cancer is in the form of a tumor or single cells, whether it is a sarcoma or carcinoma, whether it is "a very rare variety" or the most common, <u>each one</u> starts in the same <u>place</u>, one small region in the <u>brain</u>.

This information will make cancer much easier to prevent, to stop, and to cure.

All cancer starts in one organ!

All cancer <u>ends</u> in malignancy.

The cause of all malignancies is a common parasite, the human intestinal fluke. Its scientific name is Fasciolopsis buski. It arrives late in the development of a young growing tumor to make it malignant. This was first described in a book published in 1993.

A fluke is very much like a leech. The adult sticks to one spot where it produces many thousands of eggs inside our bodies.

This was never noticed before because it was not suspected and the eggs do not exit from the intestine. Commercial lab tests for parasitism search for eggs that have exited from the intestine.

You will actually be able to see your adult flukes later, when you succeed in killing them in your <u>intestines</u>, during the *3-Week Program*. The disease we call cancer is not caused by the adult flukes. That is why Fasciolopsiasis does not accompany a cancer case. This is when many adults are present, shedding eggs into the bowel and feces. But sometimes a few adults happen to be in the digestive tract...the esophagus, stomach, or colon. When they are killed and eliminated with the bowel contents, you have a chance to see them.

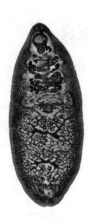

Human intestinal fluke, twice normal size, stretched out and stained (dyed) on a glass microscope slide.

Fig. 2 The cancer parasite

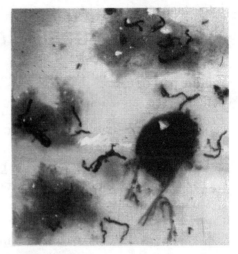

Parasites float when expelled from the bowel. "Black hairy legs" are strings of eggs that hang out when the adult bursts open and deteriorates.

Fig. 3 Five flukes in various stages of decay

You will not be able to see the flukes that are in your tumor or the rest of your body because there is no way for them to be expelled into the toilet. Dead or alive, they are stuck in your tissues.

Tiny primitive animals go through many phases in their development, somewhat like insects, with their caterpillars and cocoons. These are called **larval stages**. They are not at all like their parent butterflies or beetles. All fluke stages are too soft and tiny to show up on any scan.

Fluke stages are in the tissues, not the blood. They have gone unrecognized because only the blood is tested regularly, and the tests are chemical, not physical. Biopsies are prepared

2

by slicing the tissue very thinly. No slice of a parasite stage would ever be recognizable.

Parasites prefer to live packed into your tissues or bunched into stagnant places like vein valves or lymph vessel valves. Other blood rushes along too fast and is always patrolled by your immune system. Although a careful search of live blood would show a few of these larval stages, such a search is not a routine part of cancer research or clinical testing. Still, you may actually see an adult as you proceed through the *3-Week Program*, sweeping it out as you are doing a liver cleanse.

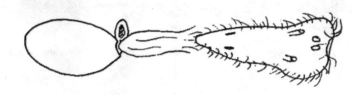

Fig. 4 Miracidia hatching from egg on left

The larval stages of Fasciolopsis buski normally produce a very potent growth stimulant, called **orthophosphotyrosine** or **OPT**. They probably make this for their own use, but only if a trigger is present. The trigger is common **isopropyl alcohol**.

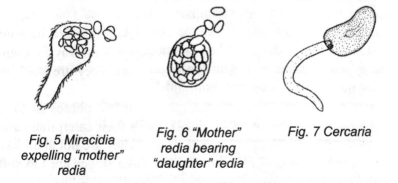

Fig. 5 Miracidia expelling "mother" redia

Fig. 6 "Mother" redia bearing "daughter" redia

Fig. 7 Cercaria

Their habitat would normally provide this alcohol since it is produced by Clostridium bacteria—those bacteria living in dying flesh and without oxygen. Animal waste is this parasite's habitat.

In people, isopropyl alcohol is provided by a lifestyle that uses it dozens of times each day, even contaminating our food. We host the same Clostridium bacteria that make isopropyl alcohol. They live in our tumors and intestines where flesh is decaying and oxygen is absent. So we have two sources of the OPT trigger: bacteria and a popular product.

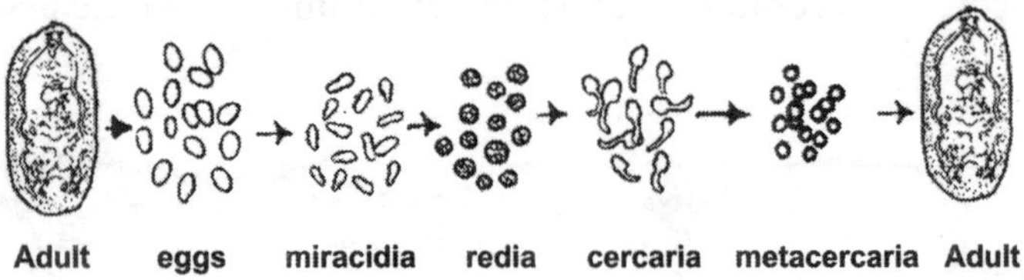

Adult eggs miracidia redia cercaria metacercaria Adult

Fig. 8 Life cycle of a fluke

When the larval stages of the fluke invade our tumors and Clostridium bacteria are present as well, we have the necessary conditions to produce OPT. It is evidence of too much growth stimulation. This is late in the life of a tumor, when mutations have already accumulated and are visible as chromosome damage. Seeing these, and the extra growth, makes the tumors appear malignant to a cytologist who examines your biopsy. All cancer patients that I analyzed by Syncrometer® and who had already been diagnosed by an oncologist had both OPT and the F. buski fluke stages in the organ with the tumor. There were no exceptions among thousands!

Fasciolopsis stages produce OPT.

It is very easy to stop this early malignancy just by killing this fluke and all its stages, and by stopping isopropyl alcohol use. Your tumor cells will stop receiving OPT, their major stimulant. But we can do more. Tumors must have the things that are needed to grow; otherwise they must stop, regardless of stimulation. Deoxyribonucleic acid (DNA) is one. Our

4

tissues only make as much of this as they need. How could they be so deluged in DNA as that the Syncrometer® sees it easily? It is being made by the same Clostridium bacteria. Clostridium produces DNA similar to our DNA. DNA flooding is not seen in the presence of other bacteria, like staphylococcus or streptococcus. Its similarity to our DNA is a unique feature. It allows sharing. Killing all Clostridium colonies will stop providing the tumor with extra DNA to grow on.

> Clostridium bacteria provide isopropyl alcohol and DNA.

Killing both Clostridium and the fluke will also stop production of Human Chorionic Gonadotropin (HCG), the **hormone** that protects the tumor. It is a human pregnancy hormone, the same hormone as protects the human fetus from attack by the mother's immune system![12] This subtle imitation of pregnancy was already noticed before 1900. The Syncrometer® shows that the cercaria stage of Fasciolopsis, together with isopropyl alcohol (from Clostridium), stimulates the *hypothalamus* to make HCG. In a human mother, the *placenta* makes HCG to start the *trophoblast* stage of the fetus. Now the tumor will get similar protection, a fact noticed by early therapists, but unheeded by later scientists. We will see the continued role of our hypothalamus gland in cancer.

The details of getting rid of a malignancy in a very short time are given in the first book, *Cure For All Cancers*, written in 1993 and updated in 1998. This method is still valid, but does not go beyond clearing malignancy.

In this book we will clear the tumor, too.

At the time the earlier book was written, it was thought by scientists, myself included, that the malignancy <u>was</u> the entire cancer. That the benign state was tolerable.

---

[12] *A Clue to Cancer,* Newsweek, Oct. 23, 1995, p. 92

Yet, further experience showed me that it was <u>not</u>. Tumors could grow in spite of being non-malignant by oncologists' standards, although slower. They did not necessarily shrink or die. They had a life of their own.

With this new insight my next research was devoted to finding the true beginnings of all tumors rather than malignancies since they obviously were a different kind of growth and provided the starting point for every malignancy.

Eventually the true beginning of each tumor was found. It will put us in awe of the body's great complexities. No story could be more riveting. It all begins in one organ, the <u>hypothalamus in the brain</u>, as we shall see in Chapter 2.

The Middle Period

We will soon learn what happens <u>initially</u>, to give us the beginning of a tumor.

We already know what will happen <u>finally</u>, to give us a malignancy.

But what happens between these times? Do all those people who have started a tumor reach the endpoint where the tumor becomes malignant?

They do not!

Early beginnings are often seen with a Syncrometer® in young children if a parent has cancer. But not all of these children go on to develop cancer. Even though the whole family of a cancer patient carries the intestinal fluke parasite and even though the whole family develops early beginnings of tumors, some will get cancer, and some will not. Something quite decisive must happen to some of the family members and not to the others to make the difference.

Knowing what makes this difference is very, very important.

Research designed to unravel such a mystery is called epidemiology.

Epidemiology

It was obvious far back to antiquity that the general health and appearance of a person made no difference. The decisive factor whether or not you get cancer was much more subtle.

The field of epidemiology grew very strong in the middle of the last century. Different religions, different occupations, different regions of the country, all had different cancer rates. Was it tea and coffee drinking, pork eating, cooking habits, the air, stress levels? Even the heights of chimneys in England were measured, in desperation, to shed light on this mystery.

As promising as all the collected facts and figures looked, nothing could be made of it, nothing could be identified as <u>the</u> deciding factor that leads us to this disease. Yet, the effort was not wasted. Many carcinogens (things that could cause cancer) such as soot from these chimneys were discovered. And the failure of every cancer victim's immune power was also discovered.

Immune Power

Immune power was a mysterious concept at first. Researchers could see that animals would not let a transplanted tumor grow in them unless the immune system was first knocked down (by radiation, for example, the very "treatment" being used today). People who had to have their immune power reduced to accept an organ transplant got many more cancers than others. Special animals were raised who were missing immune power in order to do cancer research. Special chemicals were developed to destroy immune power at will.

The loss of personal immune power is not visible. You may be a strong, healthy person in the prime of life and yet be losing your immune power. Clinical doctors, researchers and victims of cancer themselves were all aware of this. But the scientific tools available to investigate this were only biochemistry and immunology. These methods are much too slow and much too costly to do such research in a timely way. It would take hundreds of years, if ever, to find the difference between persons who get cancer and those who do not using these techniques.

Eventually all epidemiology seemed hopeless because everything, even good, nourishing food, seemed to have carcinogens and cause mutations. At the same time chemicals from industry were being dumped into our food and homes in truckload amounts, making "good nourishing food" a false concept, and obscuring epidemiological differences. Just as hopes hit bottom, a ray of light shone in.

It was quite by accident that a new technology was born. It held the promise of doing all this difficult and expensive research in a fraction of the time needed before, and for a fraction of the cost.

The device using this technology is called a Syncrometer® (see page viii).

The Syncrometer® is <u>momentarily</u> attached to the body with pressure (a probe). It could verify the close association between getting cancer and losing immunity. It could find precisely what the immune system's defects were. It could find the causes of these defects. And finally, it could find what the epidemiological factors are that bring these causes to some people and not to others.

It all pointed to the water.

What did the Syncrometer® detect?

The water coming to your kitchen faucet decides whether you will get cancer or not.

The water has the power to destroy your immune system as quietly as a stealth aircraft and just as surely. It also has the power to allow recovery and to do it quickly.

The Secret of Water

Water should be pure and free of bad bacteria; it should bring us minerals, some oxygen, a proper magnetic polarization (to be discussed later) and it should even taste good. The Federal Drug Administration (FDA) and Environmental Protection Agency (EPA) have shared the responsibility for good water quality and have done their utmost to keep it so.

They could not prevent the universal contamination of our water with hundreds of solvents, metals, pesticides and other chemicals. They could not prevent the tragedy that we now see in an explosion of illnesses beginning in childhood.

Yet, it is not <u>these</u> multiple contaminants that makes the difference we are searching for. These are present in <u>most</u> waters and consumed by <u>most</u> people. In spite of being undesirable, these do not make the decisive difference between immune system destruction or its preservation, between getting cancer or not.

Water is <u>usually</u> treated with aluminum to help it filter clear of sediment as it is passed through sand beds. It is then disinfected with chlorine gas. This is done in nearly all water treatment plants. Chlorine gas bubbled through water produces assorted harmful and even carcinogenic chemicals, but, again, <u>most</u> people have been drinking such water and do not get cancer. After the water leaves the treatment plant it is tested for its "free" chlorine level at certain checkpoints, because this level tends to get lower and lower. A certain level needs to be kept up, about 1 part per million (ppm) of active chlorine. This is what kills bacteria. Little measuring kits for free chlorine can be bought at hardware stores and pool supply stores.

Adding more chlorine <u>gas</u> on a small scale, if the free chlorine were low, would be prohibitively expensive at these numerous small checkpoints. Chlorine gas is also very dangerous to handle. Consequently, technicians have been trained to calculate how much <u>liquid chlorine</u> (bleach) needs to be added at any one checkpoint. This is much less expensive and dangerous. They have been taught which bleach has the EPA registration number and the National Standards Foundation (NSF) stamp to legalize its use in drinking water, and where to buy it. It comes in double strength concentration, large bottles, and 4 bottles to a crate, a most unwieldy package! It also comes in larger containers for manufacturer's use and other big consumers. A plastic crate is the only legal way to transport this rather hazardous fluid because it contains 12% chlorine instead of the 6% that we are accustomed to handling.

The bottles must always be carried in this crate and returned that way, not suited to engineers and workmen who must often speedily repair some water department pipes.

All the detailed requirements were expected to lead to a carefully protected process of adding a food-grade bleach to the public drinking water. But it did just the opposite.

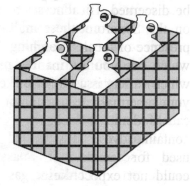
Fig. 9 Crate of bleach bottles

Somewhere a myth got started. It stated that "bleach is bleach" and any bleach would do. It would justify stopping at the corner store for a bottle of bleach. Before there were many kinds of bleach on the market, perhaps purer than now, such a myth did little harm. Now that many kinds of bleaches are on the market, it does a great deal of harm. The new bleaches arriving in the supermarkets in the past few decades have changed considerably. Some have "whiteners and brighteners" added. Many have other additives. It was already known generations ago that adding "bluing" to your laundry made it appear "whiter". Old-fashioned bluing was a cobalt compound, a heavy metal. Actually, current laundry bleaches have a huge assortment of dyes, and the heavy metals include barium, lead, lanthanum, nickel, cadmium, chromium, cobalt, ruthenium, and yttrium, for example. There is no set recipe for these, suggesting they are some other industry's wastewater. The dyes, too, are not fixed and could come from a textile manufacturer's effluent. They were never meant to be drunk— only applied to clothing and bathrooms.

The Syncrometer® typically finds about 20 heavy metals in a sample of modern bleach. All have many azo dyes, asbestos, and shocking solvents. Shocking, because PCBs and benzene solvents are well known to cause cancer. Compare this to the legally designated, NSF-grade bleach (see table on page 12).

Through a simple-minded error of using laundry bleach instead of NSF-grade bleach, your water can receive the stamp of cancer. Just which brand of bleach is being used can easily be discerned. Bleach varieties only resonate with themselves on the Syncrometer®. So if you test water samples for the presence of local supermarket varieties of bleach, you can tell which one you are inadvertently drinking. You can also find which variety is used in your pool or spa and on the produce in your supermarket.

Modern bleaches contain dyes. Being used for laundry, we could not expect these to be safe, edible dyes. The Syncrometer® detects those already banned 50 years ago in food and some legally allowed, even now. They include Fast Garnet, Fast Green, Fast Red, Fast Red Violet, Fast Blue, Dimethylaminoazobenzene (DAB, or butter yellow), Sudan Black, in fact the entire list on page 603. Maybe they are simply pollutants of the major blue (for bluing) dyes used. Maybe they are the wastewater of a dye-making industry. I don't know the sources of these dye ingredients, the heavy metal ingredients.

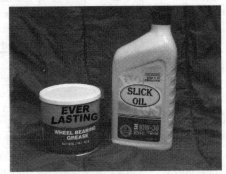

Wheel bearing grease and motor oil are added to your drinking water, not accidental pollutants.

Fig. 10 Examples of wheel bearing grease and motor oil

There are no strong pollution controls over a product like laundry bleach. The Syncrometer® finds PCBs and benzene in every bottle and asbestos in many, but not all. Plain motor oil and wheel bearing grease are also regularly present.

Undiluted bleaches tested by Syncrometer®					
Toxin	popular laundry bleach	NSF-grade bleach	Toxin	popular laundry bleach	NSF grade bleach
acetone [S]	Neg	Neg	molyb-denum	Pos	Neg
aluminum	Neg	Neg	motor oil [S]	*Pos	Neg
antimony	Pos	Neg	neodymium[L]	Pos	Neg
arsenic	*Pos	Neg	nickel	*Pos	Neg
asbestos	*Pos		niobium	Neg	Neg
azo dyes	Pos	Neg	north polarization	Neg	Pos
barium	*Pos	Neg	palladium	Pos	Neg
benzene [S]	Pos	Neg	PCB [S]	Pos	Neg
beryllium	Neg	Neg	platinum	Neg	Neg
bismuth	Neg	Neg	praseody-mium [L]	Neg	Neg
boron	Pos	Neg	rhenium	Pos	Neg
bromine, gas	Neg	Neg	rhodium	Neg	Neg
cadmium	Pos	Neg	rubidium	Neg	nt
cerium [L]	Pos	Neg	ruthenium	Neg	Neg
cesium	Neg	Neg	samarium [L]	Neg	Neg
chromium III & VI	Pos	Neg	scandium [L]	Neg	Neg
cobalt	Pos	Neg	selenium	Neg	Neg
copper	Pos	Neg	silicic acid	Neg	Neg
dodecane [S]	*Pos	Neg	silicon	Pos	Neg
dysprosium[L]	Pos	Neg	silver	Neg	Neg
europium [L]	Pos	Neg	south polarization	Pos	Neg
Fe$_2$O$_3$*, ferrite	Pos	Neg	strontium	Pos	Neg
Fe$_3$O$_4$, magnetite	Neg	Pos	tantalum	*Pos	Neg
formalde-hyde [S]	Neg	Neg	tin	Neg	Neg
gadolinium[L]	Pos	Neg	tellurium	Neg	Neg
germanium	Neg	Neg	terbium [L]	Neg	Neg
gold	Neg	Neg	thallium	Neg	Neg
holmium [L]	Pos	Neg	thulium [L]	Neg	Neg
indium	Pos	Neg	toluene [S]	Pos	Neg

Undiluted bleaches tested by Syncrometer®					
Toxin	popular laundry bleach	NSF-grade bleach	Toxin	popular laundry bleach	NSF grade bleach
iridium	Neg	Neg	tungsten	*Pos	Neg
isopropyl alcohol [S]	Neg	Neg	uranium	Pos	Neg
lanthanum [L]	Pos	Neg	vanadium	Pos	Neg
lead	Neg	Neg	wheel bearing grease	Pos	Neg
lithium	Neg	Neg	xylenes [S]	Pos	Neg
lutetium [L]	Neg	Neg	ytterbium	Neg	Neg
manganese	Neg	Neg	yttrium	Neg	Neg
mercury	Neg	Neg	zinc	Neg	Neg
methanol [S]	Neg	Neg	zirconium	Neg	Neg

nt = not tested   L = lanthanide   S = solvent

* The two iron compounds and polarizations are not toxins. An asterisk means the level detected was exceptionally high. See also page 251.

Fig. 11 Toxins in bleach

Maybe all this does little harm rubbed against your skin (though perhaps it contributes to skin diseases) after doing the laundry. But added to your drinking water, these 5 toxins: **PCBs, benzene, asbestos, heavy metals and azo dyes**, together become the "fingerprint" of cancer. They will be in your saliva, lymph, cerebrospinal fluid, and tumors together.

Legitimate food-grade bleach, the kind stamped with the NSF mark and given a registration number has none of these 5 categories.

> The difference between these bleach varieties in your water makes the difference between those who get cancer and those who do not.

Of course the FDA, EPA and Department of Agriculture who are in charge of disinfectants and sterilization methods cannot be expected to accept results obtained with a Syncrometer®. The Syncrometer® is not an FDA-approved device nor will it be for some time to come. Automation of the device must come first. The keen interest of our agencies would help to arrive at this.

Regular analytical laboratory tests are approved and could be used by anybody to validate the Syncrometer® results. I have already done this, finding the heavy metal analysis to be the most reproducible and least expensive. I recommend this test for anyone who gets cancer, or wishes to prevent it and wants to confirm the extraordinary heavy metals in their drinking water. See the list of laboratories on page 604.

Testing for PCBs and benzene by labs is more expensive and much more unreliable than for metals. Often no results are obtained by a lab because of the tendency for grease to stick to the sides of the container. PCBs and benzene are greasy. They came with the motor oil and grease in the bleach. Just pouring out the water sample into the labs' own containers or sucking up a portion of it leaves these toxins behind! They miss being tested, especially when plastic bottles have been used in sampling. Grease sticks to the container the way it sticks to a dishpan if no soap is used.

Asbestos and azo dyes cannot be tested at all because no commercial labs have been found that can do this. Even research labs can only detect asbestos spears above a certain (10 micron) length. Most asbestos in water is shorter than this and gets missed. When a pollutant gets missed, it ruins the epidemiological study. Even the short asbestos bits are easily found by Syncrometer®. The smaller spears are probably the most harmful ones because they can be eaten whole by your white blood cells. The number of longer spears allowed is 7 million per quart!

In spite of these difficulties some simple tests can be done by <u>anyone</u>, to test for laundry bleach in their water. Since PCBs and benzene are in grease and oil, they slowly rise to the top of standing water and can be seen and felt as a greasy film. But great care must be taken to sample the water carefully and to view the surface correctly. If only one day's water sample is used, you could miss the results completely as would happen if a commercial or official lab were to come to test your water.

Bleach is added to your drinking water intermittently, according to "need". Often it is once a week. So you should sample your water for 7 days in a row to be sure you are testing the bleach addition in a meaningful way. See details on page 579.

The 5 toxin categories occur <u>together</u> in the popular bleach varieties. If you find grease in your water you will find all 5 toxin categories, too, if you are testing by Syncrometer®. You can then assume it is not NSF-bleach that was used in your water and that you do have laundry bleach water. Hurry to correct this! In a cancer patient, the body has reached its limit of detoxifying ability and these toxins stand out clearly, including the bleach brand, because they have been accumulating in you. In healthy people, maybe none will be seen since they are actively detoxified by the body or stored in a future tumor.

All the cancer patients seen in the last 5 years, including many not seen but merely tested had these 5 toxins and a popular laundry bleach variety in their drinking water. The same set was seen in their saliva, lymph, organs, and tumors. This comes to a very large number of patients, possibly a thousand. Not a **single** cancer case was missing this "laundry bleach fingerprint" in their bodies. But a few patients had the evidence only in their tumors or lymph, not saliva. These persons had recently moved to a new home and luckily found good water. Cancer victims in Europe showed a different brand of laundry bleach I have named *European laundry bleach*. This is particularly high in azo dyes, motor oil and wheel bearing grease, but without PCBs and benzene. The manufacturing plant given for it was American. Cancer victims in Central America, India, UK, and all HIV victims in Africa showed the same bleach brands as in the USA. Victims in Mexico showed a Mexican brand of bleach with the USA brand included.

There were no exceptions among cancer patients, making this a compelling statistic. Of course, family members of cancer victims may not have cancer yet although they are using the same water. Their risk is much higher than others but maybe they will move away before it happens. Moving to a residence in a clean-water district should and does remove the risk of cancer developing. Now it is understandable how a parent with cancer could raise a family where only some children get cancer. They all moved to different residences. It only takes a few weeks to lower the level of all these toxins in your body if you are still healthy. Each patient seen by us was asked to obtain water samples from friends and relatives until a clean-water district was found. Judging by such water samples there are about as many water departments using the legitimate bleach as using the wrong bleach. This ratio was much better just 5 years ago. The bad bleach habit is spreading.

Why is bad bleach used? Because of the myth, no doubt. Maybe convenience and cost are considered. The answer is not known.

As thorough and demanding as our regulatory agencies have been with water regulations, the control has not extended to the end-of-the-line processes. Which grade bleach to use for periodically cleaning the small tank where bleach and water are premixed before pumping it to the large tank, which oil and grease to use for the pumps themselves and

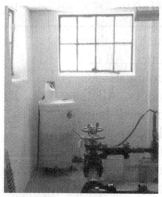

Bleach is first added to a small tank of water (in the corner), using pump at center front to make a premix.

Fig. 12 A water department pump house

which kinds of pumps to use are not specified. And which bleach to use when repairing water pipes and digging wells is not specified. Nor is it specified when giving cautionary advice about cutlery, kitchen counters and sinks. It is human nature to reach for the quickest, easiest, cheapest brands of bleach. Our agencies have trusted the water departments' GMP (good manufacturing practice) for all these details. We must not trust any department, regardless of its good intentions. They mean no harm, certainly, but drinking water must be guarded to the very last detail of its delivery process. Good to the last drop must be literally interpreted. The record of procedure must be provable in detail with a log, dated and signed, as for any manufacturing business. Now it is not.

Thank you, Syncrometer®, now we know the problem.

Cancer Prevention

The first step toward prevention of cancer is to test your water for the presence of laundry bleach. The statistics are very clear. No case of cancer in a series of many, many hundreds, if not thousands, of patients, was without the presence of laundry bleach in their tumors and drinking water. No case was omitted. All of the patients had already been diagnosed by their oncologists. There was no error from assuming cancer wrongly. All the cancer patients brought water samples that contained laundry bleach. We looked further. All of our failures, patients who later died and had sent us a water sample beforehand, had moved back to bad water. It was done innocently, since they believed the water to be good. And all patients who returned because their cancer had returned at home had been using bad water again. Still further, all follow-up patients who were doing well at home had switched to NSF-bleached water, rainwater or well water. The picture is clear. How could you get cancer unless you had laundry bleach water? The probability seems to be less than one in a thousand (assuming I did a thousand tests).

Cure or Remission?

The first step in curing your cancer, once it is found, is to change your residence. Without this, there will be no chance of curing your cancer permanently. A clinical or alternative treatment may give you quick success, at first, as any band-aid would to a painful wound, but not a permanent cure…only remission.

17

Of course, you must move to a location that is bleaching the water correctly. When you do this, precancerous growths and very early tumors will probably clear themselves. But when <u>you</u> do this, already diagnosed with cancer, will <u>you</u> be cured permanently? This depends on removing the 5 toxins from your body. <u>It is these 5 that destroy your immune power</u>. Taking immune boosters is a minor, very temporary help. Only taking the toxins <u>out</u> of your body can bring back your immune power. Fortunately, we have found ways to clear them all out in about 3 weeks. The body is a miraculous living machine. Once you rescue it from its 5 worst enemies, and nurture it with a few critical supplements, it rewards you with a cure. The "magic" substances are organic germanium, organic selenium, and organic vitamin C. We will discuss these later.

We might imagine that filtering the water, distilling it, or treating it in some "purifying" way could clean it and remove these 5 toxin categories. We might imagine that carrying in clean water for drinking and cooking purposes would be sufficient. It is not. All patients got a cancer recurrence after trying one of these "shortcuts". At first, their health merely declined. Later they got cancer again.

Guard your first success, whether you got it using natural means or by the usual clinical means. You cannot change the water department's policies or people's habits. Move. After finding good water in another water district, move immediately. The water you drink exchanges with all your body's water in 2 days! This is much faster than the rate for food. Don't delay this because it is the most significant and fast-acting part of the cure. In 3 weeks you can be a different person.

What guarantee do you have that the water you switch to will stay good? None! But habits get ingrained for responsible or irresponsible behavior. Over a 5 year period I have only seen three switches in water bleaching policy by any water department.

When your immune power goes down, the number and variety of parasites goes up; the number and variety of bacteria and viruses also goes up. Parasites bring us their own viruses and some are **oncoviruses** (tumor-causing viruses). They bring their own bacteria, too. Parasites are not newcomers for people. We have had them for millennia because they came from rats, mice, chickens, rabbits, pigs, cows, horses, dogs, all animals we have lived with for these same millennia. In theory, we should not get animal parasites. But in immunodepressed conditions we do.

Losing immune power happens stepwise; first it affects the kidneys, then the organ with a tumor. We will see later, why this organ is "chosen". Without immune power in a particular organ, there is no normal "housekeeping" done there. No metals nor solvents coming in with the bad bleach water are removed. No azo dyes, nor asbestos slivers are removed. Even the chlorine itself, in the form of hypochlorite, accumulates. Both metals and chlorine are strong oxidizers. The whole area becomes over oxidized from toxic metals and chlorine accumulating there. The area becomes a "toxic dumpsite" for the body, complete with living invaders. Eventually, there is no organic selenium, organic germanium, or reduced vitamin C left for the white blood cells to use. It has all been oxidized, and is now useless and even toxic. More immunity damage will come from the PCBs and benzene accumulated. Finally, as oxidized **iron** is formed and accumulates, the toxic zone switches to a south polarized zone. This is mainly due to **nickel**, one of the heavy metals being drunk. Iron oxidized to the ferrite, Fe_2O_3, has a **south polarization**. Nickel can oxidize the iron in your body and start this pathological process. It will spread.

We will discuss the meaning of magnetic polarization later. Meanwhile, we can see that the accumulation of toxins and parasites will go faster and faster. The more toxins have accumulated to lower your immunity, the more parasites and **pathogens** (bad bacteria and viruses) will grow. The more invaders grow, the sicker the organ gets, letting in more toxins. The kidneys will be affected first. Will there be a limit? Can the body protect itself from being <u>completely</u> invaded and

19

turned into a <u>systemic</u> waste site? Is that why the body wraps the tumor in a tough coat—to limit its invasion? Why aren't we consciously aware of all this?

With a paralyzed immune system in the tumor zone where so many unwanted things have accumulated, the body's only recourse is **detoxification**. This is a very heavy burden for some small organ or tissue. The large liver and kidneys were meant to do most of this. A smaller organ normally relies on its white blood cells (immune system) to eat most of the toxins or enemies that arrive. And, of course, detoxification does not kill anything, such as parasites, bacteria or viruses. It only does detoxifying-chemistry, whereas the immune system could do both.

The accumulation of heavy metals in the tumor zone has left it in an oxidized state.

The body's metabolism normally shuttles between **oxidized** and **reduced** states, back and forth continually, to make energy for the life process. It must not get stuck in any one state.

Reducing action to counteract over-oxidation is a method we will use to help the body free itself from its stuck position.

But let us stop for a minute. Isn't food, ordinary food the reducer meant to do this? Meant to bring the oxidized state back to the reduced state? Why can't our metabolism get us unstuck from iron overoxidation and magnetic consequences? Are we missing essential factors to make it all possible? Are these factors destroyed by the toxic accumulation? We do not yet know. Meanwhile, we will use vitamin C and sulfur compounds, time-honored supplements that are reducers. Making it possible to reduce iron again, in the cyclic way that it should, helps the most. It will correct the magnetic polarization at the tumor sites and kidneys, so cycling becomes automatic again.

Review

1. Every cancer has a distinct beginning, middle period, and end. These are the same for all cancers. The true beginning was only discovered in 2000. We will discuss it in the next chapter.

2. The middle period sees the tumor growing and accumulating many things that would normally be excreted or eliminated. This is due to large-scale destruction of the immune system by drinking laundry bleach in the water. Five specific pollutants are responsible: PCBs, benzene, asbestos, certain heavy metals, and azo dyes. It allows nickel to accumulate in the kidneys first, changing their magnetic polarization to south, which is ineffective for excretion.

3. The end is malignancy; caused by the larval stages of the human intestinal fluke, which flood the tumor with orthophosphotyrosine, OPT. The large amount of OPT in the tumor zone is evidence of intense stimulation of the enzyme systems that attach a phosphate group to tyrosine groups in proteins. This accelerates cell division called **mitosis** explosively.

4. By killing this fluke, and its stages, the excessive production of OPT is stopped. HCG production is stopped, too.

5. Clostridium bacteria also play a role in every cancer. By killing Clostridium bacteria and stopping personal use of isopropyl alcohol, excessive amounts of isopropyl alcohol disappear along with excessive DNA. Excessive HCG, DNA, and OPT are the hallmarks of malignancy. By stopping these we can gain the time necessary to stop the beginnings—the tumor-making process—which always starts at one place, the **hypothalamus** in the brain.

6. By switching to a clean water source we stop the accumulation of PCBs, benzene, asbestos, heavy metals and dyes. Each of these must now be eliminated from the body to regain immunity.

7. All the accumulations in the tumor must be cleared away. Then the tumor can shrink.

Clearing away the critical 5 toxins that arrived in your drinking water returns immune power. Then we can get help in clearing <u>all</u> the accumulations. Our white blood cells will repay us with their help. But the tumor cells have a task, too.

We will see that for tumor cells to disappear, they must be able <u>to digest themselves, be digested by your digestive enzymes</u> and <u>be eaten by your white blood cells</u>. These three steps can be monitored with the Syncrometer® to be sure they are happening. Nothing must remain.

The *3-Week Program* eliminates all 3 phases of cancer. The first and last are easy and brief. The middle is the most challenging and takes your devotion and determination.

Let us go back to the beginning now and see how easy it would be to prevent a tumor from ever starting. There will be an order to the events.

> The events leading to a tumor form a chain with distinct links.

It is a fascinating, though deadly, series of events that leads to the first tumor. An extension of the chain then leads to additional tumors.

We now will see the scientific way to prevent all cancers. We can begin to abolish this disease from people, our pets and our domestic animals. The beginning itself has 3 steps. They will lead to the **tumor nucleus** that supplies all tumors, growing anywhere in the body.

CHAPTER 2

THE BEGINNING OF ALL TUMORS

Step 1

In one small corner of the hypothalamus gland, a quiet explosion is taking place. Tiny bits and pieces are flying away from it. Cells of the hypothalamus are landing in the blood, in the lymph, in the saliva. They float alongside the red blood cells, white blood cells, and platelets, in the blood, quite undisturbed.

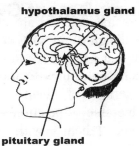

hypothalamus gland

pituitary gland

Fig. 13 Master glands in the brain

We might think these cells should die, separated this far from their parent organ, but they do not. Nor do white blood cells eat them. White blood cells, being your immune system, should somehow eliminate them. But your white blood cells have been trained to <u>protect</u>, never to eat, or even attack, cells that belong to your very own body. <u>Dead</u> cells of your own would be quickly devoured. Are these exempt because they stay alive? Will they never die? Are they doing any harm?

Step 2

Not far away, in a small part of the pituitary gland, another tissue explosion is taking place. The pituitary is just a tiny marble hanging down from the hypothalamus in the floor of the brain. This is just above the roof of

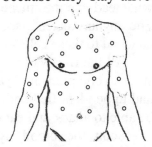

Fig. 14 Our body fluids distribute the tiny bits of hypothalamus

your mouth. The pituitary explosion is independent of the hypothalamus event. They could happen before or after each other.

Now two organs are doing this very strange thing—coming apart, letting bits of themselves come loose, to float away in the body's fluids. How long will the tiny bits live? No white blood cells will eat them unless they are dead. To kill them, **complement** has to arrive.

Complement C₃

An arm of our immune system is called **complement**. There are many actors in this arm, called C_1, C_2, C_3 and so on. Each contributes to the daily drama. They round up certain bacteria, get them into a vulnerable position and pierce them with their daggers. We must remember that bacteria are a thousand times bigger than complement molecules. This achievement is spectacular.

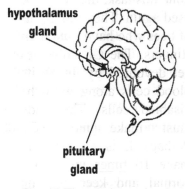

hypothalamus gland

pituitary gland

Fig. 15 The pituitary gland hangs below the hypothalamus

The job of dispatching the renegade hypothalamus and pituitary cells is, evidently, the complement's. The Syncrometer® sees C_3 attached to these cells at first.

All the runaway cells get stuck to complement C_3 and pierced. It seems the live runaways had to be identified and "prepared" for the white blood cells to be able to attack and eat them.

Soon the blood, lymph, and saliva are all cleared of wandering hypothalamus and pituitary cells.

Remember, the Syncrometer® is the electronic detection device that lets us identify our own tissues, parasites, or chemicals **very accurately** inside ourselves. We can watch events happening and where they are happening. Opportunities for discovery are almost endless. Details on how to build one and use one are given in the *Syncrometer® Science Laboratory Manual* by this author. Nobody is too old to learn to use this powerful scientific tool.

But then another flood of runaway cells arrives, and another, as if hailstorm after hailstorm had loosened them and set them free. It can be difficult for complement C_3 molecules to keep up with its skewering task. Once these molecules have done this task, they can't be used again. They remind us of bees who have used their stingers. The C_3 molecules get devoured by the white blood cells along with the disabled cells. The body must make more C_3. Perhaps it is expected to make 10 times more than normal and keep this up day after day, or perhaps a hundred times more.

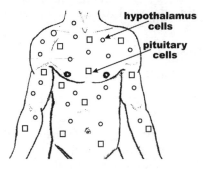

Fig. 16 Now both hypothalamus and pituitary gland bits are afloat

Soon your body can't keep up with the big demand for complement C_3! Then both kinds of brain cells float side by side undisturbed. Will they communicate with each other? They normally do, when they are in their own glands in the brain.

Hypothalamus and Pituitary Cells Join

Maybe they often bump into each other as they float. Maybe they normally attract each other. Maybe they are just sticky. Suddenly the Syncrometer® sees tiny duplexes, part hypothalamus and part pituitary. They fused!

Now duplexes as well as single cells are circulating. Undaunted, complement now attacks the duplexes too, trying to take them all out of the circulation as well as the single cells. There is more demand for C_3.

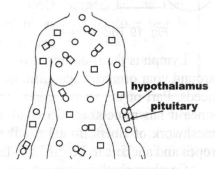

Fig. 17 Diagram of single cells and duplexes afloat in the body's fluids

Step 3

Just above the navel and a tiny bit to the right is the "head" of the pancreas. From here it stretches around to your left side. The same sinister force is beginning to act. A tissue erosion begins. Pancreas cells begin to float free in the body fluids.

Suddenly, a "snowball" forms. The duplexes that were formed before now stick and fuse to the new loose pancreas cells to make triplets. They are in this order: the pancreas cells stick to the pituitary, not to the hypothalamus portion. Complement tries again to kill all triplets as well as duplexes and single cells.

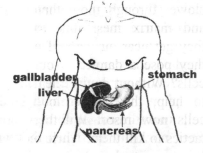

Fig. 18 The pancreas will contribute the third tissue

Finally, there is no more complement. Single cells of all three organs, their duplexes and their triplets, fill the body fluids. The

26

Syncrometer® finds them in the saliva, blood, **lymph** and **cerebrospinal fluid**.

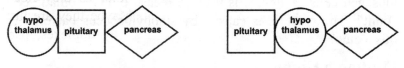

Fig. 19 This is the triplet.......................Not this...

Lymph is the fluid that is not in your arteries or veins; it is around your organs, bathing them and taking care of their daily needs. Part of the space around organs is called the "**matrix**" since it has more than just fluid. Close to our cells there is a meshwork of fibers lashed about the cells and each other like ropes and anchors to keep everything securely in place.

Cerebrospinal fluid is a lymph for the brain, bathing it and taking care of its daily needs. It reaches down the center of the spinal cord. Then it flows out and around to reach the brain again, round and round.

The renegade tissue bits float through organ after organ by means of our arteries and veins, lymph and cerebrospinal fluid (CSF). They travel much slower through the lymph and matrix meshwork as they get near our cells. Do they pose a danger to our cells? Without complement to help, the white blood cells now resort to other

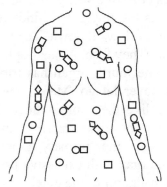

Fig. 20 Single cells, duplexes and triplets everywhere

tactics to kill them. Nitric oxide is used as a chemical weapon. It is present whenever complement C_3 has run out. But all these tactics are "too little and too late". They do not control the tide of tissue bits awash in the body.

Why did it happen? How did it happen? What will happen? Was it due to inflammation? Why were these organs inflamed? Why were there no symptoms?

27

Cow's milk always has udder (breast) cells in it. When **mastitis** (udder infection) strikes her she has many more loosened cells. A device is used to measure this "somatic cell count". The mastitis is caused by staphylococcus bacteria. Is this a clue?

Finding a Home

Sooner or later, a fourth organ will follow the trend and begin its micro-explosion. Unless we know what is causing these, we cannot stop them. We will study this soon.

Now, cells of a fourth organ are released to join all the others in the circulating body fluids. Whether it is the prostate, breast, or another organ, new loose cells are being added to those already afloat and traveling.

The fourth organ has a difference from the other three. It is making glue. Sticky substances are being made along with fine threads, called **fibronectin**, **laminin**, and **cadherin E**. These glues ooze like sticky mucous. They could form a trap.

As the tiny triplet finds itself floating through this organ, the glue slows it down. The triplet suddenly sticks to the fourth organ. They fuse. A quadruplet is made!

The fourth organ has triplets stuck to it all around. They will never let go. Many new "quads" are already swimming away like the triplets did before. But many stay stuck right there in the sticky matrix of the fourth organ. This fourth organ will make the "primary tumor". The triplet only gets attached to an organ with excessive fibronectin and laminin threads and with cadherin E, the glue.

But why was so much glue produced? It is, after all, normal to have some—and normal to have some laminin and fibronectin. It only happens when totally different, quite independent parasites are living nearby. Wherever these parasites exist, all these are overproduced. It is probably for their own purposes—not to get washed away easily. But the triplet gets caught in it, like a moth in a spider web, and then fuses itself to the fourth organ cells.

It (the triplet) will provide the growing point of the tumor, so I call it the **tumor nucleus**.

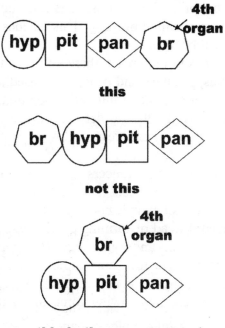

this

not this

nor this is the arrangement

hyp = hypothalamus; pit = pituitary;
pan = pancreas; br = breast

Fig. 21 The primary tumor forms

The parasites are common Fasciola and Ascaris, not others! Fasciola and Ascaris parasites increase, too, as the immune system is destroyed by laundry bleach. It is part of the increased parasitism always seen with immunity destruction.

Fasciola is another fluke, fairly easily killed, like Fasciolopsis. Ascaris is a roundworm, harder to kill, it seems, than flukes. And the gluey trap substances, fibronectin, laminin, and cadherin E can be digested. Our ordinary digestive enzymes produced by the stomach and pancreas can digest them in days. We will do this, but why did our digestive organs not do this automatically?

The Primary Tumor

When you or your doctor find your first tumor it is called the "primary tumor". Which organ it is does not matter; it is your first one, so is called primary. This decides all the others because they will be its offspring.

If the tumor is in the breast, there will be a tumor nucleus of hypothalamus, pituitary and pancreas—fused to breast cells. Every tumor so far searched (hundreds upon hundreds) has the same nucleus. And the order is always the same: hypothalamus, pituitary, pancreas, followed by the organ that develops the primary tumor.

Even non-tumorous cancers like the leukemias or eosinophilia or thrombocytosis, have the same tumor nucleus in the bone marrow or lymph nodes or spleen. These cancers remain dispersed instead of forming solid masses. And masses that form away from an organ, like Hodgkin's and plain abdominal masses have the same tumor nucleus attached to lymph node cells that have gotten themselves wrapped up by a filaria parasite here. The growing force for each is the same tumor nucleus.

Soon there will be genuine tiny tumors wherever the tumor nucleus has fused with the organ cells. They cluster together, making it look like "one cell started it all". But the tumor nuclei are numerous.

Now starts the Middle Period when the tumor begins to accumulate things and grow. Now immunity destruction by laundry bleach will play a more visible role. And several new actors will join this tragic drama.

Would it not be an easy matter to prevent the first step from ever happening? Because there is an orderly sequence in this snowballing behavior, couldn't we prevent any one of these steps and already achieve our goal? There will not be just one way to prevent cancer, but at least half a dozen ways. It will be possible to stomp out this disease to completion—for our pets, and for domestic animals, too. To accomplish this we must know what causes these organs to explode.

Back at the Hypothalamus

An extraordinary chemical has accumulated in the hypothalamus gland of the brain whenever it is loosening its cells and letting them go free into the circulation. This chemical is absent when there are no cells being shed. All cancer patients have such an accumulation and it is the same chemical for each.

The chemical is called **chlorogenic acid**, a well-known plant compound! It is considered an **antigen** (or **allergen**) by "ecological allergy" specialists. It is known by botanists to be a common "intermediate" in plant growth, often taking part in the forming of fruits and vegetables. It is there naturally, although how plants grow and ripen must surely affect the chemicals produced in them. How foods are cooked could also affect this chemical. Research is badly needed.

A search of the ordinary foods people eat showed chlorogenic acid to be present in some of our popular foods. Certain less common foods contain it, too. We should certainly avoid foods containing chlorogenic acid. Here is the list:

Foods Containing Chlorogenic Acid

- potatoes, except sweet potatoes
- cow's milk and all dairy products, except goat milk
- peppers of all kinds, except jalapeño seeds
- unripe fruits of many kinds,
- watermelon
- coffee and regular tea

For potatoes very thorough cooking destroys chlorogenic acid, but frying does not. This agrees with Dr. Charles Ivy's[13] results of 50 years ago that fried food is carcinogenic in some way. He was the world's most renowned gastroenterologist. Chips are not safe, either.

---

[13] Lane, A., Blickenstaff, D., and A.C. Ivy, *The Carcinogenicity of Fat "Browned" by Heating*, Cancer, v. 3, 1950, pp. 1044-51

Dairy products and beverages are not normally cooked, but this could change.

Because there is a <u>chain</u> of events—only one chain—that leads to cancer could we not pluck out one link to stop it all? It has not been tried on a large scale but is so tantalizing a thought that I will list the links as I find them.

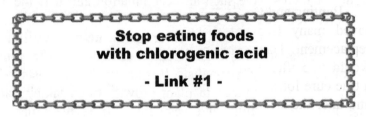

**Stop eating foods
with chlorogenic acid**

- Link #1 -

The food list for chlorogenic acid is not perfectly complete, but avoiding these gives excellent results. In five days no more hypothalamus single cells can be found in the body. The erosion has stopped. See the *Food Table* on page 36.

Is the same phenomenon causing the other organ explosions?

Back at the Pituitary

Another extraordinary chemical has accumulated at the pituitary gland, the "downstairs" neighbor of the hypothalamus gland. It is called **phloridzin** (or phlorizin), again, a plant substance. It, too, is a "phenolic" substance, belonging to the list of food antigens or allergens. Food allergists have studied it, too. In fact, it has even been found to be associated with cancer in the past, rather often, about 80% of the time![14]

Phloridzin has been studied in another connection, too, for nearly 100 years. It could give rabbits instant diabetes if they were given a small dose. The diabetes was permanent. It was a popular way to do research on diabetes in the 1940s and 50s. It was not suspected that phloridzin was actually a cause of <u>our</u>

---

[14] Ber, A. MD, FRCP, *Neutralization of phenolic food compounds in a holistic general practice.* <u>J. Orthomolecular Psychiatry,</u> 1983 4th quarter p. 283

<u>own</u> diabetes, even though it could be obtained from apples, a popular human food! Eating too much sugar was suspected, instead.

The Syncrometer® detects phloridzin accumulation in the pancreas of every diabetic. It is right at the tiny islands of tissue called "islets of Langerhans", where insulin is made.

Banting and Best[15], the discoverers of insulin in the 1920s, saved many lives of diabetics. It was not a cure but a replacement. They could not have guessed that basic research would stop after their departure so that doctors are still without a true cure for diabetes. The connection to phloridzin in foods, and later the arrival of a parasite, the pancreatic fluke and the solvent, wood alcohol, would have excited them greatly.

So for two reasons we should not be eating phloridzin in our food. It is part of cancer development and it leads to diabetes.

Foods Containing Phloridzin

- apples, except Red Delicious and Golden Delicious, both very ripe
- pork, ham and derivatives
- soy products including oil
- unripe fruits of many kinds
- bananas with any tinge of green at the ends
- cauliflower, kohlrabi (all raw)
- cashews, dark green zucchini (all raw)
- amaranth, millet (uncooked)

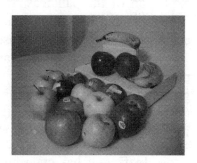

Fig. 22 Pick your apples carefully

---

[15] Banting MB, F.G. and Best BA, C.H. *The internal secretion of the pancreas* <u>The Journal of Laboratory and Clinical Medicine</u>,Vol. VII 1922

We must avoid phloridzin in our foods to stop fragmenting the pituitary gland in the brain (and protect the islets of Langerhans in the pancreas).

After avoiding all foods on the phloridzin list for five days, we again find no single cells or fragments of the pituitary gland in the blood or lymph. Success is swift. Neither duplexes <u>nor</u> <u>triplets</u> can be found. We have stopped the formation of tumor nuclei as we had hoped.

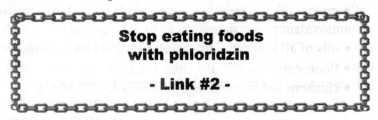

**Stop eating foods
with phloridzin

- Link #2 -**

Back at the Pancreas

Still another chemical is responsible for the microscale explosion of the pancreas. It is **gallic acid**, another phenolic substance coming from food. All cancer patients have an accumulation in their pancreas.

Its presence on all our grains in the USA makes it the most pervasive of the three food antigens. It is not native to the grains though. We place it there by spraying our grains with it (!) for its antioxidant, anti-mold, (preservative) action. We put it <u>in</u> the oils on supermarket shelves for the same preservative effect. Only a few foods have it naturally. Many milk varieties, many chickens, and most eggs in the USA have it. Others don't, like eggs from Mexico. I am guessing this depends on the feed used. It explains why cow's milk has it while goat milk does not (goats shun processed feed such as "rations" and "supplements"). It could explain why chickens are so full of tumors; they are primarily grain eaters. And perhaps why other **alternative therapists** have taken chicken and eggs off the cancer patients' diet. One therapist, a bacteriologist, Virginia Livingston M.D. founded an institute based on the concept that the cancer "bug" came from chickens (and eggs).[16] We will see more evidence for this, later.

Gallic acid, too, has been studied by allergists. It causes many allergic symptoms, especially muscle spasms and very painful cramps, but its role in cancer development was not suspected and it does not cause pain in the pancreas.

Foods Containing Gallic Acid

- grains of all kinds, treated for longer shelf life with antioxidant preservatives
- oils of all kinds, treated to prevent rancidity (antioxidant)
- flour, enriched and bleached
- chickens fed supplementary rations and their eggs
- cows milk and dairy products
- most maple syrup

How to grow and handle foods so they do not have these three food allergens will hopefully become one of our Agriculture Department's high priorities. How to avoid eating them will be our highest priority.

> **Stop eating foods
> with gallic acid or propyl gallate**
>
> **- Link #3 -**

Foods tested by Syncrometer® for these three food antigens are listed in the *Food Table* below. Foods with other antigens are also listed. We will soon see what role they play.

After your tumors are gone you may use certain tips and "loopholes" to regain some of these foods but not sooner. By then you will have acquired some new tastes and will be able to diversify your food better than before.

---

[16] Livingston-Wheeler, MD, Virginia and Addeo, Edmond G., *The Conquest of Cancer, Vaccines and Diet,* New York, F. Watts, 1984, Chicago, Advanced Century Pub. Co. 1978

Food Table

Use this table to identify which foods are safe for you to eat. Find the food you are interested in, for example, almonds. They are *Positive* (*P*) for acetaldehyde, meaning they <u>do</u> contain it. Another example is avocados. They are *Negative* (*N*) for all food phenolics tested, meaning they do <u>not</u> contain them. Foods that are *P/N* means they can be either.

Foods do not always give consistent results. Ripeness, handling methods, and growing methods can make a difference to the phenolic content of food. Test yours to be certain[*].

Sometimes I find a food that acts as an allergen, but I have not identified the substances involved. Those foods are shown in capital letters, for example, CORN.

PIT stands for phenylisothiocyanate, a food phenolic.

The three columns that are shaded are the three that cause the tumor nucleus to form. They are always a top priority.

Thallium is a popular pesticide in foreign countries. It has been banned in USA, even for rodents. Unfortunately, they can expect leg pain, nervous system diseases, and birth defects now. (See *Dangerous Properties of Industrial Materials* 7th ed. by N. Irving Sax and Richard J. Lewis Sr., Van Nostrand Reinhold, N.Y. 1989.)

TRY is free tryptophane, an amino acid. NGF is nerve growth factor. Mo is molybdenum.

D-mannitol is a sugar isomer that appears after processing.

All honey and corn products have air pollutants: beryllium, strontium, vanadium, chromium in metal form.

---

[*]Syncrometer® testers, please accumulate your findings with as much detail as possible. It will be a timeless treasure.

Food Table

FOOD PHENOLIC ALLERGENS / FOOD OILS

Legend: N = Negative, P = Positive, N/P = both Negative & Positive

FOOD ITEM	Apiol	ASA (aspirin)	Asparagine	Acetaldehyde	Caffeic acid	D-Carnitine	Cinnamic	Chlorogenic	Coumarin	Gallic acid	Limonene	Malvin	Menadione	PIT*	Phenylalanine	Phloridzin	Quercitin	SHRIMP	ONION	Tyramine	Umbelliferone	Food Oils (Linoleic/Linolenic/Lauric/Myristic/Oleic/Palmitic)	Notes
agave, syrup	N	P	N	N	P		P	N	N	N	N	N	N	N	N	N	N	N	N	N	N	both gone if boiled	has fructose, which is changed to mannitol by boiling
alfalfa sprouts	N							N		N						N			N				
almond	N			P				N		N						N			N			have mandelonitrile	
aloe vera																P			P				
amaranth	N							N		N						N			N			gone if cooked	
anise seed	N				N	N	N	N	N	N	N	N	N	N	N	N	N	N	N	N	N		
apple, Golden & Red Delicious	N							N		N						N						phloridzin present if unripe; test for thallium	Granny Smith has caffeic
apple, others	N	N	N	N	N	N	N	N	N	N	N	N	N	N	N	P	N	N	N	N	N	phloridzin gone if cooked	
apricot, raw, very ripe	N	N	N	N	N	N	N	N	N	N	N	N	N	N	N	N	N	N	N	N	N	no naringenin, NGF; has phlor if dried	
arrowroot flour	N	N	N	N	N	N	N	N	N	N	N	N	N	N	N	N	N	N	N	N	N	no naringenin, NGF, mannitol	
artichoke	N							N	N	N						N			N			cooked	
asparagus	N		P					N		N						N			P			cooked	

Legend: **N = Negative**, **P = Positive**, **N/P = both Negative & Positive**

FOOD ITEM →	avocado	banana	banana, frozen	banana, small	barley, cooked	barley, raw	basil, fresh	bay leaf	beans, green	beans, pinto, lima, cooked	bee pollen	beef, cooked	beef, range fed	buffalo	beet greens	beet, raw	beet, cooked
Palmitic oil	N	N	N	N	N	N	N	N	N	N	N	N	N	N	N	N	N
Oleic acid oil	N	N	N	N	N	N	N	N	N	N	N	N	N	N	N	N	N
Myristic oil	P	black center has Bacillus cereus; test for thallium	N	N	N	N	N	N	N	N	N	has F. buski	has F. buski, no oils	N	has no mannitol	has no mannitol	has NGF, mannitol
Lauric acid oil	P	N	N	N	N	N	N	N	N	N	N	N	N	N	N	N	N
Linolenic oil	N	N	N	N	N	N	N	N	N	ONION gone if slow cooked twice	N	N	N	N	N	N	N
Linoleic oil	N	N	freezing removes phloridzin, tyramine, and Bacillus cereus	has no Bacillus cereus	has manganese metal	has organic manganese	N	N	cooked	N	has naringenin, phenol	N	N	N	N	N	N
Umbelliferone	N	N	N	N	N	N	has piperine	N	N	N	N	N	N	N	N	N	N
Tyramine	N	P	N	N	N	N	N	N	N	N	N	N	N	N	N	N	N
ONION	N	N	N	N	N	N	N	N	N	P	N	N	N	N	N	N	N
SHRIMP	N	N	N	N	N	N	N	N	N	N	N	N	N	N	N	N	N
Quercitin	N	N	N	N	N	N	N	N	N	N	N	N	N	N	N	N	N
Phloridzin	N	P	N	N	N	N	N	N	N	N	N	N	N	N	N	N	N
Phenylalanine	N	N	N	N	N	N	N	N	N	N	N	N	N	N	N	N	N
PIT*	N	N	N	N	N	N	N	N	N	N	N	N	N	N	N	N	N
Menadione	N	N	N	N	N	N	N	N	N	All develop ONION if cooked at high temperature	N	N	N	N	N	N	N
Malvin	N	N	N	N	N	N	N	N	N	N	N	N	N	N	N	N	N
Limonene	N	N	N	N	N	N	N	N	N	N	N	N	N	N	N	N	P
Gallic acid	N	N	N	N	N	N	N	N	N	N	N	N	N	N	N	N	N
Coumarin	N	N	N	N	N	N	N	N	N	N	N	N	N	N	N	N	N
Chlorogenic	N	N	N	N	N	N	N	N	N	N	N	N	N	N	N	N	N
Cinnamic	N	N	N	N	N	N	N	N	N	N	N	N	N	N	N	N	N
D-Carnitine	N	N	N	N	N	N	N	N	N	N	N	N	N	N	N	N	N
Caffeic acid	N	N	N	N	N	N	N	N	N	N	N	N	N	N	N	N	N
Acetaldehyde	N	N	N	N	N	N	N	N	P	N	N	N	N	N	N	N	N
Asparagine	N	N	N	N	N	N	N	N	N	N	N	N	N	N	N	N	N
ASA (aspirin)	N	N	N	N	N	N	N	N	P	N	N	N	N	N	N	N	N
Apiol	N	N	N	N	N	N	N	N	N	N	N	N	N	N	N	N	N

Legend: N = Negative, P = Positive, N/P = both Negative & Positive

FOOD ITEM (columns, left → right):
1. bok choy, raw
2. boneset herb
3. Brazil nuts
4. bread, bakery
5. bread, (Mex) bolillo
6. bread, supermarket
7. bread, health food store
8. bread, machine, or homemade
9. broccoli
10. Brussels' sprouts
11. buckwheat
12. burdock root
13. butter, organic
14. butter
15. buttermilk
16. cabbage, raw
17. cactus, raw
18. cantaloupe
19. cardamom

Oil-row notes (by food column):
- bok choy, raw — gone if very fresh
- boneset herb — no naringenin, NGF
- Brazil nuts — P (Lauric acid oil)
- bread, bakery — has mannitol
- bread, (Mex) bolillo — no mannitol, bromine or live yeast
- bread, supermarket — has mannitol, bromine, live yeast
- bread, health food store — has live yeast
- bread, machine, or homemade — no live yeast or gallic acid
- broccoli — gone if cooked
- Brussels' sprouts — cooked
- buckwheat — cooked
- burdock root — no naringenin, NGF
- butter, organic — has HGH
- cabbage, raw — PIT gone if cooked
- cactus, raw — has ASA if cooked
- cantaloupe — no MELON allergen

(Oil rows listed: Palmitic oil, Oleic acid oil, Myristic oil, Lauric acid oil, Linolenic oil, Linoleic oil)

Substance	1	2	3	4	5	6	7	8	9	10	11	12	13	14	15	16	17	18	19
Umbelliferone		N		N					N		N	N	N				N	N	
Tyramine	N	N		N	N				N		N			N		N	N	N	N
ONION	N	N			N	P	P	N	N	N	N	N	P	P		N	N	N	N
SHRIMP	N	N		N	N				N		N	N	N			N	N	N	N
Quercitin	N	N			N				N		N	N	N				N	N	P
Phloridzin	N	N	N	N	N	N	N	N	N	N	N	N	N	P	N	N	N	N	N
Phenylalanine	N	N		N	N				N		N	N	N			N			N
PIT*	N	N			N			P	P		N	N	N			P	N	N	N
Menadione	P	N			N		P		P		P	N	P			N	N	N	
Malvin	N	N		N	N				N		N	N	N			N	N	N	N
Limonene	N	N			N				N		N	N	N			N	N	N	
Gallic acid	N	N	N	P	N	P	P	N	N	N	N	N	N	P		N	N	N	N
Coumarin	N	N		N	N				N		N	N	N			N	N	N	N
Chlorogenic	N	N	N	N	N	N	N	N	N	N	N	N	P	P		N	N	N	N
Cinnamic	N	N		N	N				N		N	N	N			N	N	N	N
D-Carnitine	N	N			N				N			N		N	N		N		
Caffeic acid	N	N		N	N				P		N	N	N			N	N	N	N
Acetaldehyde	N	N	P		N				N		N	N	N			N	N	N	
Asparagine	N	N			N				N		N	N	N			N	N		
ASA (aspirin)	N	N			N				N		N	N	N			N	N	N	
Apiol	N	N	N		N	N	P	N	N	N	N	N	N	P	N	N	N	N	

Legend: N = Negative   P = Positive   N/P = both Negative & Positive

FOOD ITEM → (compounds ↓)	carrots, raw	cashew, raw	cauliflower	celery	chard, Swiss	cheese, cottage, other	cheese, goat	cheese, organic	cherimoya	cherries, Bing, ripe, black	cherries, red	cherries, yellow	chicken, cooked	cilantro, fresh	cinnamon	cloves, whole	coconut	collards
Palmitic oil		no umbelli if peeled	both gone if cooked		has no mannitol	most cheeses have *Bacillus cereus, pituitary, hypothalamus cells, vasopressin, HGH, TSH, FSH*				have phloridzin if unripe	have chlorogenic and phloridzin if only red		has lauric acid, MYC oncovirus, E. recurvatum fluke		N		P	
Oleic acid oil		no phlor if roasted													N	N	P	
Myristic oil															N	P	P	
Lauric acid oil															N	N	P	
Linolenic oil															N	N	P	
Linoleic oil															N	N	P	gone if cooked
Umbelliferone	P			N	N	N							N	N	N	N	N	
Tyramine	N			N	N	N							N	N	N	N	N	
ONION		N		N	N	N	N				N	N	N	P	N	N	N	N
SHRIMP	P			N	N	N	N						N	N	N	N		
Quercitin				N	N	P	N						N	N	N	N		
Phloridzin	N	P	P	N	N	P	N	N/P	N	N	N	N	N	N	N	N	N	N
Phenylalanine	N			N	N	P		P		N			N	N	N	N		
PIT*	N		P	N	N		N			N			N	N	N	N	N	P
Menadione				N	N		N			N			N	N	N	N		
Malvin	N			N	N		N			N	P/N		N	N	N	N		
Limonene				N	N		N			N		P	N	N	N	N		
Gallic acid	N	N		N	N	P	N	P	N	N	P	N	N/P	N	N	N	N	N
Coumarin	N			N	N		N		N	N			N	N	N	N		
Chlorogenic	N	N		N	N	P	N	P	N	N	P	N	N	N	N	N	N	N
Cinnamic	N			N	N		N			N			N	N	P	N		
D-Carnitine				N	N								P	N	N	N	N	
Caffeic acid	N			N	N		N						N	N	N	N		
Acetaldehyde		P		N	N								N	N	N	N		
Asparagine		N		N	N								P	N	N	N		
ASA (aspirin)				N	N								N	N	N	N		
Apiol	N	N		N	N	P	N		N	N	N	N	N	N	N	N	N	N

Note (chicken, cooked): range fed has no gallic, MYC, SV 40, malvin

N = Negative P = Positive N/P = both Negative & Positive — FOOD ITEM	Apiol	ASA (aspirin)	Asparagine	Acetaldehyde	Caffeic acid	D-Carnitine	Cinnamic	Chlorogenic	Coumarin	Gallic acid	Limonene	Malvin	Menadione	PIT*	Phenylalanine	Phloridzin	Quercitin	SHRIMP	ONION	Tyramine	Umbelliferone	Linoleic oil	Linolenic oil	Lauric acid oil	Myristic oil	Oleic acid oil	Palmitic oil
comfrey leaf or root, dried	N	N		N	N			N	N	N	N	N	N	N	N	N	N	N	N	N	N						
corn	All corn varieties and products: in husk, cooked, popped, organic have incorporated major air pollutants: strontium, beryllium, chromium, vanadium																										
coriander	N	N	N		N			N	N	N	N	N	N	N	N	N	N	N	N								
cranberries	N	N	N	N	N		N	N	N	N	N	N	N	N	N	N	N	N	N	N	N	have hippuric acid					
whipping cream, heavy: supermarket	N	N	P				N	N/P	N	P		N	N	N	P	N	N	N		P		has lactose and galacturonic acid					
• org, kosher	N	N	N	N	N		N	P	N	N	N	N	P	N	N	N	N	N	N	N	N						
• Lala (Mex)	N	N	N	N	N	N	N	N	N	N	N	N	N	N	N	N	N	N	N	N	N	no lactose, or piperine					
clover, red	N	N	N	N	N	N	N	N	P	N	N	N	N	N	N	N	P	P	N	N	N						
cucumbers	N	N	N	N	N	N	N	N	N	N	N	N	N	N	N	N	P	N	N	N	N						
cumquat, raw	N	N	N				N	N	N	N	N	N	N	N	N	N	N	N	N	N	N	has no naringenin					
dates, dried	N							N	N	N						N						have acetic acid					
dextrose	N	N	N	N				N	N	N		N				N			N			has CORN (air) pollutants					
eggs USA, raw or cooked	N	N	N	Hypothalamus and pituitary cells as well as SV 40 and MYC oncoviruses are present in most USA, raw or cooked eggs, but they can be destroyed with HCL, 3 drops each.						P		P	N	N	N	N	N	N	N	N	P						
eggs (Mex)	N				N			N		N	N	N		N	N	N	N	N	N	N	have no hypothalamus, pituitary, SV 40, MYC						
eggplant	N			N			N	N	N	N	N	N	N	N	N	N	N	N	N	N							P cooked

N = Negative P = Positive N/P = both Negative & Positive

FOOD ITEM	Umbelliferone	Tyramine	ONION	SHRIMP	Quercitin	Phloridzin	Phenylalanine	PIT*	Menadione	Malvin	Limonene	Gallic acid	Coumarin	Chlorogenic	Cinnamic	D-Carnitine	Caffeic acid	Acetaldehyde	Asparagine	ASA (aspirin)	Apiol
elder leaf	N	N	N	N	N	N	N	N	N	N	N	N	N	N	N	N	N	N	N	N	N
epasote (soup flavoring)	N	N	N	N	N	N	N	N	N	N	N	N	N	N	N	N	N	N	N	N	N
eucalyptus (all parts)	N	N	N	N	N	N	N	N	N	N	N	N	N	N	N	N	N	N	N	N	N
fennel, seed (leaves have ONION)	N	N	N	N	N	N	N	N	N	N	N	N	N	N	N	N	N	N	N	N	N
fenugreek	N	N	N	N	N	N	N	N	N	N	N	N	N	N	N	N	N	N	N	N	N
fig, raw, dried (has acetic acid)		N	N	N		N						N	N	N							N
fish, fresh or canned (has Fast Garnet, Fast Red, Fast Red Violet dyes)		N	P	P		N						N	N	N							
flax seed, oil			P	N	N	N	N	N	N	N	N	P	N	P	N		N	N	N	N	N
flour, wheat (Linolenic oil P; no bromine or gallic if unbleached)		N	N	N	N	N	N	N	P	N	N	P	N	N	N	N	N		N	N	N
flour, white (unbleached)		N		N	N	N	N	N	N	N	N	N	N	N	N	N	N	N	N	N	N
flour, rye (has no menadione)	N	N	N	N	N	N	N	N	N	N	N	N	N	N	N	N	N	N	N	N	N
garbanzo beans, cooked (develops ONION at high temperature)	N	N	N/P	N	N	N	N	N	N	N	N/P	N	N	N	N	N	N	N	N	N	N
ginger (has hippuric acid and mandelonitrile)	N	N	N	N	N	N	N	N	N	N	N	N	N	N	N	N	N	N	N	N	N
garlic, raw		N	P	N	N	N	N	N	N	N	N	N	N	N	N	N	N	N	N	N	N
grapes, red, blue (no benzoic or citric acid or fructose)	N	N	N	N	N	N	N	N	N	P	N	N	N	N	N	N	N	N	N	N	N
grapes, green	N	N	N	N	N	N	N	N	N	N	N	N	N	N	N	N	N	N	N	N	N
grapefruit (caffeic gone if tree ripened)						N					N	N		N			P				
grain, Kamut						P						P		P							
guayaba		N			N	N		N	N	N	P	N		N	N		N	N			P

Legend: N = Negative, P = Positive, N/P = both Negative & Positive

FOOD ITEM	Apiol	ASA (aspirin)	Asparagine	Acetaldehyde	Caffeic acid	D-Carnitine	Cinnamic	Chlorogenic	Coumarin	Gallic acid	Limonene	Malvin	Menadione	PIT*	Phenylalanine	Phloridzin	Quercitin	SHRIMP	ONION	Tyramine	Umbelliferone	Linoleic oil	Linolenic oil	Lauric acid oil	Myristic oil	Oleic acid oil	Palmitic oil
gum, chewing	P						P	N		N		P				N			P			has mannitol					
hamburger					N		N	N	N	N		N		N	N	N		N		N		has pyrrole					
honey	N							N	P	N						N			N			has fructose					
horseradish	N	N	N	N	N	N	N	N	N	N	N	N	N	N	N	N	N	N	N	N	N						
hydrangea	N	N	N	N	N	N	N	N	N	N	N	N	N	N	N	N	N	N	N	N	N		root	P			
Jalapeño seed								P		P				N		P							all gone if ripe				
Jamaica flower							N	P	N	P	P	N	N	N	N	P	N	N	P	N	N		popular Mexican drink				
jicama, raw	N				N		N	N	N	N	P	N	N	N	N	N	N	N		N	N						
kipper snacks	N							N		N						N			P				has pyrrole, NGF				
kiwi	N	N	N	N	N	N	N	N	N	N	N	N	N	N	N	N	P	N	P	N	N		has no mannitol				
kornrabe herb																N		N					kills SV 40, tumor nucleus				
kohlrabi, raw								N	N	N						N		N									
lard																N						N	N	P	N	N	N
lamb	N	N	N	N	N	N	N	N	N	N	N	N	N	N	N	N	N	N	N	N	N	N	N	N	N	N	N
leeks, raw								N		N						N			P								
lecithin, soy	P							N		N						N											
lemons	N	N	N	N	N	N	N	N	N	N	P	N	N	N	N	N	N	N	N	N	N		have citric acid				
lentils, cooked	N	N	N	N	N	N	N	N	N	N	N	N	N	N	N	N	N	N	P	N			gone if slow cooked				
lettuce, iceberg	N	N	N	N	N	N	N	N	N	N	P	N	N	N	N	N	N	N	N	N			has menadione if wilted				
limes, all					P		P				P	P															
mango	N									P						P			N								

* PIT = pit

Note (honey row): all honey has incorporated air pollutants: strontium, beryllium, chromium, vanadium.

Legend: **N = Negative**, **P = Positive**, **N/P = both Negative & Positive**

Column notes (appear as annotations above certain FOOD ITEM columns):
- melon — *has MELON antigen*
- milk, goat, raw — *no HGH, TRY, casein, piperine, or free cells*
- milk, goat — *has mannitol, TRY*
- milk, cow, all kinds — *has hypothalamus, pituitary cells, TRY*
- oats, cooked — *has manganese metal*
- oil, almond / canola / corn / cottonseed / olive — *all these oils had malonic and maleic acids, whether "pure" or not*
- oil, peanut, pure / oil, safflower — *antigens gone if pure*

Antigen	margarine	maple syrup	melon	milk, goat, raw	milk, goat	milk, cow, all kinds	mint, fresh	mustard seed	nectarines	nutmeg	nuts, Hazel	oats, cooked	oil, almond	oil, canola	oil, corn	oil, cottonseed	oil, olive	oil, peanut, pure	oil, safflower
Palmitic oil															N				
Oleic acid oil															N	N			
Myristic oil														P	N	N			
Lauric acid oil														N	N	N			
Linolenic oil															N	N			
Linoleic oil														N	N	N			
Umbelliferone			N		N					N	N								
Tyramine		N	N			P	N			N	N								
ONION	P		N	N	N	N	N	N	N	N	N	N	P	P			N	N/P	N
SHRIMP	P	N	N				N		N	N	N								
Quercitin			N				N		N	N	N								
Phloridzin	P	N	N	N	N	N	N	N	N	N	N	N	P	P			P	N	N
Phenylalanine	P	N		N		P	N		N	N	N								
PIT*				N			N	P	N	N	N								
Menadione			N				N		N	N	N					P			
Malvin		N	N	N			N		N	N	N								
Limonene			P	N			N		N	N	N								
Gallic acid	P	N/P	N	N	N	N/P	N	N	N	N	N	N	P	P	P		P	N	N
Coumarin		N		N			N		N	N	N	N							
Chlorogenic	P	N	N	N	N	P	N	N	N	N	N	N	N	P			P	N	N
Cinnamic		N		N			N		N	N	N								
D-Carnitine										N	N								
Caffeic acid		N		N			N		N	N	N								
Acetaldehyde			N				N		N	N	N		P						
Asparagine							N		N	N	N								
ASA (aspirin)		P/N	N	N			N		N	N	N								
Apiol	P	N	N	N	N	N	N	N	N	N	N	N	P	P	P	P	P	N	N

Legend: **N = Negative · P = Positive · N/P = both Negative & Positive**

FOOD ITEM	Apiol	ASA (aspirin)	Asparagine	Acetaldehyde	Caffeic acid	D-Carnitine	Cinnamic	Chlorogenic	Coumarin	Gallic acid	Limonene	Malvin	Menadione	PIT*	Phenylalanine	Phloridzin	Quercitin	SHRIMP	ONION	Tyramine	Umbelliferone	Linoleic oil	Linolenic oil	Lauric acid oil	Myristic oil	Oleic acid oil	Palmitic oil
oil, sesame	N/P							N/P		N/P						N/P			N								
oil, soy, pure	P							P		P						P											
oil, sunflower	N							N		N						N			N								
oil, vegetable	P									P						P											
okra, cooked	N	N	N	N	N	N	N	N	N	N	N	N	N	N	N	N	N	N	N	N	N						
olive leaf, dry	N	N	N	N	N	N	N	N	N	N	N	N	N	N	N	N	N	N	N	N	N	all absent if fresh					
olives, black	P			N	P			N	N	N	N	N	N	N	N	P	N	N	P			ONION gone if cooked					
onion, raw	N			N		N		N	N	N	N	N	N	N	N	N	N	N	P	N	N						
oranges, supermarket	N	N	N	N	N	N	N	N	N	N	N	N	N	N	N	N	N	N	N	N	N	have naringenin					
oregano, dry	N	N	N	N	N	N	N	N	N	N	N	N	N	N	N	N	N	N	N	N	N	no naringenin					
papaya, ripe	N	N	N	N	N	N	N	N	P	N	N	N	N	N	N	N	N	N	N	N	N	no naringenin					
parsley, raw	N	N	N	N	N	N	N	N	N	N	N	N	P	N	N	N	N	N	N			both gone if boiled					
pasta	N	N	N	N	N	N	N	N	N	N	N	N	N	N	N	N	N	N	N								
peaches, ripe	N	N	N	N	N	N	N	N	N	N	N	N	N	N	N	N	N	N	N	N	N	no naringenin, NGF					
peas, green, split, yellow	N	N	N	N	N	N	N	N/P	N	N/P	N	N	N	P	N	N/P	N	N	N			have ONION after cooking					
peanuts, raw in shell	N	N	N	N	N	N	N	N	N	N	N	N	N	N	N	N	N	N	N	N	N	have ONION if roasted					
peanut butter, old fashioned			N		N		N	N		N		N				N	N	N	P	N/P		smooth ground has nickel and chromium					
pears, ripe	N	N	N			N	N	N	N	N		N	N	N	N	N	N	N	N	N	N	have limonene if cooked					
pecans	N		N	P				N		N						N			N								P

Notes appearing across the oranges, supermarket row: "caffeic not present in homegrown oranges; Mandarin & tangerine have no naringenin; have no naringenin"

Legend: N = Negative P = Positive N/P = both Negative & Positive

Column notes (oils / Umbelliferone header area):
- peppers, all: gone if cooked
- pineapple: raw or cooked
- plantain, fried: N — both gone if ripe
- plums, black: have phlor if under ripe
- potatoes, well cooked, baked: test for malonic acid
- potato, sweet, or yam: no piperine, NGF
- potato chips: has mandelonitrile, test for malonic, apiol
- pumpkin: gone if cooked
- pumpkin seed: has Mo if roasted
- radish, red: no naringenin, NGF
- radish, white: SHRIMP gone if cooked
- raisins, all: have mannitol
- rice, USA, cooked: Mexican varieties have no coumarin
- sage, dried: gone if cooked

	peppermint	peppers, all	pineapple	plantain, fried	plums, black	pomegranate	potatoes, well cooked, baked	potatoes, fried	potato starch	potato, sweet, or yam	potato chips	pumpkin	pumpkin seed	quassia herb	radish, red	radish, white	raisins, all	raspberries	rice, USA, cooked	rosemary	sage, dried
Palmitic oil																					
Oleic acid oil																					
Myristic oil																					
Lauric acid oil																					
Linolenic oil																					
Linoleic oil																					
Umbelliferone		N		N	N					N			N		N		N		N		N
Tyramine	N			P	N								N		N		N		N	N	N
ONION	N	N	N	N	N	N	N		N	N		P	N		N		N		N	N	N
SHRIMP	N			N	N	N			N	N			N		N	P	N	N	N		
Quercitin	N			N	N					N	P	N	N		N		N		N	N	N
Phloridzin	N	N	N	P	N	N	N	P	N	N	P	N	P	N	N	N	N	N	N	N	N
Phenylalanine	N		N	N	N	N				N			N		N		N		N	N	N
PIT*	N		N	N	N					N			N		P		N		N		N
Menadione	N		N	N	N					N			N		N	P	N		N		N
Malvin	N		N	N	N					N			N		N		P		N	N	N
Limonene	N		P	N	N					N			N		N		N		N	N	N
Gallic acid	N	N	N	N	N	N	N		N	N	P	N	N		N	N	N		N	N	N
Coumarin	N		N	N	N					N			N		N	N	P		N		N
Chlorogenic	N	P	N	N	N	N	N	P	N	N	P	N	P		N	N	N	N	N	N	P
Cinnamic	N		N	N	N					N			N		N		N		N	N	N
D-Carnitine	N			N	N					N			N		N		N		N		N
Caffeic acid	N			N	N					N			N		N		N		N	N	N
Acetaldehyde	N			N	N					N			N		N		N		N		N
Asparagine	N			N	N					N			N		N		N		N		N
ASA (aspirin)	N		N	N	N					N			N		N		N		N	N	N
Apiol	N	N	N	N	N		N		N	N	P	N	N	N	N		N		N	N	N

N = Negative P = Positive N/P = both Negative & Positive — compound \ FOOD ITEM	salmon, fresh canned	sardines, oil	sardines, water	seafood, fish, shrimp, crab	sesame seed	soybeans	soy beverage	spinach, raw	squash, all	strawberries, org., supermkt	sugar, icing	sugar, org. USA	sugar (MEX)	sunflower seed	tahini, organic	tapioca, cooked	tea, regular	thyme, dried
Palmitic oil	test for dyes, SHRIMP	have NGF	have NGF	no SHRIMP in first 6 hours after catch		all soy products have apiol	apiol	has oxalate, use little	gone if cooked; no naringenin, NGF, mannitol	has fructose, CORN, mannitol	has mannitol; test for CORN	test for CORN	zulka azuca estandar and azucar estandar (CALIMAX) dark have no mannitol	raw		has PIT if undercooked		
Oleic acid oil																		
Myristic oil																		
Lauric acid oil																		
Linolenic oil														N	P			
Linoleic oil				P										N	P			
Umbelliferone					P													P
Tyramine					N				N					N	N		N	
ONION	N	N	N	N	N	N	P	N	N	N				N	N	N	N	N
SHRIMP	N	P	P	P					N					N	N	N	N	N
Quercitin					N				P			N		N	N		N	N
Phloridzin	N	N	N	N	N	N	P	N	N	P	N	N	N	N	N	P	P	N
Phenylalanine									N					N	N	N	N	N
PIT*									N			N		N	N	N	N	N
Menadione									N			N		N	N	N	N	N
Malvin						P			N	P		N		N	N	N	N	N
Limonene									N			N		N	N	N	N	N
Gallic acid	N	N	N	N	N	P		N	N	N/P	N	N	N	N	N	P	P	N
Coumarin					N	N			N			N		N	N	N	N	N
Chlorogenic	N	N	N	N	N	P		N	N	N	N	N	N	N	N	P	P	N
Cinnamic					N				N	P		N		N	N	N	N	N
D-Carnitine					N				N			N		N	N	N	N	N
Caffeic acid					N	P			N	P		N		N	N	P	N	N
Acetaldehyde					N				N		N	N		N	N	N	N	N
Asparagine					N				N					N	N		N	N
ASA (aspirin)					N				N		N	N		N	N		P	N
Apiol	N	P	N	N	N	P	P	N	N	N	N	N	N	N	N	N	N	N

N = Negative P = Positive N/P = both Negative & Positive FOOD ITEM	Apiol	ASA (aspirin)	Asparagine	Acetaldehyde	Caffeic acid	D-Carnitine	Cinnamic	Chlorogenic	Coumarin	Gallic acid	Limonene	Malvin	Menadione	PIT*	Phenylalanine	Phloridzin	Quercitin	SHRIMP	Tyramine	Umbelliferone	Linoleic oil	Linolenic oil	Lauric acid oil	Myristic oil	Oleic acid oil	Palmitic oil
tomatoes, raw or cooked	N	N						N	N	N	N/P	P				N/P		N				malvin gone if cooked 5 min.				
tomato, cherry	N		N	N	N	N	N	N	N	N	N	N	N	N	N	N	N	N	N	N		malvin if blemished		N	N	
tuna, canned	N							N		N						N		P					in water			
tuna, canned	P							N		N						N		P					in oil		P	
tuna (kosher), Albacore, Tongol, Skipjack, canned in water has no SHRIMP																										
turkey, free range, organic	N	N	N	N	N	N	N	N	N	N	N	N	N	N	N	N	N	N	N	N	N	N	N	N	N	N
turkey, regular						P		N	N	P						N					P					
turmeric, pwd	N	N	N	N	N	N	N	N	N	N	N	N	N	N	N	N	N	N	N	N				N		
uva ursi, pwd	N	N	N	N	N	N	N	N	N	N	N	N	N	N	N	N	N	N	N	N	N	N	N	N	N	N
vanilla	N		N					N	P	N						N										
walnuts	N	N	N	P	N	N	N	N	N	N	N	N	N	N	N	N	N	N	N	N		P				
walnut, Black, hull tincture	N		N	N	N		N	N	N	P	N	N	N	N	N	N	N	N	N	N				N		
watercress	N																				tablets have coumarin					
wheat, sprouts	N	N	N	N	N		N	N	N	N	N	N	N	N	N	N	N	N	N	N						
wheat germ	N	N	N	N	N	N	N	N	N	N	N	N	P	N	N	N	N	N	N	N	gone if nitrogen					
wheat, cooked	N				N		N	N	N	N	N	N	P	N	P	N	N	N/P	N	N	packed					
yogurt, all varieties	P			N/P	N/P		N/P	P/N		P/N		P		P/N	P	P/N	N/P	N/P	P		has mannitol					
zucchini	N	N	N	N	N	N	N	N	N	N	N	N	N	N	N	N	N	N	N	N	cooked					

Allergens Destroyed by Ozonation (ozonate 10 minutes; then close container and wait another 10 minutes to complete the action; see page 518)

- casein
- CHEESE
- estradiol
- estriol
- estrone
- PIT
- quercitin

Allergens Destroyed by Boiling (keep up a rolling boil for 5 minutes; add liquid to thick foods like beans or porridge to help it boil; microwaving is not satisfactory)

- caffeic acid
- chlorogenic acid
- gallic acid
- menadione
- ONION
- phloridzin
- quercitin
- SHRIMP
- umbelliferone
- PIT

Special Attractions

Food antigens can be especially attracted to certain organs, just as bacteria or medicines are. Such attractions are called **tropisms**. We have many examples. For instance, herbs expected to help the eye or throat should have a tropism for these organs, to be truly useful. Bacteria with tropisms are, for example, tuberculosis for the lungs, and staphylococcus aureus for the skin and breast. The three allergenic food substances are specifically attracted to the three eroding organs.

Chlorogenic acid has a tropism for the hypothalamus. When a tiny bit of potato is chewed, raw or fried, we can detect chlorogenic acid in the hypothalamus in seconds, before it could have reached the liver!

Even when free hypothalamus cells have already settled in a different organ, where they are living as part of the tumor nucleus, chlorogenic acid is immediately there.

When a tiny bit of the wrong apple is nibbled, phloridzin goes immediately to the pituitary gland. In less than a minute it can be detected in free pituitary cells passing through some organ. And a tropism exists for the islets of Langerhans too; it is the same…phloridzin!

Gallic acid has a tropism for the pancreas, not the islets of Langerhans where your insulin is made. It is there in three seconds after putting a bit of gallic acid-containing food in your mouth. Again, it arrives before it could have reached the liver where detoxification would occur.

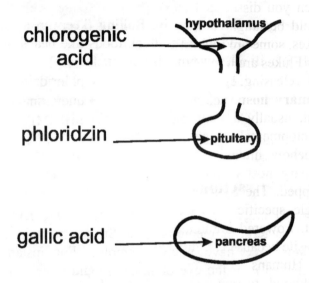

Fig. 23 Food antigens go to specific organs

The tropisms of chlorogenic acid, phloridzin, and gallic acid are the same for all of us, whether or not we have cancer or allergies or other illnesses or are completely well. What matters for our health is how long it stays in the target organ. It depends on parasitism, as we will see.

CHAPTER 3

OUR PARASITES

Humans, like other animals, have always had parasites, both outside and inside our bodies. It is easy to see in animals when you dissect a frog or fish in a college classroom. You would be taught that every organ has its parasite. Some are flukes, some are roundworms, some are tapeworms.

Flukes are like little leeches, stuck in one spot, just feeding and releasing eggs. The animal with the adult fluke is the **primary host**. The animal with the larvae is the **secondary host**, usually a snail. Inside the snail the larvae go through developmental stages that suits the parasites' need to, somehow, hitchhike from animal to animal till it can reach its primary host again. This has changed since immunity has dropped. The Syncrometer® finds that instead of requiring a single, specific snail, many snails can be used as the secondary host. Lowered immunity allows shortcuts to be taken by the parasite because the vigilance of the immune system is gone.

Humans go through infancy, childhood, teenage, and adulthood, to reproduce and arrive at infancy again. All with the same purpose: to survive and thrive. Our parasites survive with us, but how they will thrive depends on our health. They do not thrive when we are healthy. It is the less healthy animal that is the most parasitized in Nature.

In times of plentiful, nourishing food and clean water for animals, parasites do not take over the host animals. But if food is scarce, and the water source is crowded with other animals, their general health declines and parasites thrive instead. Poor health and parasitism go hand in hand.

The roundworms look a lot like earthworms without feet, or means of travel. A roundworm just wiggles and molts its skin off a number of times to grow till it is an adult. Our common roundworms are **Ascaris**, **Strongyloides** and **heartworms (filaria)**. Cats have learned to spit up their

Ascaris by eating grass. Puppies, too, are taught to eat "dog grass" to entangle their stomach Ascaris and spit them up. But humans, with all their intelligence, seem to be doing nothing to keep their parasitism in check.

The Syncrometer® shows that we all, from early childhood, harbor Ascaris eggs and larvae, the young hatchlings that go through molts. These tiny wormlets give us seizures, eczema, lung disease, and the common cold.

Parasites even live in other parasites. They have their own bacteria and viruses. The bacteria themselves have viruses. And, at least one bacterium, common Salmonella, has **prions**.

Ascaris brings us **Chicken Pox** and **mumps**, **Herpes 1** and **2**, **Coxsackie viruses**, and **Adenovirus** (the common cold). It brings us **Mycobacterium avium** that causes night sweats. We didn't notice these connections in the past because these diseases are commonplace and the parasites so tiny and quiet.

It takes a special astuteness to be suspicious of commonplace things. Ancient and primitive societies had special astuteness. Why did the Hebrew nation ban pork in the diet? Did they notice that herdsmen of swine often had epilepsy, skin disease and other health problems?

Modern American citizens have some astuteness, too, having recognized that smoking cigarettes often leads to lung cancer.

Strongyloides bring us **migraine** headaches and the very beginning of all tumors, as we will see. Which problem they bring depends on where they colonize and what we, the host, are eating.

Heartworm (Dirofilaria) may even be more prevalent than Ascaris, and is a major contributor to <u>all</u> heart disease. Since our lives are ended in heart disease more than any other way, heartworm should really have our greatest attention. So far, the Syncrometer® has found it not just in the heart, but everywhere we have fluids. Our eyes even have tiny threads of filaria suspended in their fluids. The chest with its lymph fluids around the lungs has heartworm bits. The belly with its **peritoneal** fluid has its short bits. If any of these short pieces of Dirofilaria manage to escape both the immune system and your digestive enzymes so that it can grow long, it produces a snarl. Such a snarl is the starting point for **Hodgkin's Lymphoma**, **abdominal tumor masses**, and possibly, even the brain "tangle" in Alzheimer's disease.

For animals it is the availability of clean food and water that decides if they are heavily parasitized and short-lived.

For humans it is also the food and water that decides our health and whether we are heavily parasitized and destined to a life of low energy and lots of medicine.

> For humans, unclean food and water has brought immunodepression.

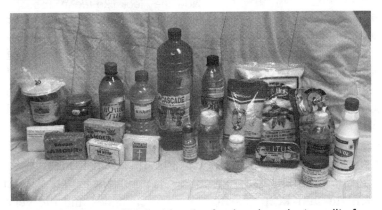

The local water quality decides the food and product quality for that region. Two out of all these African products did <u>not</u> have PCBs, benzene, azo dyes, heavy metals, motor oil, wheel bearing grease, and whatever else comes with laundry bleach. They were the <u>imported</u> jam and pasta. At extreme right is bleach meant to be added to food!

Fig. 24 African products bring the same 5 immunity depressors

Water has brought 5 critical immune system depressants: PCBs, benzene, asbestos, azo dyes and certain heavy metals. Food has brought the same five, through food processing that uses the same polluted water to accomplish it all.

Humans now have 4 very common flukes, besides Fasciolopsis: the sheep liver fluke, the lung fluke, the pancreatic fluke and human liver fluke. Don't believe that the sheep liver fluke is for sheep alone. Hosts can be substituted when immunity is down so that we can become the "accidental" host or "incidental" host, already known for decades. Less common flukes are becoming more common, too, such as Gastrothylax, Acanthocephala, Echinostoma revolutum, and Echinoporyphium recurvatum. You may see any of these now while you are killing parasites with a vigorous program that induces a brief diarrhea. Get a strong

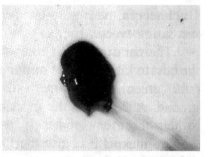

Plump F. buski was passed with urine into catheter bag. This avoided the osmotic pressure shock that ruptures flukes when passed into plain water, so no "hairy leg" egg strings hang out. Now they look like the microscope slide specimen. Body distended and glistening shows a well-fed specimen. Pointed head end aims down. Tissue at right is adhering blood clot.

Fig. 25 Intact F. buski resting on eyedropper

flashlight and keep plastic cups and utensils in the bathroom, as well as Lugol's iodine, so you can see your own parasites safely and identify them.

Heartworms have gained ground in us by growing longer, even inside the bowel, so their clear glass-like threads make loops in the bowel contents, easy to recognize. And

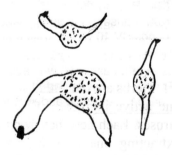

Appears as black dots (mid region) in toilet bowl, about ¾ inch long.

Fig. 26 Acanthocephala drawn from life

54

Onchocerca, very similar to the threads of heartworm is increasing everywhere, too.

The parasite-killing recipe given in earlier books is by far the best to kill flukes. It is a combination of Black Walnut hulls (still green), wormwood leaves and cloves, very freshly ground. A slow, easy to manage pace is given in earlier books to help those who must be cautious about new treatments. If you are inexperienced with herbs, you should try a very small dose first and work up to the really effective doses.

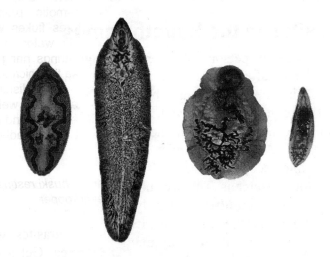

L to R: lung fluke (6X); sheep liver fluke (3X); pancreatic fluke (5X, causes diabetes, nucleates our cancerous tumors and brings SV 40 virus); and human liver fluke (5X).

Fig. 27 Four common flukes

Herbs are our greatest gift on this planet! They do not have <u>one active ingredient</u> that kills a parasite or kills bacteria or viruses. Each herb has <u>many active ingredients</u>. The concept of extracting one principle compound, and making its "sister" chemical (analogs, derivatives) is seriously flawed. An active ingredient, such as l-ascorbic acid, for example, has its "sisters" right with it in Nature! Potency of an herb does not depend so much on the amount of active ingredient you eat. Potency is increased much more by eating all the natural "sister" compounds, which means, the herb intact. Rose hips have much more potency than l-ascorbic acid. The Syncrometer® shows that several nuts or a few rose hips can accomplish much more than plain germanium capsules or pure vitamin C.

For this reason and because herbs belong to you, being your own true treasure, I have chosen herbs wherever possible to deparasitize yourself, kill bacteria and viruses, and maintain your health in a regular way. This is besides electronic and other ways I will discuss later.

Parasites in the Hypothalamus

In a healthy person chlorogenic acid goes straight to the hypothalamus after eating it. But in five minutes, at most 20 minutes, it is gone. It has been detoxified, digested, or removed.

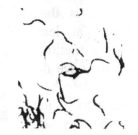

In a cancer patient it never disappears. A tiny wormlet is present, microscopically small. It is Strongyloides stercalis. This wormlet belongs to the **roundworm** family, not the flukes, nor the tapeworms. Its larval stages have **molts**. Molting brings special molting chemicals. Perhaps it is one of these that

Fig. 28 Strongyloides drawn from a microscope slide

interfere with the removal of chlorogenic acid from the hypothalamus. Maybe this wormlet <u>needs</u> this food antigen to molt or accomplish other purposes. The worm is never there unless chlorogenic acid is there.

Parasites in the Pituitary

Phloridzin, too, goes directly to the brain, lodging in the pituitary gland even in healthy persons. But it is there only for minutes. Then it has already been removed.

In a cancer patient it is always there. This irritating allergen is present constantly—yet only if the common human liver fluke is there. Somehow this parasite prevents the removal of phloridzin or, again, perhaps it needs it. The human liver fluke is a small parasite, less than ¼ inch long even when it is stretched flat. Its scientific name is Clonorchis sinensis. A new name, Opisthorcis, has been given to Clonorchis species recently.

Human Liver Flukes and Cancer

Human liver flukes are very common, and like Strongyloides, they become more plentiful as we age. It is not surprising that they play a role in cancer. In fact, scientists in Asian countries have often proclaimed their theories that this fluke actually is the chief cause of cancer, at least, liver cancer. After a traditional liver cleanse you may see dozens of these in the toilet bowl, but having shrunk to $^1/_8$ inch to $^1/_{16}$ inch in length, they go unnoticed. The association between this fluke and liver cancer has been studied for decades.[17] The fact that it plays a role in <u>every</u> cancer would be more obscure, without the technology of the Syncrometer®.

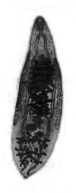

Stretched to ¼ inch on a microscope slide and stained with dyes, its organs are clearly visible.

Fig. 29 Clonorchis (Opisthorcis), the human liver fluke

The smallest piece of apple, a wedge the size of a penny, brings phloridzin to the pituitary gland in the brain, and some to every other bit of pituitary in the body, such as bits traveling in the blood and lymph. It only persists, though, if Clonorchis is present.

---

[17] *Infection With Liver Flukes* (IARC) Summary & Evaluation, Vol. 61, 1994; (p.121) Last updated 08/26/1997

Parasites in the Pancreas

The food allergen, gallic acid, has accumulated in the pancreas in cancer patients. Again, there is an associated parasite; this time it is the pancreatic fluke, with the scientific name, *Eurytrema pancreaticum*. This is the same parasite that brings us diabetes. It is very common, probably due to our consumption of non-sterile dairy products. Cow's milk and cheese always have eggs and larval stages of the pancreatic fluke. Its essential role in the initiation of cancer could not have been guessed because milk drinking and cancer seem quite far apart. Without Eurytrema, gallic acid does not accumulate; in fact, it is gone in minutes! Nor does the pancreas begin its micro-explosion.

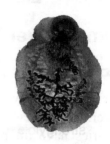

Fig. 30 Eurytrema, the pancreatic fluke photographed from a slide

3 Parasites, 3 Allergens and 3 Target Organs

All three parasites must be present to make the three food allergens pile up at the three organs involved in starting a tumor. Without them no sticky "snowball" could form to become the tumor nucleus.

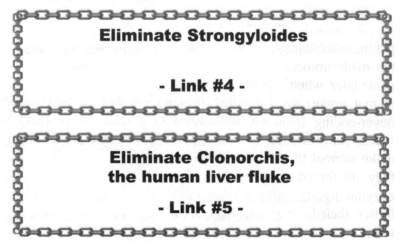

Eliminate Strongyloides

- Link #4 -

Eliminate Clonorchis, the human liver fluke

- Link #5 -

Not only should we avoid the foods with these allergens, we should kill the parasites responsible for it all. We will have 3 more links to perfect prevention of cancer.

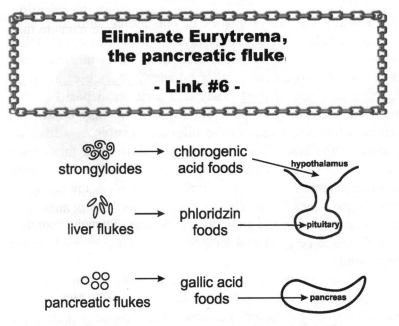

Fig. 31 Three events start the tumor nucleus

A Special Allergy

We are <u>all</u> damaged by eating foods we are allergic to and we all respond the same way. Our organs fight back when they get these substances by making **prostaglandin E2** (PGE2). It is not made immediately—not the first few times we eat it. It is made later, when a south pole force, perhaps nickel, has arrived at that organ. No matter which food allergen is causing the never-ending irritation, the organ cells respond by making PGE2. After this the cells no longer seem to stick together to make normal tight tissues. Maybe (and this is only a theory) they are forced to spill their enzymes, like **collage<u>nase</u>**. This enzyme digests collagen in its neighborhood. Then cells would loosen their hold on neighbor-cells and set themselves free to roam.

59

Allergies make PGE2.

The Age Factor

Hosting all three parasites in our bodies until they have reached a high enough level to invade these three organs takes some years. They may begin their invasion at the liver, and then continue to colonize other organs <u>if you are eating their favorite or essential food</u>. They will seek out deposits of this food left there by your poor digestion. There may be another colony of Strongyloides at the **migraine center** or **addiction center** of the brain. The Syncrometer® shows that this causes the absence of **acetylcholine** here. Acetylcholine is a major **neurotransmitter** (nerve compound) that connects your brain's messages to the rest of your organs. These messages, controlling tension and anxiety, are blocked. The addiction lets acetylcholine be <u>produced</u> temporarily. Addiction needs much more study.

Young people have had less immunity damage, less allergy damage, and also less exposure to these parasites than middle-aged and older persons. This could explain the tendency to see cancer in older people. But young people, even babies, could easily "inherit" these parasites since some can cross the placenta. Inheriting parasites from birth could pose as a "genetic disease". It does not necessarily mean the baby will be heavily parasitized. Everything depends on the baby's food, water, and family habits. What counts most is keeping the baby's immunity strong after birth. Most important is not giving the baby laundry bleach in its food and water.

Immunity to certain parasites is often seen in one or two members of a family while the others are more heavily parasitized.[18]

It would be wise to protect ourselves—and all of society—by exterminating these parasites constantly with anti-parasite

---

[18] Barriga, Omar, *The Immunology of Parasitic Infections*, University Park Press, ISBN-8391-1621-7

herbs and the traditional practice of herbal "cleaning" of the liver and kidneys. This is inexpensive and well tolerated, a practice that was relied on in primitive societies. We should hurry to save such priceless knowledge.

Starving Parasites

Just as people need vitamins with their food, parasites need quite specific things, too. Monarch butterflies need milkweed plants for their larvae (caterpillars). Other butterflies need cabbage for their larvae. How fortunate it was to discover that Fasciolopsis larvae need **onions**. They require them. When their onion stores are digested away with huge amounts of digestive enzymes the larvae leave. In a few days half of the larvae are gone. Strict avoidance of any food with raw onion-like substances (**diallyl sulfide**, **allyl sulfide**, **allyl methyl sulfide**) gets rid of them. A small deposit of **onion** will still be seen inside tumors and at the organ that has the most attraction for **onion**, the medulla plus 1 pF. This location appears to be the crevice between the medulla and base of the cerebellum on the right side. Onion seems to have a tropism for the medulla and F. buski follows. If the onion stash is at the left side of the medulla, F. buski will be seen there, too. If it is on the right side, F. buski will be seen there. But health problems come to the opposite side of the body. Cancer in the right breast, right lung or right kidney means F. buski and its onion stash are at the left side of the medulla. The role of the medulla is not yet clear.

These are the essential foods for the 3 parasites that start the tumor nucleus:

3 Essential Foods

- Strongyloides – potatoes
- Human liver fluke – oats
- Pancreatic fluke – lemons and food oils
-

The Syncrometer® finds many food oils distributed in tiny deposits in cancer patients and even in their urine. They may be essential in the human diet, but it seems the patients were eating much more than could be digested. Certainly, the patient should catch up on digestion of oil before eating more. Going off all food oils, as well as potatoes, lemons and oats, would give us the fastest way to pull these parasite links out of the chain leading to cancer. In the future you will be able to eat small amounts that can be completely digested. These will not be available then, to parasites.

It should now be possible to prevent all newly starting cancers and be free of this risk in your family.

Choose food and prepare it so it is free of any <u>one</u> of the three tumor starting chemicals or free of the essential food of <u>one</u> of these parasites. You may soon belong to the first cancer-free society that people have ever known.

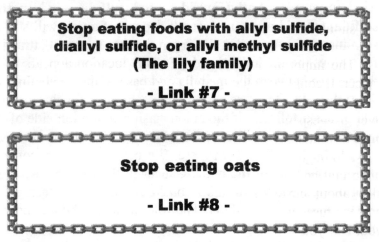

Stop eating foods with allyl sulfide, diallyl sulfide, or allyl methyl sulfide (The lily family)

- Link #7 -

Stop eating oats

- Link #8 -

Cancers that have already started and even progressed to an advanced stage need a different course of action, understandably. But the first step to be taken here, too, is to stop making any more tumor nuclei and to stop feeding our predators. In five days the effect of your new diet can be easily seen with a Syncrometer®. There will be only half as many larvae and there will be no single cells, no duplexes, nor triplet combinations of the three glands to be seen anywhere, except inside tumors. You do not need to kill or destroy the tumor nuclei. Although there are special herbs and substances that can do this (6 fresh seed recipe for example), your body will catch up with these chores by itself, now that no more tumor nuclei are being made.

Prevention of All Cancers in 5 Days

Although I do not know how phenolic food allergens bring about organ erosions except through a PGE2 effect, and I do not know how a parasite can interfere with the allergen's removal, I do know it can all be stopped in 5 days. Preventing cancer, like preventing malaria or a forest fire is very easy, certainly more powerful than curing it.

Prevention of diseases, not cure, or treatment, should be society's foremost goal.

The importance of this book is learning how to prevent cancer. It could be done in one generation, starting now.

Being able to raise a family without this sword hanging over us—especially in a cancer-ridden family—would be a huge advantage to all of society, not just the stricken families.

Although I am emphasizing prevention because it is so important and could be accomplished so quickly, this book is also about curing those already attacked. Once the tumor nucleus fuses itself to one of your organs a cancer is attacking you. But you will not know it until it is discovered much later by yourself or your doctor. By then it is in the last stage, the malignancy stage. Your immediate goal then will be to kill Fasciolopsis buski. But you should at once stop making tumor nuclei, too. This way you will stop making OPT first, the major growth factor, to reverse the malignancy, but at the same time you will stop the whole process of tumor making.

Fortunately, flukes are quite easy to kill. The first cancer book, *Cure For All Cancers*, was devoted to getting rid of them and has many details. In the present book we will simply incorporate Fasciolopsis-killing in the *3-Week Program*.

Having eliminated the end (malignancy) and the beginning of cancer (tumor nucleus formation), you can focus on the middle phase next.

The most challenging, but exciting, part of this cancer curing program will be eliminating the middle phase. This is what shrinks the tumor. It is the result of two things: getting your immunity back (to eat the tumor) and removing the tumor's oncoviruses (that extend the tumors' life). We will meet them soon. Your newly renovated white blood cells will help to unload the toxic accumulation (to shrink it further), and kill the "immortalized" bacteria that are making you sick.

In this book we will learn for the first time that the same oncoviruses that give immortality to our tumor cells also give it to our bacteria. But we will be able to kill them all with herbal enemas, described in a later chapter. After this we can enjoy shrinking our tumors instead of being invalids.

A newly formed tumor in the first, primary location begins to grow and to accumulate many items that should have been excreted or detoxified. The underlying defect is magnetic and involves the heavy metal nickel and its impact on the state of iron. The phenomenon is a toxicity. When this disables the kidneys, so that many toxins cannot be excreted, they must go elsewhere.

As laundry bleach toxins accumulate throughout the body, destroying the immune system, it permits increased parasitism, and increased bacterial and viral growth. Tumors become infected with bacteria, invaded by fungus and yeast. Each of these, in turn, becomes infected with viruses. Some of these viruses are **oncoviruses**, already known to encourage tumor growth. These oncoviruses extend the life of any cells they infect, by donating their enzymes, or even directly with their genes. These lower life forms do not have a life span. They could go on living forever if nothing killed them. Their few genes provide them with everlasting life. Infected cells benefit from this even as they suffer in other ways. Bacteria, too, are reinforced and become invincible, taking over huge areas of the body as oncoviruses infect them. They become immortalized in various ways. Human tumor cells are made long-lived and invincible the same way, also immortalized. We will soon see how this is done.

To be Sick or Not to be

Sickness strikes at this time, during the spread of immortalized bacteria and viruses. Mumps, Coxsackie viruses, Flu viruses, E. coli, Salmonella varieties, and prion proteins, besides Yeast are increasing together. This kind of infection is overwhelming. It has not been noticed before because each of them is behaving uncharacteristically. They behave differently due to their own virus infection. (We behave differently when we have an infection of some sort.) Yeast buds are particularly damaging because they consume the blood sugar of the patient, so weight is lost. The weight loss period marks the spread of Yeast. The bowel contains most of these immortalized pathogens. We will use powerful herbal methods in the form of special enemas to eliminate them.

Allergy Explosion

Meanwhile, another parasite, Fasciolopsis buski, enters the tumor zone to produce a growth stimulant, orthophosphotyrosine (OPT). A bacterium, *Bacillus cereus*, streams from this fluke, its own personal host. These bacteria produce **d-tyramine**, a special amine that can turn nearby substances from l-form to d-form, like itself. Amines are made from amino acids by the body's chemistry. Northerly zones have changed to southerly zones where the d-forms are made.

l-tyramine is a normal phenolic amine, formed from the phenolic amino acids, l-tyrosine, and l-phenyl alanine. l-tyrosine will make your l-thyroxine, your normal thyroid hormone. Your metabolism uses l-forms but Bacillus cereus makes d-forms of tyramine.

How could the d-form be contagious? Yet, all the l-amino acids in the near neighborhood have soon switched to d-forms! By interacting with other phenolic-type amino acids (those with a OH attached to their rings) to establish an equilibrium, it

65

seems possible to perpetuate d-forms in the presence of south pole forces.

The d-form process spreads from d-tyramine to the neighboring phenolics making d-thyroxine, d-phenylalanine, d-tyrosine, d-histidine, and more. The d-amino acids cannot be used by the body. The d-form of our thyroid hormone can do nothing for our bodies. We are now lacking this essential hormone. <u>It is an emergency for the tissue</u>. This should get immediate attention and it does. PGE2 is made.

The change in amino acid structure from l- to d- alerts the tissue to call in the allergy-fighting mechanism. But the situation is made much worse when food after food that we eat has many d-forms of amino acids and d-forms of phenolics. They stimulate more PGE2 because the body considers them allergens, too. We should not eat them. I believe it is the similarity between phenolic food allergens and our phenolic amino acids that allows this "creeping allergy" of l-forms to d-forms to extend to our foods. We should eat only the freshest of food that has l-forms exclusively. We should carefully avoid aged food, regardless of its chemical preservation to avoid getting more d-forms. The F. buski fluke is acting as a catalyst for this allergy explosion. This is the forerunner of metastasis. Once more F. buski plays a role in cancer...metastasis.

The allergy explosion fills us up with inflammations from PGE2. The inflammations open the doorways of our cells to bacteria and viruses. Now we get sick. Pain bacteria, bloating and gas bacteria, cough-mycoplasmas, sweats-mycobacteria, diarrhea bacteria...all these make the cancer patient miserable. We must stop the allergy <u>process</u> by killing more F. buski. To stop the allergy immediately we must stop eating the responsible phenolics.

Magnetic Switch

The accumulation of heavy metals in the tumor zone can be easily found by Syncrometer®. They cause numerous chromosome breakages and mutations. It becomes part of the diagnosis of cancer.

All body tumors have a magnetic polarization that is southerly instead of northerly by daytime. Our internal organs should be northerly except for brain and nerves. What caused the switch? The Syncrometer® sees deposits of plain iron, such as ferrite, Fe_2O_3, which is south. Plain iron comes partly from iron-containing asbestos but also from the ordinary effect of heavy metals on our iron. Nickel, specifically, changes the north form of iron, magnetite, to ferrite. Other heavy metals oxidize other organic forms of iron to useless inorganic forms. In this way they destroy enzymes that contain ferrous iron, crippling the organ's life processes. A southerly polarization invites **stem cell factor** to the location because a need for repair is being felt by the hypothalamus. We will discuss this soon.

The body has its own way of changing back the wrong polarization, using **iridium**. We will learn about this too. When the deposits of Fe_2O_3 (south) are changed back to magnetite, Fe_3O_4 (north), stem cell factor disappears again and north polarization comes back.

What's Left to Do?

After stopping the beginning and end stages of cancer, we are still left with the tumors themselves. But we know now what will shrink them:

- stop the immune destruction by laundry bleach
- stop the parasitism with its far reaching influences
- stop the allergy-PGE2 process
- stop the bacterial and oncovirus invasion that got its start from parasitism and incidentally makes you sick
- stop the toxicity effects of dyes and metals on your magnetic polarization, your kidney excretion, your water holding (effusions), and chronic disease.

The tumors may be large, numerous and growing fast. But they must stop "on a dime" when the growing force is pulled out from under them. As soon as we kill the tumor's oncoviruses, yeasts and bacteria turn back into their vulnerable selves. White blood cells can recognize them again and eliminate them in a sweep. This includes the tumor nucleus with its "super oncovirus", **SV 40**. After this the tumor cells can go into normal **apoptosis**.

Apoptosis means self-digestion. The body can remove its own cells when needed, such as at the irregular edges of a wound, but it must do this in a very precise way. It is the beginning of **healing**. The body recycles its own abnormal and sick cells to make healthy, working cells. You can see healing in action after dental work when little flaps of tissue disappear in days to repair the mouth. Healing requires stem cell factor, extra DNA and ribonucleotide reductase (RRase), the same actors as in the tumor. But the body is able to control these forces during healing, but not in a tumor. Apoptosis was blocked in the tumor but is present during healing. We will soon see how this shrinks the tumor.

Three Tumor Removers

So far, the Syncrometer® has seen 3 ways the body uses to shrink a tumor to disappearance. There may be more. It is not uncommon to see tumors disappear completely with intravenous alternative therapies, providing EDTA, which removes metals; laetrile, which kills SV 40 and other oncoviruses; DMSO, which dissolves wheel bearing grease; vitamin A, D_3, and thyroid, which are differentiators. Used together the three tumor-removing processes are at work.

One is apoptosis, internal digestion of tumor cells. It gets started after a "flag" is hoisted on the cell membrane. The flag is **phosphatidyl serine (PS)**. We can see this with the Syncrometer®. It is a task of the tumor cell.

The second is plain digestion. Our bodies let our food-digestion enzymes, lipase, pancreatin, and many others penetrate the tissues and clean them up. It is the job of the pancreas.

The third is **phagocytosis**. Our newly revitalized white blood cells; particularly CD8s and macrophages (CD14s) can simply eat all the leftovers of the tumor and take them to the bladder. It is the task of our WBCs.

We will meet all these actors again.

Monitoring your own progress in tumor shrinking with a Syncrometer® makes it an exciting adventure. Hopefully you or a friend will be motivated to learn to use it. But it is not essential. What is essential is diligence with every detail so you can be certain these 3 steps are happening, even without monitoring.

So far we have learned about the beginning of <u>all</u> tumors. Those that will become benign, not malignant, have the same beginning. We will discover the difference later.

Summary of Chapters 2 and 3:

1. Every malignant tumor has its beginning in a tumor nucleus. Even tumorless cancer begins this way.

2. The tumor nucleus consists of cells from three organs, the hypothalamus, pituitary gland and pancreas, attached to each other in that order.

3. Free-floating cells of these three organs are produced from an erosion of the parent organ. It is caused by a specific food substance and a specific parasite. The hypothalamus sets free its cells due to the presence of chlorogenic acid and Strongyloides, a minute threadworm. The pituitary sets free its cells due to the presence of phloridzin and Clonorchis, the human liver fluke. The pancreas sets free its cells due to the presence of gallic acid and Eurytrema, the pancreatic fluke. The food substances are common "food phenolic antigen" substances that cause allergies. The three parasites are common human parasites. Each is necessary and represents another link in the cancer-chain. Any one could be pulled out to provide perfect protection from cancer.

4. A "snowball" effect sticks the hypothalamus cells to pituitary cells to form a duplex. The pituitary end of the duplex sticks to pancreas cells to form a triplet. This triplet is called the tumor nucleus.

5. To start a cancer-forming tumor, the tumor nucleus fuses itself to the cells of another allergic organ. This organ is coming apart, too, so cells are available for fusing. A specific food substance causes this fourth event, too, specific for that organ, and again a food phenolic. The fusing of the tumor nucleus to an organ only happens in the presence of huge amounts of laminin, fibronectin and cadherin E. Perhaps their stickiness traps the tumor nucleus. They are excessive <u>only</u> when Fasciola and Ascaris parasite stages are nearby. They are part of the matrix that is right outside each cell, keeping it in position.

6. There are many ways to stop the whole cancer process because an orderly sequence of events is involved. Three food substances are necessary and can be avoided. Five parasites are necessary: Strongyloides, Clonorchis, Eurytrema, Fasciola, and Ascaris; these can be eliminated. Parasites can be removed with herbs and electricity, and by starving them. But none of these improvements will last if laundry bleach continues to be consumed in the drinking water, continuing to destroy your immunity. More and different parasites will arrive, instead.

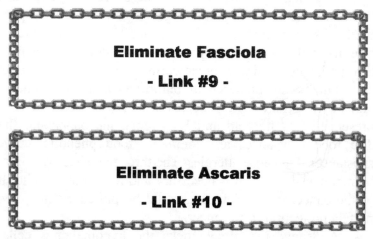

Eliminate Fasciola

- Link #9 -

Eliminate Ascaris

- Link #10 -

7. Prevention of cancer or its recurrence can be achieved in about a week by killing these parasites and correcting the diet. This is not the same as succeeding to shrink the tumors you already have, though.

8. A cancer patient has 3 different problems: a runaway growth in some organ, sickness from certain common pathogens (bacteria and viruses), and a toxicity that damages some organ. These problems get intertwined but have separate causes.

9. To stop the tumor growth, we can stop making tumor nuclei and stop setting free human growth hormone and stem cell factor from their normal controls. We will discuss this soon.

10. To shrink the tumor we can get apoptosis started, digestion started, and the immune system eating the leftovers.

11. To banish illness so recovery can be <u>felt</u>, bacteria and their oncoviruses must be killed. Since these come directly from our parasites, killing parasites comes next.

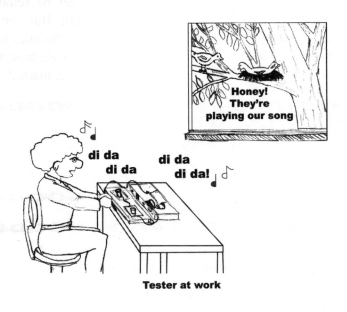

Tester at work

CHAPTER 4

KILLING PARASITES

Individual parasites are very, very fragile. Any little change in temperature, or salt concentration, or interruption of their special food supply removes them immediately. In fact, Barlow, the early researcher who had a grant to study Fasciolopsiasis in China in the mid 1920's, could not keep them alive by feeding and culturing them in any way at all. But he did not get done with his research in time for his departure date and he wished to continue his research at home in the USA. He resorted to swallowing them (counting them carefully first) and retrieving them after he arrived home (researchers can be very dedicated to the betterment of society and the search for truth). Then why are they so hard to eradicate? We still do not know their weaknesses and exact requirements. The traditional ways of killing parasites by swallowing a dose of sulfur twice a year or taking an herbal potion several times a year does not eliminate them.

In fact, no invaders can be eliminated in an immune depressed person. We must correct our immune depression. We are wallowing in the 5 immunity destroyers without recognizing them and at the same time wallowing in pet excretions, domestic animal excretions and our own excretions without even recognizing them! Our food is tainted with all of them.

Visit a pet shop and a feed store. Notice the shelves are full of medicines for parasites. Notice the refrigerators are full of antibiotics and further medicines for parasites. They are to be given repeatedly, because the situation does not improve for them. Parasitism does not go away without deeper intervention than medicine. Our animals and pets have become immune depressed with us. Our health and their health are intertwined.

We must care for their health in order to care for ours. It is nature's fairness. See *Curing Cancer in Pets* page 441.

> To prevent our cancers we must prevent immune depression in our animals besides ourselves. This will prevent parasitism for both of us.

As you learn how to regain your immunity, and how to cure your own cancer as well as your family's cancers, you will see what needs to be done for animals and the rest of society.

But your immediate tasks are to kill your own parasites— and your own bacteria—at the same time as regaining immunity. The more advanced your cancer is, the more varieties you have. They are contributing to your illness, even if not to your cancer. Killing many will not be harder than killing a few, but we will need to be mindful of detox-illness. We will discuss that soon.

The parasites to conquer are:
- Ascaris lumbricoides
- Ascaris megalocephala
- Dirofilaria, dog heartworm
- Fasciolopsis buski
- Fasciola
- human liver fluke
- Onchocerca
- pancreatic fluke
- Strongyloides

The bacteria to conquer are:
- Clostridium varieties
- Salmonella varieties
- Staphylococcus aureus
- Streptococcus G and pneumoniae
- E. coli
- Mycobacterium avium
- Bacillus cereus
- Mycoplasma pneumoniae
- Pseudomonas aeruginosa

The viruses to conquer are:
- Mumps
- MYC (oncovirus)
- RAS (oncovirus)
- JUN (oncovirus)
- FOS (oncovirus)
- SV 40 (oncovirus)

- NEU (oncovirus)
- SRC (oncovirus)
- EBV (Epstein Barre virus)
- CMV (Cytomegalovirus)
- Hepatitis B virus
- Adenovirus
- Influenza A and B

Extra invaders to conquer are:
- yeast, the bread and alcohol making kind
- prions

Once we see that small invaders come from larger invaders and these may even come from the list of parasites, we will be able to conquer them all with a few treatments instead of 30!

Once we see that each parasite has a food dependency, much like its own vitamin requirement, and each bacterium has a metal dependency, while each virus requires a trigger, we will have more ways to control each one besides killing it.

We can kill some invaders, starve some, create deficiencies for some and block reproduction for others. It is a powerful patrol, though not without its gaps in our knowledge.

In 3 weeks all these invaders can be reduced so much, you feel decidedly better, your cancer crisis could be over, and your tumors visibly shrinking.

But only if you don't get sick from the treatment itself, and cause a big delay. How can that be? Isn't this a supreme irony? How could killing parasites make you sicker than if you kept on nurturing them?

Detoxification-Illness

As soon as you kill the Fasciolopsis buski fluke, the common Flu virus and several salmonella bacteria jump away...and into you! Before killing them the Syncrometer® cannot hear any Flu frequency emissions. Immediately after killing them, within the hour, one or more varieties can be heard. The Fasciolopsis buski flukes, although quietly causing your cancer, were not making you feel physically unwell. Flu and salmonella <u>do</u> make you feel unwell, very unwell if you don't have remedies. This explains how you can feel sicker from killing the parasites than leaving them be. We must expect and prevent as much Flu and Salmonella illness as possible.

Our Prevention Strategy Will be...

...to clear one set of white blood cells before killing parasites. These are the kidney WBCs.

If your white blood cells, both the virus-eaters and the bacteria-eaters, are already cleared of their 5 immunity blockers they will snap up all the viruses and bacteria as soon as they are released so you do not feel an iota of illness. You may have killed some key parasites so that Flu and salmonella are swimming everywhere, but your kidney WBCs will be capable of catching them and throwing them into the urine and out of the body. That is why the kidney WBCs are chosen, above all the others. If your white blood cells still have dyes and heavy metals in them, on the other hand, you will not be helped by them and must rely solely on Flu virus killing and salmonella killing. Failing to do this while you are on the program can then lead to a Flu and salmonella attack. Although detox-illness is not very serious, it is demoralizing for everybody, wasting your time as well. You could lose 3 days having to get yourself well enough to continue. That is why Flu and salmonella patrol is one of your regular "housekeeping" chores throughout the program.

Besides being free of the 5 blockers, your white blood cells must be fed, too. Like any army, they must be fed constantly, not on starvation rations. They need 3 foods:

- organic germanium
- organic selenium
- organic vitamin C

If you feed them lower quality food, they will need much more of it. A teaspoon of hydrangea root or raw nuts supplies the organic germanium; an equivalent supplement would need to be huge.

A large Brazil nut, freshly cracked, brings 50 mcg of organic selenium, but can replace a dose of pure sodium selenite of 1000 mcg.

A teaspoon of coarsely ground rose hips, seeds included, supplies the vitamin C power of 2000 mg.

This is because the effectiveness of a natural substance does not just depend on an "active ingredient". There are extra factors involved, making the <u>whole</u> food more effective.

If you grind these substances yourself, you must promptly eat or encapsulate them and store them in the freezer. They must only be <u>coarsely</u> ground to avoid putting nickel and chromium in them yourself. They must not be stored, nor purchased already cracked. Nuts are, of course, delicious. But the other 2 immune-cell foods are less so and can be put into a cocktail or made into a dressing (see *Recipes*) promptly.

All cancer patients have <u>starved</u> white blood cells[*], so our very first task will be to feed them. In ten minutes we can see them at work clearing their own bacteria and viruses, which they could not kill and get rid of before. After this, we can help them get rid of their asbestos, heavy metals, and dyes. They won't need help with PCBs and benzene. All these can be gone in about 5 days. Soon they can take on the larger task of clearing your organs one by one. We will help those WBCs at the kidneys first because they create an exit path for the others.

Remember that white blood cells act like relay runners. They pick up toxins from nearby and bring them to a relay station (a lymph node). They unload them on another white blood cell that takes it to the kidney white blood cells. These relay it to the bladder white blood cells and the job is done. Next, we see the toxins in the urine. They will be gone.

Levamisole clears the ferritin off kidney white blood cells. If your water is no longer bringing you asbestos, the deferritinizing will be complete here in a few days and everywhere in about 3 weeks.

---

[*] Testers, place the WBC sample beside (touching) the saliva sample, and test for organic germanium, selenium, and vitamin C. You can expect only the oxidized versions of these to be present (*Positive*).

Getting the heavy metals and dyes, all trapped in thick wheel bearing grease, out of the kidneys and their white blood cells must be done homeographically. Even this is too slow when a crisis threatens. A mere ¼ tsp. DMSO, in ½ cup cold water, drunk once a day begins to dissolve wheel bearing grease. It shows up in the urine in minutes and continues for several hours. Then it stops again. In a few days your kidneys and their WBCs are cleaned enough to permit steady detoxification without detox symptoms. But you will need to go to a foreign country for DMSO treatment. Read more about it on the Internet. See also a book by Dr. Morton Walker[*], *DMSO Nature's Healer* on how to use it for many other serious illnesses.

No amount of vitamin B_2 or coenzyme Q10 can reach inside the WBCs to remove dyes here. And no chelation treatments can pull heavy metals out swiftly and surely when only days remain. But they come out with DMSO along with the wheel bearing grease. That is why the standard treatment of IV therapists in Mexico has included DMSO for decades; its benefits are so obvious. But, of course, there must be no more grease arriving. Your success will depend on whether you moved to a clean water zone.

All 5 toxins can be cleared out of the kidneys and their WBCs together, starting as soon as no more are coming into your body, that is, when food, water, dental metal and cooking pots have been cleared. It takes 4 days. Then we can start killing parasites without fear of a detoxification-illness attack.

> To prevent a Flu attack while curing your cancer, keep clearing the kidneys and their white blood cells of wheel bearing grease, dyes and heavy metals first. And feed them germanium, selenite and vitamin C constantly.

Your kidneys' WBCs will be back on patrol.

---

[*] www.drmortonwalker.com

What could be easier or more "magical"?

Now we can kill parasites in earnest, in 4 ways: with herbs, by zapping, with homeography, and by starving them. Dogs, elephants, birds, and whales use multiple approaches, too. They bite them, lick, scratch, attract helpers like birds, throw dust, go swimming, and eat specific plants. Every bit helps them, like us.

The Herbal Way

How to make your own green Black Walnut hull tincture was described in earlier books. It is best to make it yourself because you understand the water and chlorine pollution problem better than others. Use the recipe on page 552.

The Black Walnut way of killing parasites includes 3 herbs:

1. The green hull of the Black Walnut extracted in ethyl alcohol

2. Freshly ground cloves (each capsule with 400-500 mg clove) in capsules or ¼ cup bulk whole cloves. Store bought or bulk sources do not work. Immediate encapsulation after grinding does keep it potent. Beware of nickel and chromium from grinding; test them.

3. Wormwood, encapsulated (each capsule with 200-300 mg of wormwood), or ½ cup of Artemisia leaves gathered from the shrub.

These herbs must be taken together as a single treatment within ½ hour (preferably within 5 minutes). But they should not be premixed because they interact with each other to destroy their potency.

The 3 herbs kill different stages; cloves kill eggs, wormwood kills cercaria and the tincture kills adults. But altogether, many escape to start their cycle all over in an immune depressed person like yourself. This is because dying parasites release their eggs immediately, to travel in your blood to some safe, out of the way place, like your inner ear, an eye muscle, or the crevice between the cerebellum and medulla (called medulla plus 1 picofarad).

For this reason you should take your daily parasite herbs together and if possible <u>while you are zapping</u> with at least a half hour more to zap. Plain regular zapping kills eggs and stages swimming in your blood. No doubt the current is highest here. The Syncrometer® then shows they will be caught by the white blood cells (only the CD8s and CD14s can eat them, though). Remember to feed your white blood cells just before your daily parasite-killing herbs.

It is only the <u>green</u> hull that has this amazing parasite-killing power. A few days after opening a bottle it may already be much darker and less potent. Use the one-serving (2 oz.) bottle to maximize potency and results. Store in freezer after opening.

Beginner's methods, using only drops of green Black Walnut tincture, are described in earlier books. You may use those if you are just preventing cancer or have very early cancer. In an extremely advanced case, where every hour of every day is precious, we will use 1 whole bottle in a single dose or as much as you can take comfortably. <u>Always check beforehand or some days earlier what 1 tsp. of green Black Walnut tincture would do</u>, if anything, to give you some discomfort. If only the taste is objectionable, search for solutions. Add an equal amount, approximately, of heavy whipping cream, syrup, or a juice. Take the other herbs along with the tincture, but not mixed in it, then sit down to wear off the alcohol. Do not drive a vehicle or do anything complicated

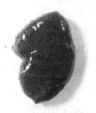

Too gorged with blood and fecal matter from a colorectal cancer victim, this Fasciola did not swell and burst as it fell into the toilet water. Fasciolas often share the ulcer with F. buski. Pointed head aims Fasciola down. A gash on the left side was the result of moving it for this photo.

Fig. 32 Photo of Fasciola

80

for a while. Take niacinamide, too, if available, to help the liver detoxify the alcohol.

In spite of this large dose, you can easily miss one or two adults attached to the esophagus or stomach or bladder. Contacting a parasite is never a certainty with any dose. That is why repetition is important.

These three herbs are not the only ones that can kill parasites, especially flukes, but it is the best I have found. The vast literature on herbal parasite-killing needs fresh study so that each nation can grow what is suited to its climate and thereby improve its general health.

A Meadow of Health

All herbs have **tropisms**. This means they go to a certain organ preferentially. Black Walnut tincture does not penetrate the brain well. Wormwood does. So if you have brain cancer or eye cancer, you should increase wormwood in each dose.

Here is a list of human organs and the herbs that go there preferentially, to kill a particular parasite (besides the Black Walnut recipe).

Organ	Parasite or Pathogen	Herb
adrenals	Echinoporyphium recurvatum	cardamom
most body organs	Fasciolopsis buski	6 fresh apricot, peach or nectarine seeds for 5 days, repeating after 5 days off
anterior pituitary	prions	6 fresh apricot seeds for 5 days, birch bark tea, fennel seed, Reishi mushroom, horseradish, licorice root powder, sage, raw nopales (cactus)
blood	Fasciola	coriander
breast	Fasciola	mullein
breast	Paragonimus	mullein
breast	*	mullein
cerebrum	Echinostoma revolutum	white thyme
cerebrum	Macracanthorhynchus	oregano oil

81

Organ	Parasite or Pathogen	Herb
cerebrum	prions	myrrh, Lugol's iodine
eye	Fasciola	wormwood
eye muscles	Fasciolopsis buski	fennel seed, anise seed), nutmeg, wormwood, watercress, 6 fresh seed recipe
hypothalamus	Strongyloides	chaparral, coriander
hypothalamus	*	wormwood
kidneys	Echinoporyphium recurvatum	BQ drops**, watercress, 6 fresh seed recipe
kidneys	*	cardamom, parsley tea, hydrangea root, ginger, nutmeg, uva ursi
lumbar spine	Echinostoma revolutum	white thyme
lumbar spine	Macracanthorhynchus	oregano oil
lung	Fasciola	BQ drops
lung	Paragonimus	mullein, BQ drops
lung	*	mullein
muscle tendon junctions (joints)	Fasciolopsis buski	6 fresh seed recipe, fennel seed, horseradish, pomegranate juice, watercress
pancreas	Eurytrema	nopales (cactus)
rectum	Fasciolopsis buski	turmeric, oregano leaf
at whole body	Paragonimus	nutmeg, coriander, Pau D'Arco

*Where no parasite or pathogen is listed, the herb simply benefits the entire organ.

**We will discuss making drops later. BQ is benzoquinone.

Fig. 33 Selected herbs and their tropisms

Other parasites play important roles in cancer, besides the intestinal fluke. Use as many of the herbs as possible to single out other parasites. Be sure your selections pass the *Food Table* test, too, on page 36.

Exact amounts of the Black Walnut tincture, wormwood, and cloves that we will use are given in the *3-Week Program*. Others are left for you. Make the strongest potions you can tolerate. Try to make them pleasant. You have nothing to lose but illness.

Zapping Parasites

Many variations in zapping technique have been discovered since the first one found around 1990.

The original technique showed that very small animals, like our parasites, could be killed with a very small voltage. But only IF the voltage is 100% _Positive_ offset, and only IF the voltage is varied up and down repeatedly.

If the varying voltage becomes _NEGATIVE_, even momentarily, it supports and maintains their lives! This must be avoided. You cannot take this for granted when you purchase a zapper. The maker must assure you that it has been checked on an oscilloscope and not even the briefest spike of _Negative_ voltage found. Preferably a picture of the zapper output on an oscilloscope should accompany the device together with an arrow pointing to the zero line. If the circuit parts used are exactly as given on page 480, there will be no error.

If the voltage is applied in pulses, to produce a "square" wave, it will affect many parasites at once so that the rate of pulsing, called frequency, is not critical. Even though these tiny animals undoubtedly have a "mortal frequency" (a frequency that kills), this rate does not need to be known or used when a square wave of electricity, **totally _Positive_**, is used.

A _Positive_ electrical force that pulses up and down not only appears to kill tiny invaders, it also seems to energize your white blood cells to go on an all-out attack on your enemies: your parasites, your toxins, your bacteria, everything, in spite of their five immunity blockers. In spite of benzene, PCBs, metals, dyes, and asbestos! For a time, your WBCs turn into Super-WBCs. That is why I recommend eight hours of zapping daily until you are well.

Remember that killing parasites, as we can do with herbs, removes the source of OPT, and oncoviruses, but this does not return immune power. Only removing the immune destroyers does that. A zapper, on the other hand, not only destroys parasites; it does so by turning on immune power, at least temporarily. Each method has its advantages.

With this knowledge you may build or purchase a zapper. It is energized by a 9-volt battery. This is too small a voltage to harm you, or even to feel, although some people can feel a weak tingling sensation. Most of the current is flowing through the blood in your arteries and veins, but a fraction of it reaches every organ and tissue in your body. Except when this organ is saturated with a liquid *insulator*. Insulators do not let current pass.

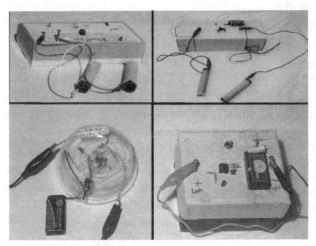

Fig. 34 Homemade zappers

Cancer victims are particularly full of insulators because they have been drinking and cooking with water that is polluted with PCBs, benzene, motor oil, and wheel bearing grease. These are insulators. They accumulate in the thin layer of fat just under the skin and surrounding internal organs. They do not let the current pass through the skin or into an organ easily.

Plate-Zapping

The zapper current does not easily penetrate a body region that is full of automotive oils and grease. Yet, cancer patients are full of them from drinking the laundry bleached water. I believe that a new kind of zapping, called plate-zapping can overcome the obstacle of grease insulation. There will now be resonance between the sample organ on the plate and the same organ in your body, giving you a higher voltage and current at that organ. For instance, by placing a sample of liver on a 3½ inch square aluminum plate in the path of the zapper current, the two similar organs (your liver and the liver sample on the plate) will be in resonance. I think this maximizes the current through your liver. The liver sample you put on the plate can be in the form of a <u>microscope slide</u>, meant for study by biology students. Microscope slides can be purchased from biological supply companies (see *Sources*) and are safe to handle.

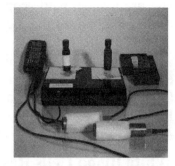

The location to be zapped is on the plate. Bottles or slides represent them. Escaping tiny pathogens can be placed here, too.

Fig. 37 Plate-zapper

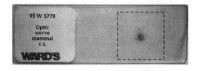

Fig. 35 Microscope slide with real tissue under glass square

Bottled Alternative

Instead of an actual sample of an organ, like on a microscope slide, it is possible to use a <u>virtual</u> copy. A virtual copy is a sample of <u>water</u> that has the frequency pattern of an organ in it. This bottle of "patterned" water can act like the slide or real sample and has the advantage of convenience and availability. The zapper circuit uses the frequency pattern in the bottle-copy to find an identical one in your body. Whether

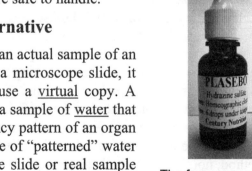

The frequency pattern of any item can be copied into water.

Fig. 36 Bottle-copy replaces the real item

you use a slide, bottle-copy or a piece of real tissue does not matter; it provides the <u>location</u> where you want to maximize the zapper effect.

Bottle-copies are easily made from slides or real organs, even by a totally inexperienced person, using a regular zapper (30 kHz or more) see page 105. Extra details are given in Experiment #96 of the *Syncrometer*® *Science Laboratory Manual* (see Parts Kit #96 in *Sources*) by this author.

White Blood Cells Respond...

With the sample of liver placed in the pathway between you and your zapper, the current has an instant effect on the white blood cells of your liver. Instantly they are energized and begin to eat the PCBs, the benzene, the heavy metals, the dyes, and the malonic acid in your liver. They even eat wheel bearing grease!

Like a fairy godmother that has waved her wand, all toxins are quickly taken out of the liver tissue and imprisoned in the liver white blood cells. They have eaten, although they could not earlier. If they have been fed themselves they can unload all this into the urine. Then they continue to eat toxins without zapper help. Gradually, conductivity returns. To speed up degreasing, we use DMSO, in tiny amounts, not to overwhelm the kidneys (25 drops of 100% DMSO tested for thallium, copper and lead). Hundreds of toxins, heavy metals, fungus spores, mycotoxins, all are eaten in one big frenzy.

However, it can all come to a screeching halt if the voltage of the battery has dropped below 9.0 volts. To do this superb job the battery must not run below 9.0 before the job is done. And it takes 20 minutes, not just seven as it does for regular zapping. Only the locations placed on the plates are zapped by this method, not the whole body as for regular zapping.

...But Only If Fed

What will happen to the gorged white blood cells after they have "eaten" all this toxic waste? Will they carefully guard against any losses on their way to the kidneys and bladder using their relay system? Will they unload their super toxic cargo in the proper place (bladder)? How do they unload their cargo? It all hinges on being fed! Only <u>selenite</u>, <u>organic germanium</u> and <u>vitamin C</u> are useful. These three enable the white blood cells to transfer their toxic load to the kidneys' WBCs, and then to the bladder and from there to appear in the urine. A Syncrometer® urine test will now be *Positive* for PCBs, asbestos, lanthanide metals, nickel, mercury and all the others identified before, even Fast Garnet, and Fast Green dyes.

If there is not enough of any <u>one</u> of these three supplements, the white blood cells simply stop; they wait as at a dock, for a day or so, then some of the toxic cargo escapes to the <u>kidney itself</u>, clogging it, changing its polarization to south, and stopping its ability to put toxins into the urine. You are back at the beginning now. The toxins escaped and will have to be "eaten" again. Much time is lost this way.

Throughout the day, the organ with a tumor should be plate-zapped in various ways: combined with arteries, combined with veins, combined with white blood cells, each for 20 minutes. These zaps are followed with zaps to clear blood, lymph and the white blood cells themselves. Or these zaps are done at the same time if you are using a double plate-zapper. And, of course, the kidneys are zapped to keep them from clogging repeatedly with the heavy metals and greases they are handling. Twenty-minute zaps can be kept up for eight hours or more.

A miracle has been done for you in one day. The battle for your sick organ has been won. Be sure you are protecting and helping the kidney white blood cells as we discussed earlier. Be patient with the after-effects due to dead parasites.

What happens to the dead carcasses of large flukes lying about like dead rats? They will soon be enveloped in mold and toxic decay. Watch what happens to a tiny dead fish at the bottom of an aquarium at a pet store. Within a day fine fuzz appears all over the surface, like velvet. In a few days if it is not scooped out, a halo appears around the dead fish. Fungus has taken over the entire fish and is now going through its own stages of development, glistening under the aquarium light. The owner will scoop it out.

Who will scoop up the dead flukes in your organs? If you had zapped flukes in the intestinal tract or liver or pancreas, they could have been pushed out through their ducts into the intestine and finally into the toilet. But most organs have no such ducts; dead parasites will have to rot on the spot, being fought over by scavenger Clostridium bacteria and its competitor, **Aspergillus** fungus. Clostridium will produce isopropyl alcohol, DNA, DNA polymerase, **thiourea** (cell division accelerator), and even turn on the **ribonucleotide reductase** enzyme that makes DNA. These contribute directly to malignancy, to make matters worse. Aspergillus will produce **aflatoxin**. Even if it has to share the carcass with **Penicillium** mold, it does not help; they both produce aflatoxin. The aflatoxins are very sinister **mycotoxins** (fungal toxins). They precede all **jaundice**. A much better solution is to digest the dead flukes before these scavengers get them.

Fifteen capsules (about five or six grams) of mixed enzyme powders can digest the dead matter coming from four hours of zapping. Eight hours require two such doses. More is better.

In advanced cancer nothing less than eight hours of zapping daily can catch up and exceed the rate of spread of disease. Zap eight hours daily until you are well. There are reports from victims who zapped without stopping for a whole month; symptoms came and went while they cleaned up their environment and suddenly the disease was gone.

The Flu Again

Remember, there is a price to be paid for killing so much so quickly in your body. When an animal is "wormed" intensively, it can get quite ill. Yet, "sick-time off" is a luxury that is not available for many cancer patients. Every day must show advances made over parasitism and immune depression. What can you expect realistically? Although the Clostridium takeover and fungal growth can be avoided with enough digestive enzymes, detox-illness cannot be entirely avoided. The discipline of prevention is too demanding. What can you expect from zapping 8 hours when you are a very advanced case? This means you have a lot of F. buski's to kill. And a lot of Flu and salmonella "bugs" will escape into you! Next morning you may awaken to see the ceiling rotate and find it necessary to hug the walls as you search for the bathroom, which seems to have moved. But your mood is just fine; it even seems a bit funny. This is the **prion** contribution to detox-illness. If your caregiver would quickly make "gold-out-of-the-hypothalamus" drops and a cup of birch bark tea, or give you Reishi mushroom, you would soon be "set right" again.

Prions are associated with gold. Remove all gold metal if you had forgotten, that very day. Birch bark tea has natural fluoride; perhaps it chelates out gold. Maybe it or Reishi (Ganoderma) mushroom act directly to kill prions.

If, instead, you begin to shiver, ache all over, cough and feel a sore throat, it is the Flu, with or without Adenovirus, the common cold. You immediately know you killed a "buski" and an Ascaris. F. buski presented you with the Flu, and Ascaris gave you the cold. You must stay warm in bed and drink Boneset tea, Eucalyptus tea and small sips of Elder leaf tea throughout the day. These can have you feeling fine again in hours. Also take a dose of Oscillococcinum at bedtime, homeopathic medicine for Flu, to feel normal next day.

But if you get a fever, nausea and diarrhea, you have salmonellas. These can be terminated with 6 doses of Lugol's, 6 drops each in ½ cup water, during the day. Salmonellas need gold, ruthenium, and molybdenum. Killing salmonellas releases the gold they have been using. Then prions can snatch it. Without gold in your body, you could not get Salmonella illness, nor prions!

If you can't test for these detox-"bugs" yourself, you must treat yourself for all of them...or miss several days of cancer curing till you are back to normal again. This time, study which parts of the *3-Week Program* protect you from each "bug". And if you forget to take your protective supplements again, this time you might be able to smile as you feel ill, while gloating over your "real" evidence of progress: detox-illness…you did reach and kill some F. buski's.

But if you get quite ill and lose weight over it, ask your caregiver to take over the responsibility of preventing detox-symptoms while you agree to dutifully sip, swallow or take whatever is put before you.

Your cancer does not get worse from a bout of detox-illness. In fact, it could even be helped by a fever. Fever-inducing "bugs" have been used successfully to combat cancer[*]. But losing weight is serious.

It is important to know that if you develop <u>any</u> after effect from zapping, however small or large, we have <u>always</u> found it to be due to Flu, Salmonella and Prions, not a worsening of the cancer, or anything harmful. For some persons, weeping plays a role in detox-illness, too. This is caused by a special Clostridium variety, C. botulinum. It appears after killing human liver flukes. If you kill very many, the C. botulinum "undertaker" bacteria can reach the hypothalamus, so weeping starts. If you are a "weeper", be sure to drink Eucalyptus tea to kill all Clostridium and take drops of oregano oil (in capsules) daily to stay cheerful while you zap and starve the flukes.

After plate-zapping the organ that made the tumor, zap the tumor itself. Follow these detailed instructions.

The Plate-Zapping Method

First of all:

1. Identify the "hot" (+) lead from your zapper. If you accidentally choose the (-) lead you will get no benefit, although it does no harm. If your zapper is not clearly marked with a (+) sign take it to any electronics shop. The technician will gladly check it for you. Ask to be shown how to use a voltmeter for this detail.

---

[*] Read about Cooley's toxins and hyperthermia on Internet.

2. Do not use a wall outlet as power source. Do not use a frequency generator without supervision by an electronics expert.

3. Purchase a voltmeter and test your batteries before beginning and after every two zaps afterward. Make sure the voltage is not below 8.9 volts at the end of each zap or it will have to be repeated. Start at 9.4 volts to be sure of this.

4. Purchase a battery charger for metal hydride batteries that will charge to 10 volts and two to four metal hydride rechargeable batteries.

You will need:

1. Zapper with continuous running capability instead of seven-minute sessions; this is for convenience only.

2. Plate box that can be attached to the "(+)" lead of the zapper with proper leads.

3. Two copper pipe electrodes and two banana-to-alligator clip leads (wires).

4. A kitchen timer.

5. Four packages of 1 pF capacitors and 1 μH inductors.

6. Microscope slides of body organs (anatomy set), and digestive tract organs.

7. Bottle-copies of any tissues that cannot be purchased as slides (see *Sources*). These are white blood cells (WBC), lymph (the fluid), and others.

Digestive System Slide Kit

Appendix	Liver
Bile duct	Pancreas
Colon	Parotid gland
Duodenum	Rectum
Esophagus lower	Stomach, cardiac region
Esophagus upper	Stomach, fundic region
Esophagus-stomach junction	Stomach, pyloric region
Gall bladder	Sublingual gland
Ileum	Submandibular gland

Jejunum   Submaxillary gland

Anatomy Kit

Brain, composite (cerebrum, cerebellum, medulla)
Bone marrow, red   Lung
Bladder   Lymph node, human
Blood, smear, human   Mammary gland (breast)
Hypothalamus   Pineal
Kidney   Pituitary gland
Thymus

Anatomy Male Slide Kit

Ductus deferens   Seminal vesicle
Epididymus   Sperm
Penis   Testis

Anatomy Female Slide Kit

Cervix   Ovary
Fallopian tube/Oviduct   Uterus
Fimbria   Vagina

Miscellaneous Specimen Kit ("B.C." means Bottle-copy)

Lymph (fluid) B.C.
Saliva B.C.
Artery combination, "A", arteries, veins, nerves B.C.
Lymph vessel combination, "L", lymph vessels, veins B.C.
Cerebrospinal fluid B.C.
Heavy metals, about 50, from amalgam plus cobalt, strontium,
        gold, antimony, uranium, chromium, radon, ruthenium
        and rubidium
Prion B.C.
Copper (atomic absorption standard)
Mercury (atomic absorption standard)
Thallium (atomic absorption standard)
White blood cells, B.C.
Dye set, assortment, B.C.
Motor oil, B.C.

Wheel bearing grease, B.C.
Tricalcium phosphate
Malonic acid, maleic acid, maleic anhydride
        methyl malonate, D-malic acid

Basic Vascular Set

Blood	WBC
Lymph	cerebrospinal fluid
"A"	"L"
Four 1 pF capacitors	Four 1 μH inductors

You do not need to purchase all the items listed. Use the schedule to guide you. You are now ready to start zapping every organ for which you have a specimen, slide or bottle.

Setting Up:

Wrap a <u>single</u> layer of paper towel around one of the copper pipes. Wet it under the cold faucet and place it under your foot, near your heel. Protect the carpet with a paper plate pushed into a plastic bag.

Connect the **Positive** side of your zapper to each plate (in "parallel") on your plate box. Then connect each plate, in parallel, to your left foot, meaning the copper pipe under your left foot. (Although the Positive current is coming to your left foot via the plate box, it doesn't really matter which foot gets the Positive current. You may alternate feet every day if you wish.)

Connect the **Negative** side of your zapper directly to your other (right) foot.

Now the current will be guided to whatever organ (location) you put on the plate.

On each plate you must choose only one location. If you choose more than one the current must divide itself between them and neither one gets enough to do a good job. However, if you put on two locations that <u>touch each other</u>, such as liver and arteries, the current goes to your liver-arteries, not foot arteries or any other arteries.

The Left Plate

Your blood and lymph system is the most important place (location) to zap, because this is the river-system that all pathogens use to spread themselves. Whenever adult parasites are killed, in any way, they release their eggs, which immediately enter the blood and lymph system. Fortunately this body fluid conducts electricity best, even when PCBs and benzene are everywhere. It is called the *vascular system*. By zapping one of the body fluids at all times, all released eggs are promptly zapped. We will use the left plate to zap the vascular system, but this is only a convention.

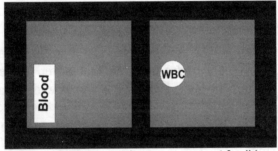

Fig. 38 Plate-zapping arrangement for #1

With regular zapping instead of plate-zapping, the current already goes mostly along the vascular system and is therefore very useful, especially after taking parasite-killing herbs. With plate-zapping you must specifically choose the vascular system to accomplish this. Simply leaving one plate empty also accomplishes this since the whole body is reached through it.

Plate-Zapping Schedule

Each zap will be 20 minutes long. Before you begin, attach your kidney magnets, (see page 247), north side touching skin, using one inch of wide tape. Set your supplements, voltmeter and charger on the table nearby. Find a comfortable chair, warm blanket, and begin.

Plate-Zapping Arrangement

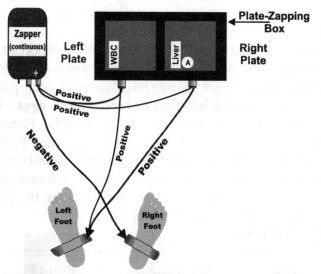

Fig. 39 Plate-zapping arrangement for #6

#1. Put the blood slide on the left plate.
Put the WBC (white blood cell) sample (bottle) on the other plate. Turn on the zapper and put your feet on the copper pipes for 20 minutes. Three 7 minute sessions are fine, too.

#2. Exchange the blood for the lymph sample (bottle). Exchange the WBC for the "A" sample (arteries, veins, nerves). Also place a 1 pF **capacitor** on the plate, but not touching A nor hanging over the edge of the plate. This capacitor somehow creates a preference for the **right side** of your body. In this case, it is the arteries, veins, and nerves on the right side of your body. Zap for 20 minutes.
Keep notes on locations you have zapped (blood, WBC) and check the battery.

#3. Keep "A" on the plate, remove the capacitor, and replace it with a 1 µH **inductor**. The inductor creates a preference for the **left side** of things. In this case, it is the arteries, veins, and nerves on the left side of your body.
Remove lymph from the left plate and place the bottle called "L" on it, and a 1 pF capacitor beside it (without touching each

95

other). Now you are focusing on zapping the lymph vessels and more veins on right side of your body. (The lymph vessels are different from the lymph fluid sample used earlier.) Zap for 20 minutes. After 20 minutes you will have completed your first hour of plate-zapping. It is unlikely that you will feel anything yet. Remember you can take a break between 20-minute zapping sessions.

#4. Keep "L" on the left plate and replace the capacitor with your 1 µH inductor. During the next 20 minutes your left side lymph vessels and veins will get zapped.

Remove "A" and the inductor from the right plate and place the bottle called "CSF" on instead. This stands for cerebrospinal fluid. It is equivalent to lymph, but bathes the brain instead of your other organs. In fact, it is the same as <u>lymph plus 3 pF</u>. Zap for 20 minutes.

#Zap	Left Plate	Right Plate
1	blood	WBC
2	lymph	A + 1 pF
3	L + 1 pF	A + µH
4	L + 1 µH	CSF

The order of these locations does not matter.

These four zapping sessions form the **basic set**. Do these every day. They consume a little more than 1¼ hours, leaving seven hours for you to advance into your other organs and tissues. Even if all you do on the first day is the basic set, you are off to a good start. You do not need to wait for a complete set of slides or supplies. Use whatever you have as soon as you have it. You may make your own organ samples, too, using animal parts from the meat market. Even a drop of blood squeezed from a slice of beef liver into a plastic zippered bag works well for a blood sample.

On the next day go back and do the basic set, first. You will do the basic set, first, every day.

We will continue zapping a part of the basic set at the same time as other organs throughout the day with a double-zapper.

#5. For the next zap, place the blood slide on the left plate again. On the right plate place the organ with your problem. For instance, the liver, if you have liver cancer, or the prostate if you have prostate cancer. It is the organ that <u>has</u> the cancer, not the cancerous part itself. We will zap that later.

#6. Replace the blood slide with WBC on the left. On the right plate add the arteries to the liver sample by touching bottle "A" to the liver sample. They must touch to make a single location, namely the liver arteries.

#7. Replace the WBC with lymph on the left. On the right, replace the arteries with the lymph vessels, bottle "L". It should touch the liver sample.

#8. Replace lymph with the arteries (A) on the left. Then ask yourself, "how can I reach more parts of the liver"? You could move to the right, 1 pF at a time, and then move down by 1 μH. Follow the scheme used for the case study on page 388. Zap each location 20 minutes.

For each new location on the right plate, choose another part of the vascular system on the left. It does not matter in what order you zap the vascular set; you could rotate them all or just a few; you could even stick to one if that is all you have.

You are sure to have an attack of detox-symptoms by now if you have not taken preventive measures. The liver is heavily parasitized. Keep your WBC-food handy on your zapping table. Keep your detox-teas and Lugol's handy, too.

Zap your organ with the tumor every day after the vascular set. Then zap the tumor itself.

The tumor does not have the same frequency pattern as the organ with the tumor. To identify the tumor we must add tricalcium phosphate to the organ. Virtually all cancer cells have tricalcium phosphate deposited in and around them. By touching the organ with the tricalcium phosphate bottle we are selecting tumor cells for zapping.

For example, to zap a left breast tumor, first place a part of the vascular set on the left plate as usual. Place a slide or bottle of breast on the right plate. Beside it, touching it, place your tricalcium phosphate sample. Place a 1 μH inductor on the right plate, too, to indicate the <u>left</u> breast tumor. It should touch nothing and not hang over the edge.

To zap the prostate gland thoroughly, zap both sides separately.

For the right side, place a 1 pF capacitor beside the slide. For a right side tumor, place the tricalcium phosphate bottle touching the prostate slide with the 1 pF capacitor nearby.

Get all the rest of your program done while you are zapping. You can even get IV's while you are zapping.

If you cannot sit, put the pipe-electrodes under you, each on a large zippered plastic bag. Move them from place to place to stay comfortable. By lying on them you will have the necessary pressure to internalize the current. Otherwise it travels along your skin. Do not switch to flat electrodes, unless you need to contact an area with a tumor just below. Flat surfaces do not make enough pressure and this makes the skin resistance higher, to cause small electrical burns. Watch flat electrodes for tiny stinging sensations so you can move the electrode before getting an electrode burn. If you do accidentally get one, do not bandage it or treat it. Merely keep the skin sterile with 1 or 2 drops straight Lugol's each day.

If you zapped the vascular set on your first day and the organ with the tumor on the second day, followed by the tumor itself on the third day, you are off to an excellent start.

If you lost no time to detox-illness you are very fortunate. But do not leave this to chance.

Next clean up all the locations of your digestive tract. Do one a day. You should have a set of about 20 digestive slides. Most of these organs do not need to have left and right sides zapped. For those, you can do two organs in one day.

If you cannot purchase slides, use raw meat samples from the marketplace. A whole chicken gives excellent substitutes for human organs. The bones can be salvaged from a cooked chicken; they do not lose their identity. Do not clean them up too carefully; you want the cartilage and tendons to stay with the joints. Small bones can be left together. Set them in a warm place to dry for several weeks, after labeling each large bone.

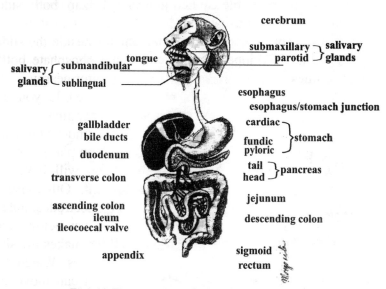

Fig. 40 The location of your digestive organs

Bones you can't identify can be used anyway. They can be stored together in a zippered plastic bag in the refrigerator.

After zapping the colon, repeat it. This time add <u>two</u> 1 pF capacitors. This targets a spot halfway down the descending colon, which I have found to be especially favored by flukes.

If you are suddenly attacked by detox-illness, write down immediately which new organs you zapped that day. They obviously had a significant number of large flukes. As soon as you are ready to continue, repeat these several times to be sure there are no parasites left there. This time be more prepared.

Expect to see parasites in the toilet bowl while zapping the digestive organs. This doesn't happen when you zap other organs, but when parasites in the digestive system die, they can leave with your bowel movement. Try to identify yours.

Fasciolas and Fasciolopsises are often an inch long but can also be much smaller. They can be distinguished by color. Their edges are ragged, like torn pieces of bread. This is due to having burst in the toilet water after falling into it. The difference in osmotic strength between their body fluids and the water outside is probably responsible for bursting. A few do not burst and resemble canned grapes. As their body tears, strings of eggs slip out, hanging loosely. Their appearance is rather translucent under a binocular microscope but when Lugol's iodine is dripped onto them, many tissues take on clearer outlines.

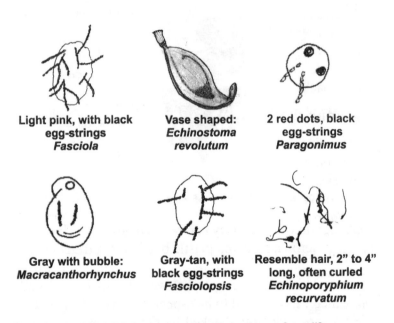

Light pink, with black
egg-strings
Fasciola

Vase shaped:
*Echinostoma
revolutum*

2 red dots, black
egg-strings
Paragonimus

Gray with bubble:
Macracanthorhynchus

Gray-tan, with
black egg-strings
Fasciolopsis

Resemble hair, 2" to 4"
long, often curled
*Echinoporyphium
recurvatum*

Fig. 41 Common parasites, drawn from life

Paragonimus is much smaller and rounder, about $\frac{1}{8}$ inch in diameter. There are actually 3 red dots, but one is much less visible. Two of them appear to be round suckers. It too is in burst condition, letting egg strings hang out. Macracanthorhynchus is easily identified by its round "bubble" at one end. It does not burst. Echinostoma has a hooked tail and

100

does not burst. E. recurvatum is tough and leathery in spite of its thinness. It resembles pieces of straw or hair. Under the binoculars one end looks rounded like a match head. Eurytrema is too small to identify from real life.

To keep toilet bowl specimens from disintegrating you should wash them in 1% salt solution (1 tsp. table salt to one pint water). This may keep one or two intact specimens from bursting, but only if you transfer them to salt water immediately. To preserve them for a few days let several drops of Lugol's solution fall right on top of them. For permanent specimens purchase 40% formaldehyde. Add an equal amount of water to formaldehyde solution in a jar. (That makes a 20% formaldehyde solution, still too strong. Add an equal amount of water again, to make a 10% solution.) Pick up suspected parasites with a plastic fork. Dump straight into the formaldehyde jar. Keep formaldehyde in a locked cabinet. Ask your pharmacist to help you, if needed.

Week Four Plate-Zapping

Depending on how many slides you have, and how long you spent on problem areas, you have been plate-zapping about three weeks. Now we are going to finish with various other locations of your body. An anatomy set is available as a slide kit (see *Sources*). Zap all locations you can acquire.

Bladder, hypothalamus, and pineal are all "single" organs, while brain, kidney, lung, lymph node, breast, and pituitary are all "left and right". These will take approximately one more week.

If you have an organ or body location that is giving you trouble, and the slides you have do not include it, **order it!** (See *Sources*.)

The complete plate-zapping program will last longer than the 3-*Week Program*. Continue steadily. Going too fast invites detox-illness. Hopefully you have seen at least a few parasites of your own, and have positive evidence of getting better.

So far we have discussed two ways to kill parasites on a grand scale: the herbal way and the plate-zapping way. But there is another, much simpler way, besides homeography.

Feast or Famine

The fastest way to get rid of any pest, like ants or mice, is to have <u>no</u> food for them. Would this principle work for internal pests, too? Does Fasciolopsis have a special food that it depends on? Insects with a complex life cycle that includes a caterpillar sometimes depend on a single plant to provide essential food factors. The Monarch butterfly is an example. It must have the milkweed plant to grow its larva. Potato beetles need the potato plant. The cabbage butterfly needs the cabbage plant. Some factor in these foods is required by the pest for its eggs to hatch or larval stages to grow. Fasciolopsis requires <u>onion</u>.

When the tiniest bit of raw onion is eaten its strong sulfide substances arrive quickly at all the Fasciolopsis stages hidden in your body. New stages can now develop and their population booms. Withholding onion is powerful. The famine we create for them cuts their population in half in about 5 days, and again in half in another 5 days. But many sources of onion are so unexpected, it is almost impossible to avoid completely. Most kitchen spices I tested and even a sample of organic butter had onion-chemicals in them! Almost every spice and flavoring has them. The only way to rout the last remnant of onion is with a diet that is also completely devoid of canned food and processed food for two weeks. And at the same time taking a supplement called MSM, which reacts and combines with any onion-chemicals left. Taking digestive enzymes helps remove tiny leftovers, too. This is the third way to kill Fasciolopsis on a large scale. And the search is on to find the essential foods of other parasites. See the incomplete table below:

Parasite Essential Foods

Ascaris lumbricoides, pet roundworm	quercitin (squash & pumpkin, undercooked)
Ascaris megalocephala, pet roundworm	D-carnitine (meat of domestic animals, not free-range, organic)
Clonorchis sinensis, human liver fluke	oats, cooked or raw
Dirofilaria, dog heartworm	lactose (milk sugar)
Echinoporyphium recurvatum	cheese
Eurytrema pancreaticum, pancreatic fluke	lemon and lauric acid (food oil)
Fasciolopsis buski, human intestinal fluke	raw onion (allyl sulfide, diallyl sulfide, allyl methyl sulfide, and other onion-like substances in the lily family)
Fasciola	wheat (gluten and gliadin); metacercaria stage requires lauric acid, food oil
Onchocerca, filaria roundworm	corn, cooked, and linolenic acid (food oil)
Paragonimus, lung fluke	lemon
Plasmodium falciparum vivax, malariae (malaria)	different stages need iron disulfide, wheat, lemon, melanin (plantain), ASA, pyrrole, and others
Strongyloides, roundworm	potatoes, raw or cooked and linolenic acid (food oil)

Fig. 42 Parasites' essential foods

When we stop eating plants with onion-factors Fasciolopsis disappears without any side-effects! No detox-symptoms occur! They must swim away!

Onions belong to the lily family. The lily family includes only a few foods: onions, garlic, leeks, chives, and asparagus. They have an assortment of onion food factors. Certain non-lily plants: cilantro, beans, peas, lentils (after cooking once), peanuts (after roasting), even aloe vera have onion chemicals. Fortunately, boiling destroys the onion factors. The solution for these vegetables is to cook them <u>thoroughly</u>. Unfortunately, canned and processed food escapes being cooked enough! Our plan will be to stay away from these foods until the cancer is conquered, however long that might be. In one week the Fasciolopsis population will be decimated. But we should kill them with direct methods, too, with herbs and zapping to speed up your recovery. Getting rid of more and more Fasciolopsis is the fastest way to get rid of food allergies as well as get your health back.

There is another way, besides herbs, zapping and nutrient withholding to eliminate parasites from your body. I believe it is the body's <u>own</u> way, although we knew nothing about it. The body normally uses benzoquinone (BQ) and rhodizonic acid (RZ), besides its own DMSO and a host of other very powerful chemicals. It makes these itself, but in extremely tiny amounts, like vitamin B_{12} or a hormone. And it uses the body's own electricity to make these, as we will see.

In cancer, as well as AIDS and other diseases, large parts of the body are no longer making BQ or RZ nor the other powerful chemical "weapons". We will find a way to help the body make them again through **homeography**.

CHAPTER 5

HOMEOGRAPHY

Homeography is a new science. It uses electronically prepared drops of water taken by mouth. It rests on the ability of water to incorporate a frequency pattern of some object or chemical or living thing and to hold it in a stable way for a very long time (years). More than one frequency or frequency pattern can be stored together.

In fact, water seems to have a large capacity to hold frequencies without getting them mixed up or weakening. These discoveries are too new to be able to answer even simple questions. What kind of energy is being held in the frequency pattern? We have seen that a purely electrical force and a static magnetic force can be held. Could a pulsing magnetic field be held and detected somehow, too? Only further research can shed light on these questions. But the electrical frequency pattern is surprisingly simple to see and repeat by anyone.

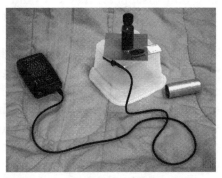

Place the bottle touching the slide or object.

Fig. 43 Making a bottle-copy

How to Make Homeographic Drops

You will need a source of *Positive* offset square waves, at least 30 kHz, close to 50% duty cycle and at least 9 volts from a fresh battery. This is what a zapper produces, so you may already have the most important item. You will also need a 3½ inch square of aluminum sheet, about $^1/_{32}$" to $^1/_{16}$" thick, called the plate. You may find the aluminum at a hardware store; just cut to size and drill a hole for a small screw in the middle. The plate is fastened to a plastic stand such as a disposable food container. A wire comes from the *Positive* output of the zapper and connects to the plate. The *Negative* output is not used. If it is accidentally used, the signal arriving at the antenna-like plate would be grounded to the *Negative* side and disappear. There would be no results.

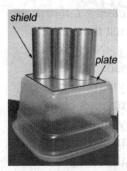

Place metal (aluminum-steel) tubes over bottles to shield them (see *Sources*).

Fig. 44 Shielded bottles make stronger copies

To use the apparatus, place a bottle of plain pure water on the plate. The bottle may be brown glass or brown polyethylene plastic. The brown color keeps out intense light, which could switch the polarization of the contents at any time. It should contain about 10 to 15 ml (2 to 3 tsp.) water. Place the item you want to copy right beside it. Surround all bottles being used with a metal tube as a shield (aluminum or aluminum-steel pipe) to make the effect stronger, although it is not strictly necessary. The two items or tubes must touch. Now zap for 20 seconds (this is not precise). The plain water now becomes a **bottle-copy**.

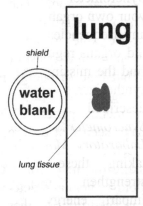

Strengthen your lungs with their own frequencies copied from a lung slide and taken as drops of water.

Fig. 45 Making organ drops

After incorporating a bone or other substance into a water sample, its presence should be, ideally, verified using a Syncrometer® or more rigorously, using a digital

106

frequency synthesizer in conjunction with a Syncrometer®. These optional details of copy-making are in the *Syncrometer® Science Laboratory Manual*. Realistically, you must be able to trust the copier.

Numerous purposes can be achieved with electronically made bottle-copies. You can use them when testing with the Syncrometer® or when plate-zapping, as we saw in the previous chapter. Secondly, the water copy itself can be taken by mouth in the form of **drops** under the tongue. How could this be useful? Depending on the variety of drops made, different goals can be achieved.

Homeographic Drops Can Strengthen

The most important goal is to clean your organs of all the toxins, pathogens and parasites accumulated there. Simply making a copy of each organ and taking this as drops many times a day accomplishes this. For a few hours the Syncrometer® sees the new frequency pattern superimposed on your own organ's pattern. For a short time you are not missing any frequencies from your own "sick" organ. Sick or merely old organs regularly miss many of their frequencies. You can find the missing ones precisely with a high quality frequency synthesizer. (This is described in the *Syncrometer® Science Laboratory Manual*). Does taking these as drops strengthen metabolism? Impart energy to that organ? The WBCs in this organ get activated, as if you had zapped this organ. The Syncrometer® sees they are soon full of their surrounding toxins. Sometimes you can feel the effect immediately.

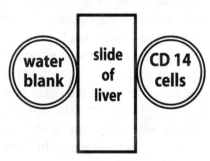

This combination makes the liver-CD14 cell pattern. Reversing them contaminates your CD14 bottle.

Fig. 46 Combinations should mimic reality

> Never take drops of a parasite or a virus or anything harmful.

Taking drops of harmful invaders would surely reach them and strengthen <u>them</u>! Use only the goals and formats given here. This is not the same as homeopathy.

The dose is six drops taken 6 times daily for two days. Drop them under your tongue just behind the lower teeth. Leave them there to slowly absorb before swallowing them. After two days reduce the dosage to 3 times daily. No food should have been in your mouth for five minutes, nor eaten afterward for five minutes.

You can combine slides or bottles (not drops) creatively to match precise locations. In the example shown we make drops of the CD14 cells in the liver. The CD14s are the macrophages, our huge white blood cells, always immobilized and coated with automotive greases in cancer victims. Taking these drops would strengthen them specifically. By touching 2 tissues on the copy plate they represent a "series" type circuit. This implies that they touch each other in real life. If they don't really touch in real life, you would leave a space between them on the plate. For example, to create the location of a mediastinal tumor which is between the upper lung and the esophagus, you would place these 2 slides on the plate, separated by a space of about ¼". The blank (for copying) touches one of these. Slides that are placed more than 1" apart are for organs that are definitely not in contact in real life. Two tissues placed at different corners act as if in "parallel" electrically. As you place them closer together, you are assuming they are partly in "series".

Many of your organs have a left and right partner. For example, you have two lungs and two kidneys. Your brain has a left and right side. In the case of the liver there are many lobes (see page 388). Your pancreas has left and right portions that are not symmetrical. The more precisely you can focus on a particular part, the more effective the drops will be.

Capacitors and inductors are electronic components with a precise amount of capacitance or inductance. By putting them on your plate, along with an organ sample, you change its electrical properties slightly. I have found by adding a 1 pF (picofarad) capacitor you can adjust a location more to the right or further up. If instead you add a 1 µH (microhenry) inductor you can structure a location more to the left or further down.

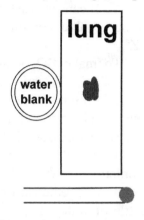

For example, suppose you know your right lung is worse than your left, and you want to zap the right lung first. You would make a bottle-copy of a lung slide with a 1 pF capacitor laid near it. The resulting drops would strengthen the right lung only. The bottle made could be used to zap the right lung only.

To make a right lung, place a 1 pF capacitor on plate.

Fig. 47 Making a Right lung bottle

You may make drops of all the organ samples you can buy or somehow locate. You may have 30 or 50 bottles to take, **giving one minute to each**. You can do this while you are zapping. There are no side-effects although you may feel new body currents in locations of disease. If you take these drops more than 6 times daily, the effect may be much stronger. And, if you give yourself detox-illness you have evidence (though uncomfortable) that you even killed large parasites. How did your body do that with only 6 drops of water?

Homeographic Drops Can Supply (add)

Homeographic drops can <u>add missing things to a particular organ</u>. The things we want most are the immune weapons benzoquinone (BQ), rhodizonic acid (RZ), glyoxal (G), and glyoxylic acid (GA). These mega parasite-killers are by far the most dramatic and versatile chemicals in our bodies, as impressive as the power of our neurotransmitters. They have the most responsible job—to kill large parasites. The cancer patient's body is full of parasite eggs and stages because there are no mega killers at most locations. Children do have them.

You can <u>instruct</u> your body to make BQ by using a homeographic combination. A different combination makes RZ.

To make BQ, which kills one of our Ascaris varieties (Ascaris lumbricoides), we must combine the organ where you wish to install it (such as the organ with a tumor or other problem), with saliva and blood all together in one blank bottle of water. The saliva and blood samples should come from a different person or an animal. Bottles have shields placed around them; slides do not. After taking these drops several times you will find BQ

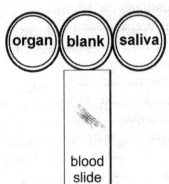

Each item touches the blank, but not each other.

Fig. 48 Making BQ in an organ

present in this organ. It will be ready to go to work for you.

One could, of course, copy some real benzoquinone into a bottle of water and take those drops. We call this "cloned BQ." These drops are quite powerful, too, but only for a short time. Inducing your body to make BQ using the combination of saliva and blood and organ is superior!

To make RZ, the organ to be replenished (your organ with a problem) is combined with saliva and lymph. The saliva can be in bottle-copy form, originally from a fairly healthy person. Bottle-copies of all these supplies can be purchased (see *Sources*), but are easily made, too. Notice that the three ingredients must not touch each other, but all must touch the blank bottle.

Why are BQ and RZ missing in the first place? It depends on the presence of Ascaris-chemicals, such as 1,10-

phenanthroline, guanidine, methyl guanidine and others. Ascaris produces a host of such abnormal chemicals. Evidently they use up BQ and RZ.

If BQ can be made abundantly, until no Ascaris or their chemicals are left, the body can continue to make its own BQ. If not enough is made and Ascaris chemicals are left over, BQ continues to be missing and now parasites can grow large, mature, and shed eggs. Parasitism continues.

As soon as you take six drops of the saliva-blood-organ bottle-copy your body starts making BQ at that organ. This destroys the Ascaris-chemicals as well as Ascaris itself at that one location. Within the day, this tissue is freed from Ascaris parasitism. You may suddenly feel like a brand new person. Ascaris was bringing you night sweats from its bacteria.

As soon as you feel better you may reduce the dosage to 3 times a day. Because of the possibility of reinfection from the environment and also from other parts of the body, it would be wise to continue taking these drops 2 or 3 times per day for weeks. Afterwards, test your ability to keep making BQ and RZ yourself.

Making G, GA and other weapons requires combining other body fluids, including bile and urine. Each combination kills a specific large parasite. Until research on these is complete take the cloned weapons themselves, which you can easily make from a master sample.

You now have a <u>very easy way</u> to remove both toxins and parasites from your most important organs with a minimum of discomfort, and to restore immune weapons. It is not unusual for a cancer patient to be taking 30 or more homeographic bottles continuously while zapping for eight hours a day.

Zapping an organ while taking drops for that same organ seems to be especially beneficial. Try to arrange for that coincidence.

111

Homeographic Drops Can Remove (subtract)

We already saw how we can put things <u>into</u> the body, by supplying it. The body will send it to the organ in need using its own discretion. We do not yet know how to direct it specifically.

But we can take things <u>out</u> of the body, quite specifically, simply by combining it homeographically with the location to be cleaned.

The most important things to take out are wheel bearing grease, azo dyes, nickel and other heavy metals. When the body's immune system can not recover fast enough to remove these major toxins in time to prevent disaster, making *take-out* bottles for them brings emergency relief in 1 to 2 days. Because of their power, you must not make a mistake with them. In the examples given, *take-out* bottles are left to the last so you can gain experience first. Do not leave such big responsibilities to others. You can reverse your jaundice, kidney failure, seizures, anemia, and other emergencies, but only if done correctly.

Homeography in Perspective

Homeography, like zapping, can be systemic in scope or focused on specific organs. Taking six drops of electronically "patterned" water mobilizes the white blood cells; that can be easily seen. It may do much more that must wait on research.

Being able to interact with the body using electrical and homeographic methods suggests that the body understands and acts with these same methods or "languages". Does a mother cat not lick her kitten from top to toe—combining saliva with nasal secretions, eye secretions, mucous, sweat, even anal and urinary secretions. Certainly a wound is immediately treated by combining it with saliva, right at the needy and bleeding organ.

Negative voltage frequencies do not have this beneficial effect, although they can be copied, too. If you are purchasing ready-made bottle-copies, be sure to specify and ask for assurance that a *Positive* offset voltage was used and <u>how</u>

much offset there was. If they don't understand the question, purchase elsewhere.

I do not understand the physics or chemistry of water sufficiently to explain these phenomena. Questions must wait. But you can harness the forces involved to "boot-up" your own immune power even when all the blockers are present. The organ chosen can begin to clean itself up provided you stop taking the toxin in. You cannot take out what you are taking in! Mobilizing the WBCs is not all that is involved. You can often "taste" the action. Sometimes you can feel the organ respond. For instance, taking kidney drops can send you directly to the bathroom. You can even get a mild detox-illness. Perhaps the electronic language of adding and subtracting frequencies (called heterodyning) or riding along on other frequencies (called modulation) is native to life. Water, being the unifying chemical for life has its electrical charges, which then make it susceptible to voltage influences. Only more research can help us understand.

You must be very careful not to set your drops near a magnet. The magnetic field destroys them. Always keep magnets in their own container, to separate them.

The first drops to make should be the "protective set" for the lymph and kidneys. These are both organs. The lymph needs cleaning more than other fluids and often rewards you with pain relief instantly or extra energy. The kidneys will be the first to get help for their white blood cells. Take these drops continually, for weeks, at least until you are done plate-zapping.

Making Drops

The Water

Use only distilled-filtered water (see page 226) to make drops. It is the cleanest. And it only stays clean if you store it in a non-seeping container! Well water nearly always has a bleach or other disinfectant added. Do not trust untested water. Bleach, whether the laundry type or NSF (good) type, still gives you sodium hypochlorite, which will get highly activated by the homeographic procedure. Don't use any chlorinated water. You cannot filter water or "let it stand" and expect to get rid of chlorine. Only boiling it, at a rolling boil for five minutes, can get rid of it. Test for chlorine with a kit available at pool supply stores. The drops you make and the drops you buy should be tested for bleach regularly.

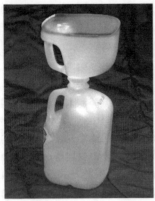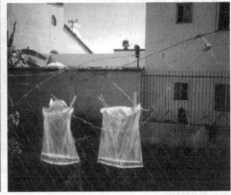

Fig. 49 Collecting rainwater

To clean and store rainwater for drop-making, collect it in an opaque polyethylene bottle, preferably a used one that had held distilled water in it at the supermarket. Make a funnel out of another such bottle or purchase a stainless steel one. All others will seep very toxic metals into your rainwater. Test its conductivity with an indicator (see *Sources*). It should be zero. Also test for strontium, PCBs, beryllium, vanadium, and chromium, the common air pollutants. If these are absent, you are very fortunate. It is healthful, you can drink it and make drops with it.

Place each rainwater collector in a bucket that is suspended in the air, or weighted down by a rock on your lawn. You may also use plastic bags of the zippered kind that can be suspended with clothespins. Do not leave your collections open and unattended. Air pollutants can fall in. If any one is present, you must filter it out, see page 587.

The Rain Filter

Wait for ½ hour of raining before starting to collect so that smog particles, bits of foliage and dust will have rained down. Test it first for pollutants. If there are none, you still need a coarse filter, which you can make yourself. A carbon or regular filter would remove the beneficial elements while adding its own toxic ones. Cheese cloth and cotton wool from vitamin bottles can be washed under the faucet several times and squeezed dry, then boiled in tap water for 5 minutes at a rolling boil. Rinse with your own purified water. After this, there should be no chlorine residue and no conductivity detected in any rinse water. Use it as a loose fitting cork in your homemade funnel to filter the rain as it comes down. Store extra filters in a double zippered bag in the freezer. The water collected can be stored, as is, in the refrigerator, ready for drop-making. Do not pour it into some other bottle.

The Bottles

Buy ½ oz. amber glass bottles with caps that have a polyethylene protected surface inside (see *Sources*). Do not buy droppers for them. The rubber end of the dropper seeps heavy metals and malonic acid. You may buy

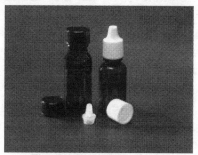

Fig. 50 Amber glass and polyethylene bottles and lids

a separate polyethylene drop dispenser (pipette) used by chemistry students (see *Sources*). Keep each pipette with its own bottle. One wrong dip would destroy the bottle! Also buy ½ oz. amber polyethylene bottles with 2 kinds of caps: a flat one and a dropper variety complete with nozzle (see picture).

DO'S and **DON'TS. Do not switch bottle caps or nozzles. You may reuse a bottle if you rinse it 3 times with pure water and also rinse the nozzle and cap 3 times. Even one drop of a different frequency destroys a new bottle of drops. Since you have no way of testing whether a bottle is**

potent or blank, be extra careful not to confuse bottle parts. This is also the reason for taking drops one minute apart. New drops must not touch old drops in your mouth.

Do not combine bottles. Do keep bottles out of direct sunlight. Do not carry them in your pocket. Do not rubber band them together while they are being copied. Do not touch them during copying. Do turn off the zapper before touching them to remove them. If you made a mistake or have some doubts, rinse everything and start over.

Organ Drops

Each organ you take as drops will show activation of its WBCs specifically; no other organs are activated. The most important organs to activate are the kidneys. In fact they are so important you should always **take kidney drops first**, along with kidney white blood cells when beginning any drop-taking session.

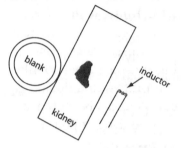

Fig. 51 Making a bottle of the Left kidney

To make your kidney protective set, to strengthen them, copy your slide or bottle of kidney tissue. Make a Right kidney bottle and a Left kidney bottle. Then make Right kidney WBCs and Left kidney WBCs.

Making Dyes-Out-Of-Kidney Set

It is failure of the kidney white blood cells to keep the kidneys clean that "clogs" them and forces the toxins to accumulate somewhere else in the body, just where there is no immune power.

We will make *take-out* drops for each kidney and its WBCs to bring back normal kidney action.

Fig. 52 Making a bottle of Left kidney WBCs

116

The power in *take-out* drops is so huge that nobody should make them before reading this entire section on homeography. And nobody should take them if the source of their dyes, heavy metals and wheel bearing grease have not been found and eliminated. In other words, you can't *take-out* those things you are still taking in! That is why cleaning up water, diet, dentalware and cooking pots come first. Nor can you clean large areas like the blood, the bones, the skin. It is meant for tiny amounts.

Take-Out Dyes From Right Kidney

Purchase a bottle of mixed azo dyes. Also purchase individual dyes: Fast Green, Fast Red, Fast Blue, Fast Red Violet, Fast Garnet, DAB, and Sudan Black. You may soon need them.

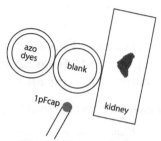

Fig. 53 Take-out dyes from Right kidney

Place the dye sample on one side of the blank bottle, on the left by our convention. Place the organ to be cleared, namely kidney, on the opposite side, on the right by our convention[*]. Place metal tubes over all bottles. Add a 1 pF capacitor to the plate, not touching anything. Zap for 20 seconds with *Positive* offset voltage. Label your newly made bottle "*take-out* dyes from Right kidney".

Take-Out Dyes From Right Kidney White Blood Cells

Place blank at center. Place dyes on left side of blank. Place kidney slide on right side of blank, adding a 1 pF capacitor. Next, place white blood cells beside kidney, touching it. Use a WBC bottle or homemade slide, but not your own WBCs. NOTE: if you used a kidney bottle instead of slide

---

[*] You may make more than one bottle at a time. Another blank bottle can touch the center blank on both sides. Every bottle can only touch the center bottle and every bottle should have its metal sleeve. If the slide gets too close (less than 8 mm) tilt it and make only one extra bottle.

117

and also a WBC <u>bottle</u>, the WBC frequency will have to pass through the kidney bottle to reach the blank and will remain there. The kidney bottle now has the WBC frequency in it. So relabel your kidney bottle "has WBC". You can avoid this by using a kidney <u>slide</u> or sample from meat shop (placed in zippered plastic bag). If you wish to use your kidney bottle, make **a copy of it beforehand. This would**

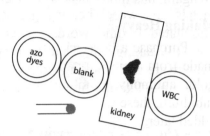

Fig. 54 Take-out dyes from Right kidney WBCs

keep one safe from accidental contamination and is highly recommended for all your purchases.

Take-Out Dyes From Left Kidney

Place blank at center. Place dyes on left side of blank. Place kidney slide on right side of blank. Place a 1 µH inductor loose on plate, not touching anything.

Take-Out Dyes From Left Kidney White Blood Cells

Place blank at center. Place dyes on left side of blank. Place kidney slide on right side and WBCs touching it. Add 1 µH loose on plate.

You now have a set of 4 *take-out* bottles for dyes from the kidney set. These can save your life when you are already on life support means with less than a week of life left for you. But they won't save your life if your very life support supplies contain dyes as they would if they were manufactured by a company that uses laundry bleach to disinfect its biologicals or if these supplies included colored plastic. Such dilemmas are common. Use your judgment. The rule is never broken that you cannot take out what you are putting in.

The whole *take-out* action is complete in 4 days, taking them 6 times daily for the first 2 days and 3 times daily for the next 2 days. Copy each bottle by cloning it before it is less than half full. Continue once a day for 2 more weeks. Store the remainder. If you are in a new emergency situation, take them all again, this time every hour the first day.

Making Heavy-Metals-Out-of-Kidney Set

Purchase a bottle-copy of mixed heavy metals. Mine was made from a piece of unused amalgam plus cobalt, strontium, gold, antimony, uranium, chromium, radon, ruthenium and rubidium; these were missing in my piece of amalgam, so were added later.

Make your own with a chip of old amalgam from any, including your own, extracted tooth. Drop it into pure water in an amber ½ oz. bottle. To take all these out of your Right kidney, again place the blank in the center. Place the heavy metal bottle on the left side of the blank. Place the Right kidney on the Right side of the blank. Just before pressing the switch button, read the line-up as a final check, like this, from left to right, "Take heavy metals-out-of-Right kidney", and check each item as you read it. Ask yourself, "Am I contaminating any of my bottles?" If so, make a copy you can discard later. Then zap 20 minutes.

Any piece of amalgam will be missing some heavy metals. Combine all the metal jewelry you were wearing, including watchband, earrings, necklaces, and dentalware you saved in one zippered plastic bag. Copy it all together. Then make *take-out* drops for your kidney set.

Finish making and taking the heavy metals-out-of-Right kidney and Right kidney WBCs, Left kidney and Left kidney white blood cells.

Making Wheel Bearing Grease-Out-Of-Kidney Set

Since wheel bearing grease traps motor oil, dyes, metals, malonic acid and solvents and slowly releases them in your vital organs, this may be the most important take-out-set. <u>Be careful not to try to take this grease out of other locations before taking it out of the kidney set</u>. It could relocate itself.

Purchase a can of wheel bearing grease at any automotive supply store. Copy it into a bottle of water, placing a shield over the blank as usual. The large size of the can will make part of it hang over the edge. Copy it only into one bottle at a time (not several). Label it.

Make wheel bearing grease (WBGr)-out-of-Right kidney, WBGr-out-of-Right kidney WBCs, WBGr-out-of-Left kidney, WBGr-out-of-Left kidney WBCs. Also WBGr-out-of-lymph.

You now have 4 sets:

- a kidney set to help and protect them
- dyes-out-of kidney set
- heavy metals-out-of-kidney set
- wheel bearing grease-out-of-kidney set and lymph

Making Extra Drops

Copy the LYMPH bottle so you can take drops of lymph as well as zapping lymph and *take-out* bottles from lymph.

Copy the peripheral BLOOD slide so you can take drops as well. Label it CIRCULATION or BLOOD.

Copy the CD14s; take drops.

Copy the CD8s; take drops.

Make dyes-out-of LYMPH.

Make NICKEL-out-of CD8s.

Make NICKEL-out-of-CD14s.

Make heavy metals-out-of-LYMPH.

Make methyl malonate-out-of-kidney set, taking drops to rescue kidneys from failure.

Next, make DAB (dye)-out-of-WBCs. This is a single bottle. Having DAB in the white blood cells causes the alkaline phosphatase to be much too high. Having cobalt in them causes low alkaline phosphatase. Check yours. Hurry to take out DAB or cobalt or both. But where will they go after being taken out? They should go to the kidney WBCs. But if the kidneys have not yet been cleared of dyes or heavy metals, it will do no good. You must wait till you have taken the kidney drops for 4 days. Then take DAB out for 4 days only, then stop. If alkaline phosphatase is too low, take cobalt out, too, for 4 days. You may take them together, as a set, one after the other.

Next make Sudan Black (dye)-out-of-RBCs. Having Sudan Black in your RBCs causes the LDH to be much too high. If LDH is too low, there is cobalt in them. Make cobalt-out-of-RBCs.

Next make Fast Green (dye)-out-of-CD8s and Fast Garnet-out-of-CD4s.

If the globulin is too low, or too high, take all the wheel bearing grease, dyes and heavy metals out of the B-cells. B-cells are also called CD37 cells.

You can make your own RBCs and platelets by structuring them electronically like this:

RBCs = WBCs + 1 μH

platelets = WBCs + 2 μH

megakaryocytes = WBC + 4 pF

If the total bilirubin is over the range given as normal on the blood test, take copper, cobalt, chromium and nickel out of all liver parts. Make separate bottles for each metal for a stronger effect than the heavy metal combination. (Follow the example on page 388.) Also make a bottle of heavy metals-out-of-each-liver part. There are at least 10 liver parts. You have only days to accomplish this before jaundice begins. After 2 days of such metal removal the fungus, Aspergillus, and its relative, Penicillium, will be in decline. You can now take aflatoxin-out-of-all-liver parts. After another 2 days you can take bilirubin-out-of-blood for 4 days. Then you are ready for a new blood test.

These are extra life-saving features of homeography. You can see that for jaundice you must find the sources of these 4 heavy metals; you must stop drinking and eating them or you will have your jaundice back very soon. Sources of these 4 heavy metals are few: food, drink, dentalware, dishes and supplements. Use extreme measures when a crisis is before you. (Eat only natural food, drink only rainwater, remove all synthetic dentalware, don't use dishes or cutlery, don't take any supplements.) After it is over, search for the metals.

Prevent Mistakes

Because *take-out* drops are very powerful, consider the effect on you if you should make a mistake.

LABEL ALL BOTTLES YOU MAKE;
put on details

Taking protective drops (same as organ drops) that are accidentally blank or got mixed up could never harm you. But making and taking salmonella drops could. Never even make bacteria drops or parasite drops or virus drops to prevent any such error. Don't make them for zapping either. Zapping them has no value. They might be gone for 15 minutes and then be back! You have them because you are feeding them unknowingly, while your WBCs aren't working.

Never make drops that take out bacteria, parasites or viruses. They could only be out for minutes anyway since they reproduce in the neighboring organs all the time. And, again, you are inadvertently feeding them while the WBCs are disabled.

Consider the hazard of making a mistake in a *take-out* bottle for dyes or heavy metals. If, by accident, your final bottle only had kidneys or WBC or RBCs, they would now be "organ drops", not harmful. But if your final bottle had only dyes in it or heavy metals, having missed the organ, I believe you could certainly harm yourself. It would be equivalent to taking the dyes or metals for about ½ hour. For this reason, do not purchase *take-out* bottles, ready-made. Make them yourself. Even you will occasionally make a mistake. But stopping each *take-out* bottle after 4 days gives a measure of safety. If you sense an error, rinse bottles and start over.

The Problem Organ

Next, make drops of organs with problems.

First make the organ with the tumor; for example, if you have cancer in the Right lung, the organ with the problem is the

Right lung. Always make drops for both members of a set though, like Right and Left lung.

Lungs are quite large. It would be useful to reach bronchi, bronchioles, and alveoli, specifically.

Use these relationships:

lung/trachea = bronchus. The slash means these two test samples touch each other.

bronchus + 1 μH = bronchiole

bronchiole + 1 μH = alveolus

Make drops for all organs with any problem, like liver for jaundice (make the whole set), bone marrow for leukemia, adrenals for high blood pressure, and so on. Make drops for their WBCs, too.

Remember that zapping an organ at the same time as taking drops for it has an exceptionally powerful effect. Try to do this.

Always take the kidney drops first, before others in any drop-taking session.

No Drops for the Tumor

You will NOT be making tumor drops. It would be harmful, I believe. You do not want to strengthen the tumor.

But zapping it is supremely powerful. To single it out <u>for zapping</u>, attach a substance, **tricalcium phosphate**, to the organ slide (see page 97).

You do not need to make a bottle of the tumor since you can construct it easily on the plate for zapping. This adds a protection against ever taking drops of a tumor. Place your tricalcium phosphate sample touching the organ.

How often should you take drops? Whenever you start new drops, take them very often the first day, even every hour if possible. This increases the chance of treating it quickly because there is a cumulative action; 6 times a day is the minimum for a new organ.

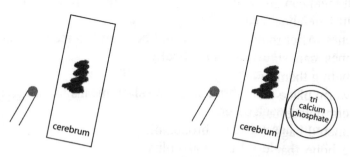

Zapping the Right cerebrum (at left) and Right brain tumor (at right).

Fig. 55 Zapping a brain tumor

Whenever intensive *take-out* treatment is planned, be sure you can take enough organic germanium, selenite and vitamin C (rose hips) too. Imagine you could build a house in <u>one</u> day. It would be a very busy building site. You dare not run out of one frequently used supply, not even nails. Imagine the cost of missing water or electricity for an hour.

After two days of intensive treatment, most of the action is done. You should go down to 3 times daily for 2 more days. After this all *take-out* drops should be stopped but continue protective or *organ drops*. Continue these once a day. Hopefully you made copies and labeled all your bottles. So, if you had a new emergency, you could repeat it all, quickly.

Keep a daily log of zaps done and drops taken, along with a note about symptoms felt, if any, at each organ.

Next, make drops for every organ that is involved in your illness. For example, you may have:

a. pain at right hip
b. a new lump

Pain at Right Hip

Pain at bones is a very common experience. But how do you know which bone it is? How could you find exactly which bone to zap and make drops for? Chances are excellent that a chicken has such a bone. Its frequency pattern would be close to yours. Purchase chicken parts that include this bone. Cook till meat can be removed. It should not be completely removed; cartilage and attached tendons and gristle should be left on the bones. After removing meat, separate the large bones, but small bones can stay together. Place on paper towels to air dry, labeling them first, including left or right side. After 3 weeks in a warm place they should be fairly dry. (You do not need to dry them before using them.) Then put larger bones in their own zippered bags. Several smaller bones can share a bag. To find the bone that matches your painful bone, you would need a Syncrometer®*. But if you can guess which bone has your pain, you can copy the bone into 2 bottles, one for zapping, and one to dispense drops. Keep your bone set in the refrigerator.

A Lump

A lump visible under the skin often cannot be given an organ name using slides or specimens. Even a small lump on the face can be impossible to give a location on your plate.

To be able to zap these precisely, you can make a **paper skin copy** of them. The frequencies of energy coming from the body leave through the skin and can be caught in water placed there.

The copy will <u>not</u> be for drop-making since it is your own (not from a healthy rat or monkey). But it will serve for analysis by Syncrometer® and for zapping. Label it: ZAP ONLY.

Paper Skin Copy

Cut a circle out of white, unfragranced paper towel to fit over the lump. Carry a small amount of pure water with you to the couch where you can lie down for 10 minutes. Place the paper over the lump and pour enough water on yourself to hold the paper against the skin everywhere. Wait 10 minutes. Pick it up with your fingers inside a zippered bag or with metal

---

* Testers, search for Streptococcus pneumoniae (pain) bacteria in bone locations, using chicken bones. Place bag of bones beside patient's saliva sample. Search for Strep pneu, OPT, etc. If *Positive*, test each bone.

tweezers. (Gloves could shed heavy metals.) The same way, stuff the paper into an empty amber glass test bottle or a plastic zippered bag. The damp paper should touch the bottom of the bottle. Shake it down till it reaches the bottom of the bottle. That is why you should use glass…to be able to see it. A zippered bag should be folded so the paper sample is only one plastic layer away from the plate. Do not add water. Close, label it; for example: <u>Below Left Eye</u>. Use this bottle or bag to zap. In this way you can zap (but not take drops) any location on your body where you can feel a lump.

A New Lump

It is demoralizing and panicking to see a new lump appear or an old one grow again after you have been shrinking several others. It brings home the painful truth that you still have toxins coming <u>into</u> your body when you thought you had found them all and detoxified enough. Tumors that are not shrinking are still receiving growth stimulators and are still accumulating toxins.

ALL problems are current.

Growth and accumulation makes tumors enlarge. Growth comes from SCF and HGH at first and from Yeast and Staph with RAS oncovirus later. Apoptosis can be blocked by just a few parasites, and the white blood cells can be disabled because they are <u>only</u> full of nickel. Test yourself for these.

When some tumors refuse to shrink, or new ones grow, jump into action. Not to zap, take drops and otherwise obliterate the new growth, but to find the source of allergens and heavy metals. Chances are best that your food has phloridzin, chlorogenic acid and gallic acid in it. And that your dishes and food are giving you chromium to feed both yeast and Staph.

Immediately improve your compliance. Do not use any loopholes in the diet* or items you thought you "were getting away with". Don't risk an untested new supplement, or somebody else's cooking. Repeat the whole program. Results should be much quicker this time. Without a Syncrometer® you must over-comply if you are very advanced. You <u>must</u> find what is stimulating the new growth.

Review your dental work. Get a blood test and interpret the results item by item using the *Blood Test Results* on page 311. Most often a stubborn lump is due to a small mistake, like using a prized product, a favorite cup, or a new supplement. If the new lump shrinks you guessed right. Notice that you have more power in your hands than the finest cancer institute. Use it to detect these simple causes. Soon there will be more patients with experience like yours to help you.

Losing Weight

If you lost weight during the dental work, you can see how critically poised a cancer patient's weight control is. A single meal lost is important. I do not know the mechanism that supports weight gain or weight loss. What helps most is keeping a clean hypothalamus. Make a *take-out* bottle for heavy metals (including gold) at the hypothalamus.

Take out chromium from lymph and from the organ with the tumor. This starves yeast in the tumor and skin by depriving it of its main metal need. Yeast consumes your blood sugar so you lose weight. First of all, avoid eating chromium.

Make a bottle-copy of hydrazine sulfate. Take 6 drops 3 times a day till you feel hungry for each meal. Then stop. Try to gain back all the weight you lost.

---

* Testers, search for SCF, HGH, gallic acid, chlorogenic acid, phloridzin, Fasciolopsis cercariae, CEA, Yeast, HCG, RRase, thiourea, heavy metals, laundry bleach, dyes, wheel bearing grease in the saliva.

The More the Merrier

It is so easy to make and take drops that there is no reason not to do a lot more! In fact, even if you have the real herbs make drops from them and take these too! Here are the ones I recommend the most:

- whole cloves
- coriander seed
- fennel seed
- fresh apricot seeds, cracked yourself (old ones do not work)

- Lugol's iodine, self made
- nutmeg pods
- rhodizonate (RZ)
- wormwood, (c/s)
- benzoquinone (BQ)

Use only tested herbs. If they contain thallium you will be giving yourself that! Do not copy powders. If they contained nickel, you would be giving yourself this!

Taking the real substance or oils might require prescriptions, and would pose dangers if too much were taken. Taking the bottle-copies is safe and inexpensive. You can learn which ones seem to help you. If you give yourself detox-symptoms, wait till you are recovered, then take it again and again till you get no detox-symptoms.

Zapper Alchemy

Freshly cracked apricot seeds and freshly picked Eucalyptus leaves are somewhat perishable—so just stuff them into a half-ounce glass bottle (no water used), or zippered bag, and copy them for posterity! Label it *master*.

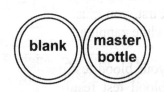

Fig. 56 To clone a sample is simple copying

Taking drops of such copies gives you <u>some</u> of the effectiveness of the real thing; in general, about one-fourth. Clone your *masters* for drop taking and copy the copies before they are half consumed in order to continue getting strong copies.

Summary of Chapters 4 and 5

1. To prevent flu symptoms you should delay killing parasites till heavy metals, dyes and wheel bearing grease are out of the kidneys and their white blood cells. This could delay you 4 days while you make and take drops that support your kidneys, remove their toxins, and start feeding their WBCs. At the same time, do your cleanups and dental work.

2. Removing metal from the mouth and throwing away seeping cookware helps so much with this kidney detoxification that we place it first in the program.

3. Killing parasites the herbal way is system-wide but can miss hard to reach places like the brain, lymph valves, and small crevices. Regular zapping at this time kills the escapees.

4. Killing parasites the zapping way should be done by plate-zapping if you are advanced, since PCBs, motor oil, and wheel bearing grease saturate many important organs preventing them from conducting all the zapper current. For plate-zapping and regular zapping sit with your feet on the zapper's copper tubes. Follow a schedule of organs to be plate-zapped. This lets you restore immunity to one organ after another.

5. Killing parasites the homeographic way can be done by depriving them of needed metals using the *take-out* drops. First, you must remove all sources of metals. You can do it all while zapping.

6. You can make *take-out* drops for certain things spotted on your blood test results that are leading to an emergency. Your blood test results for alkaline phosphatase, LDH, T.b., T.p., RBCs, WBCs and others can't improve unless specific toxins are removed from specific organs. Then they improve in days.

7. You can supply yourself with anything, briefly, by taking it as drops. You can even copy medicines and get some effectiveness...about one-fourth. But it has its hazards. Medicines, supplements, and herbs are extremely polluted. Finding one without dyes, bleach, solvents or heavy metals would be almost impossible. Taking the drops anyway would

be taking magnified doses of the toxins, too. Copy only tested items. To protect yourself, take them only 4 days.

8. Killing parasites with the starvation method is easiest, but you must be thorough.

9. You can't kill parasites successfully while at the same time feeding them their required food factors. Look them up in the tables given.

None of these successes will be permanent unless you find and remove the <u>sources</u> of your heavy metals, dyes, malonic acid and critical allergens. After you are well, your tolerance will improve as long as you are in correctly disinfected water. Tolerance depends on detoxifying ability.

It will be a fascinating adventure as long as you are succeeding, even while it is a life and death struggle. No challenge in a Greek myth could have been more adrenalizing. You will need a friend to care for you, help you make drops, help you zap for hours each day, help you get your supplements down, help you wash and treat your food, help you cook from scratch, and, finally, share your successes.

Such a friend is an angel from heaven. Reward him or her with your smiles and determination to do everything right. And if you do get detox-illness strike off 2 calendar days to rest and to think: why did I not prevent this? Then support your <u>caregiver's</u> morale. When your sickness or cancer improves even slightly, mention it. It helps everybody. Express your desire to live to your caregiver and your appreciation, because you need still more help. Early good results are only part of the goal. Getting completely well is the whole. Such a standard has never been set clinically because it was impossible to achieve. But now you can achieve it.

CHAPTER 6

SHRINKING TUMORS

A tumor <u>grows</u> and a tumor <u>accumulates</u>. These are its most unique and destructive properties. Just outside the tumor, only millimeters away, growth is normal. We can study the normal cells with a Syncrometer® and compare each detail with the tumor cells so close to it. Soon we will understand the difference.

Normal organs regulate their own size. They are made of millions of cells. Growing cells make an organ bigger. Self-digesting cells make an organ smaller. Self digesting is called apoptosis (see page 68).

Increasing and decreasing are equal for a healthy organ in an adult. We can study growth and self-digestion in the normal organ and compare that to the abnormal tumor nearby and understand exactly what needs to be corrected.

Accumulation Still Baffling

The accumulation property is more mysterious. Why thousands of toxins are coming to one organ instead of to the kidneys for excretion has only theoretical explanations. Removing the five that block immunity will be our practical solution. This will bring back the help of the white blood cells whose job it is to remove the accumulation. The white blood cells are the strongest force we have to remove anything. And if the kidneys are helped this way first, by cleaning their white blood cells, the kidneys will take over the whole job of cleaning the body again. Then toxins will flow to the kidneys and out of the body with urine excretion instead of into some organ. The liver and other organs will follow this pattern next.

Other scientists and therapists have used the same strategy. Huge amounts of kidney stimulating herbs, liver stimulating techniques, and help with detoxification achieved the same success.

Nordenstrom[19], a radiologist, saw evidence of an electrical or magnetic force surrounding the tumor on the x-rays of tumors he took. My studies show south polarization, a magnetic force, at the tumor zone when north is normal. Fully understanding the implications of this must wait for the future.

But stopping growth is less mysterious and even more crucial than removing accumulations, so we will study growth first. We can study it in normal tissue and the tumor so nearby.

Human Growth Hormone

Our pituitary gland, the very one involved in making the tumor nucleus, makes many hormones. One of them is human growth hormone, HGH. It is supremely important. The Syncrometer® sees that it is produced regularly for <u>healing</u>, especially at night. Then it is promptly excreted, even in the night. Maybe it is too dangerous to salvage or keep till morning. It is extremely powerful, so it is very carefully controlled—by the hypothalamus gland right above it. See the drawing below and page 24. After all, we must not become eight feet tall or have extra long teeth or too short fingers. The pituitary gland is not allowed to release its HGH into the body until a **releasing hormone** arrives, made by the hypothalamus.

This is the case for other hormones, too. Each one must get its final permission, its releasing hormone, from the hypothalamus. It is like having both an accelerator and brake in a car. They are placed side by side to control speed. But it is the driver who will choose which one to use, not the foot.

It is the whole brain that decides which control the hypothalamus will choose. These are some of the hormones made by the pituitary gland:

- Human Growth Hormone (HGH)
- Thyroid Stimulating Hormone (TSH)
- Follicle Stimulating Hormone (FSH)
- Luteinizing Hormone (LH)

---

[19] Search Bjorn Nordenstrom, radiologist, on Internet

- Prolactin

These hormones are the accelerators for our organs.

Each hormone stimulates a particular organ, but not too much. The hypothalamus can put on the brakes by stopping releases and staying in charge.

These are the releasing hormones sent out by the hypothalamus to control the pituitary:
- Growth Hormone Releasing Factor (GHRF or GRF))
- Thyrotropin Releasing Hormone (TRH)
- LH/FSH Releasing Hormone (GnRH)
- Luteinizing Hormone Releasing Hormone (LHRH or LRH)
- Prolactin Releasing Factor (PRF)

Notice that each hormone has its matching releasing hormone.

This system works well for us. The brain surrounding these two glands <u>knows</u> whether more of a hormone is needed or not. Messages from our organs are constantly coming to the brain telling it what is needed next. These are our "master glands" because they work to respond to our most basic needs. Maybe it should not be so surprising that all cancers start right here. They are in charge of growth.

Hypothalamus cells that have left the parent organ during its micro-explosion are far away from the brain.

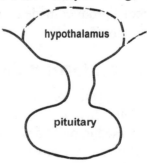

Fig. 57 The hypothalamus controls the pituitary gland

They cannot receive messages from the brain. They keep right on making releasing factors, without a stop, some more, some less. The pituitary cells <u>must</u> receive them because they have become attached to the hypothalamus cells by fusing. In a duplex or triplet they are like Siamese twins, forced to do things together. They will be forced to make and release HGH without a stop. We will find high levels of HGH in the tumors of every cancer patient. They will be high enough to find in the saliva and urine day and night.

Still mysterious, but vital in this picture, too, is **stem cell factor (SCF)**. The hypothalamus gland appears to make it, especially at night in healthy people. It, too, gets excreted at night. But again, it should be under tight brain control and it is not in cancer patients.

Stem Cell Factor

How can a seed grow into a tree? How can a whole human being, made of some trillion cells grow from one male cell and one female cell, fused? What does fusion do? Is it more than just adding chromosomes?

Each original cell (egg and sperm) came packed with a little bit of a substance called stem cell factor. Plant seeds use the identical substance, as found by the Syncrometer®.

It is kept strictly where cell division is wanted, nowhere else. It also comes with a tiny bit of **iridium complex**, perhaps a special product made to accompany SCF. We will learn more about this soon.

How an Organ Grows

An organ like your liver or prostate is made of very many tiny cells, easy to see under a microscope. They remind us of bricks used to build a wall and, actually, the whole building.

But cells are alive, connected to each other, and after a life of hard work, such as 10 days for some and months for others, they are aged and dying. Their cell voltage has run down. But just dying would be quite toxic to the rest of the body. It would decay and be a burden to the body. This is called **necrosis**. Wounds inflict this kind of damage. The aged cell is therefore not allowed to just die. It is carefully taken apart beforehand, disassembled in an orderly way, so that nothing toxic is produced and so useful things can be recycled. This is the process of **apoptosis**. Still, after this there is a <u>hole</u> in the organ structure where the aged cell was. It needs to be filled. If such holes were not filled, the organ would soon get smaller and smaller. Is replacement missing more and more as we age? We do seem to get smaller and smaller after middle age. Has this become unregulated in a cancerous tumor so the organ gets bigger and bigger instead?

It was thought until quite recently that any neighboring cell, where a hole had been left, could simply divide itself into two, then the one extra cell could fill the hole. This is <u>not</u> how it happens. To divide, a cell must stop its work schedule because chromosomes can't be duplicating themselves and making proteins (being translated) at the same time. A cell has to prepare in an elaborate way for its own division. It must acquire more proteins and extra DNA first. It takes about a day to go through one cell division (bacteria can do it in 20 minutes). After this it must prepare again to go back to its normal work, called **metabolism**. It is inefficient to shift from metabolism to cell division and back again repeatedly.

The body, and plants too, have a different scheme. Each organ has a few cells set aside. They are spread throughout the organ. Their only job is to divide when called upon. There is no delay. They are always ready; they have what is needed. It does not interrupt the work schedule of others. These are called **stem cells**[*]. How do they know when to divide and let the new cell slip into the hole? Stem cell factor reaches them to give them this vital message. Stem cell factor is only sent when there is a need. It is only sent to <u>southerly-polarized locations</u>.

It seems, from Syncrometer® studies, that only the hypothalamus makes stem cell factor; other organs, of the ones studied (most of the brain), did not. While the hypothalamus cells are in the brain, in their normal place, stem cell factor is made according to a demand from some damaged organ. This organ has a spot that has turned southerly. The damage itself

---

[*] Testers, search for placenta or umbilical cord, in any organ to identify the stem cells.

has caused iron oxidation, this seems to be the way that magnetization switches to southerly, naturally. Oxidized iron is Fe_2O_3, common ferrite, and ferric substances. The brain learns about it immediately, in less than a second from the time you cut yourself. The injured region, now being southerly-polarized, invites stem cell factor.

SCF brings with it a "welcome wagon" of iridium and other trace minerals. Now new cells can be made. In a wound new cells are needed. But away from the brain, when hypothalamus and pituitary cells are afloat, it is not based on need; they continue to make SCF and HGH <u>all the time</u>. The Syncrometer® detects them all around the tumor and wherever a tumor nucleus has been "planted". They are even attached to bacteria and viruses!

SCF will surely reach some nearby stem cells in the organ where the tumor nucleus has landed[*]. Stem cells in the neighborhood could be expected to respond by dividing. I can still only speculate about how this happens. In fact, it may even be the stem cells themselves that are chosen for the fusions. It may be the stem cells that make the entire tumor. This could even be the reason why tumor cells never mature (differentiate) into non-dividing, working cells. Only more research can make these details clear.

Cysts—Another Kind of Growth

Sometimes a mass can be seen on an ultrasound or scan that is not a malignant growing tumor. It appears to have grown for a while, then stopped and gotten encased by the body in a smooth thick coat. It is obvious to a radiologist that it is "only a cyst". What made it start and stop growing?

A cyst starts out the same way as a dangerous tumor. Bits of hypothalamus have come loose. They have fused with cells from the pituitary gland that were also loose. These duplexes swarmed about, free to join another organ. One such duplex

---

[*] Testers, construct "stem cells in an organ" by touching placenta to the organ slide. Umbilical cord slide works well, too. Search for SCF here.

has joined a third organ because Fasciolas and Ascaris stages are nearby. The Syncrometer® spots them easily. Lots of fibronectin and gluey threads are present to make the third organ a sticky trap. Now there is a tiny transplant of cells made of hypothalamus, pituitary and the third organ. But it is not the pancreas.

> A cyst in the kidney has a "nucleus" made of hypothalamus, pituitary, and kidney cells. It is missing the pancreas portion. It does not have a true tumor nucleus.

The hypothalamus portion sends out its releasing factors, its SCF and iridium complex. We will discuss this complex soon. The pituitary portion sends out HGH and its whole troop of hormones as demanded by the hypothalamus. The organ's cells begin to respond by dividing.

The organ also responds to the new hormones being poured into it. It may respond to **prolactin** if the cyst is developing in the breast. This makes the breast produce fluid. The kidney can respond to **vasopressin**, which would raise the blood pressure. The prostate can enlarge with excess male hormones in response to excess FSH. An organ, whether it is the ovary or prostate, always tries to make proper use of all hormones arriving there. All these responses can change the organ that received the tiny transplant, giving it too many "receptors" and even enlarging it.

In spite of all this, the newly growing mass does not grow endlessly in a runaway manner like a cancerous tumor. Just what force the body exerts or which chemical it produces to stop its growth is a mystery. It should be studied. Apoptosis in a cyst is not totally blocked the way it is in a tumor. The numerous oncoviruses (viruses that start tumors) are missing in the cyst. Natural cell death by apoptosis can keep up with cell growth. But is that all? An endpoint is reached for the cyst when the body finally encases it, so no more toxins or bacteria can enter and accumulations must stop. It is undoubtedly meant to protect your body, even in cancer. It is now fairly harmless, but only fairly. A real tumor nucleus, complete with a pancreas portion could still be formed, could easily land in the same location and change everything.

The difference in the cyst is the absence of the pancreas cells and a virus that comes with pancreas cells. It is called SV 40.

SV 40 stands for simian virus #40.

The Secret of Pancreas Cells

The presence of pancreas cells in the tumor nucleus makes the difference between forming a cyst or forming an ever growing tumor. Does the pancreas cell provide something unique that makes the body powerless to restrain the growing force in the tumor nucleus? In stem cell factor? In HGH? In the iridium complex? Does the pancreas cell bring something that removes the limit on cell division that every human cell should have? Does it bring a block on apoptosis so cells can never terminate and digest themselves as normal aged cells do? These were things the Syncrometer® searched for and did not find. What it found in the pancreas cells were merely SV 40 viruses! But they were not alone. Attached to its "coat tails" were a series of oncoviruses, much like skaters holding hands, pulling each other along. And all of them, the whole troupe, were outside the pancreas cells, too. Our tumor cells had let them in, in whatever organ they were. The organ with the tumor could let them in, but not others. Nearly all bacteria, which are also cells, would let them in. Some attachments are even to other regular viruses, like Flu and mumps, all sticking together. They formed a gang. Small gangs of viruses are arriving in the organ where the tumor nucleus has attached itself, and in all the local bacteria. Their leader is SV 40.

The Secret of SV 40

This virus has already been researched extensively. It is called an oncovirus because it can start tumors when it is given to animals; *onco* means *tumor*. How can it do this? We will soon see.

The Syncrometer® sees that the virus arrives in the body with the pancreatic fluke and escapes quickly to infect the pancreas[*]. Then it enters the blood. Once in the blood it can reach any organ quickly. Soon SV 40 can be detected all over the body. But it does not start tumors in all these locations. Nor does it bring a special symptom. It seemingly can't get into most places. The body cells are keeping it out. It can only get in at one site, besides at bacteria. It will be the primary tumor site. Why there?

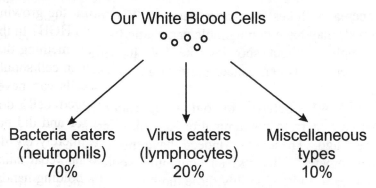

Fig. 58 Our white blood cells are specialized into classes

Our special immune cells, **lymphocytes**, normally eat and kill viruses. They are ready for these SV 40s. They can all be eaten very quickly. But to kill them the lymphocytes need organic germanium and organic selenium (or selenite) and vitamin C. The minerals make up their killing-enzymes. The vitamin C (preferably organic, as in rose hips) has an unknown action, but my speculation is that it protects the minerals from oxidation. A cancer patient's lymphocytes are deficient in

---

[*] Testers, search for pancreas / SV 40 in the lymph; and SV 40 in the pancreas organ.

these, being full of azo dyes, wheel bearing grease, mercury, and nickel instead (specifically these, not other heavy metals). The cancer patients' germanium and selenium minerals have become oxidized by these heavy metals and by chlorine, from the polluted drinking water, as have the iron molecules inside the lymphocytes. The killing enzymes don't work. The Syncrometer® finds no peroxidase, for instance. The iron in this enzyme was oxidized. Oxidized minerals become plain metals, plain germanium, plain selenium, plain ferrite (Fe_2O_3), plain ferric phosphate, and all quite toxic to these same enzymes. When the deficient lymphocytes cannot kill the SV 40 oncoviruses, which they have eaten, the viruses break free again, to continue their body invasion. They invade quickly and multiply quickly.

The Syncrometer® detects SV 40 wherever there are pancreatic flukes in cancer patients. Yet, other people (and cows!) may have innumerable pancreatic flukes, in diabetes for example, without showing the SV 40 virus! What is the difference between cancer patients and others? We will soon see.

SV 40 is believed to come to us from certain monkeys in Africa and from contamination of polio vaccine given to us years ago. These may indeed have been sources. But the Syncrometer® detects an ongoing source, the common pancreatic fluke. Possibly these monkeys had pancreatic flukes then, as many animals do now. Parasitism must be millions of years old. **Horses**, **dogs** and **cats** that have contracted cancer today, have the pancreatic fluke with its SV 40 viruses just as we do. Chickens in the market place (in USA) have them, although we do not pronounce them cancerous, or even dangerous!

SV 40 viruses, like other viruses, must be triggered to emerge. In animals or in humans they can be triggered by one food phenolic substance, gallic acid. This is the same substance that acted like an allergen and eroded the pancreas to make the tumor nucleus. It can do two things: erode the pancreas, and trigger the SV 40 virus out of the pancreatic fluke. Diabetics are not full of gallic acid as cancer patients are. Chickens used as human food in the market place (in USA) are full of gallic acid. Other animals with cancer are full of gallic acid, like human cancer patients. This conclusion is based on small numbers of horses, cats, dogs and chickens (not like the hundreds upon hundreds of humans tested) but there were <u>no</u> exceptions. It seems rather probable that the trigger for releasing SV 40 viruses from pancreatic flukes is the same for animals and humans. It is gallic acid...the common preservative, called propyl gallate!

The Secret of Oncoviruses

SV 40 is the most important of our oncoviruses because it starts gangs forming. That is why I call it the **cancer virus**. There are many more viruses that routinely invade us. But none of them attack us, as we thought, "out of the blue". They come from our parasites. Parasites, being large, have their own bacteria and their own viruses! That is why biological pest-control works. All large animals that get tumors, like horses, cows, chickens, dogs and cats, have many of the same viruses. The Syncrometer® can identify them using a bit of their own DNA that is unique. If the Syncrometer® finds a bit of a virus gene in a parasite or in us, I might assume the virus is there, not just the gene. And when the gene has spread throughout the body I might, again, assume the virus is present and spreading, not just a gene. That is how the Syncrometer® research was done—with oncogenes. But my research leads to the conclusion that they represent real viruses—oncoviruses.

Common oncoviruses in humans besides SV 40 are RAS, FOS, MYC, JUN, SRC, and NEU (also called ERB). Besides these we have Flu, mumps, CMV, Hepatitis B, EBV, and Adenovirus which may not be true oncoviruses but which frequently participate in a cancer patient's illness. We will soon see how.

The Syncrometer® shows that each of these enters us from a parasite or other invader that actually lives in us. In the following table are listed the oncoviruses seen in all cancer patients, some more, some less, all more frequent in the organ involved in the cancer because that is where the parasite also lives.

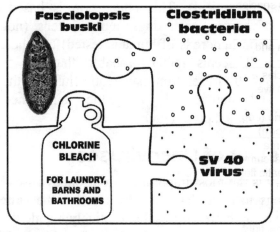

A cancer parasite, cancer bacteria and cancer virus are the three main actors.

Fig. 59 The cancer puzzle

Together, the oncovirus gang keeps cancer cells growing endlessly (immortalized) and makes bacteria appear resistant to anything we use against them (also immortalized), such as antibiotics.

In the table below is given the name of the parasite that brings each oncovirus and the trigger required to activate the virus genes. This lets you stop triggering it immediately.

Parasites Bring Oncoviruses

Parasite	Oncovirus * it carries	Virus trigger	Kill parasite with
Ascaris lumbricoides	NEU	linolenic acid (food oil)	starvation, horseradish,
Ascaris megalocephala	NEU	linolenic acid (food oil)	cysteine, levamisole, ripe

---

* Oncovirus genes are underlined.

142

Parasite	Oncovirus * it carries	Virus trigger	Kill parasite with
Ascaris megalocephala	mumps	casein (dairy food)	jalapeño seeds, BQ & RZ
Ascaris species	Adenovirus	myristic oil, death of parasite	
chicken and eggs**	MYC		avoid
Clonorchis (human liver fluke)	Hepatitis B	umbelliferone (carrots)	starvation, BWT ***, 6 fresh seed recipe
Dirofilaria (dog heartworm)	FOS	oleic acid(olive oil, other oils)	starvation, levamisole, BWT
Eurytrema pancreaticum (pancreatic fluke)	SV 40	gallic acid	starvation, BWT, 6 fresh seed re-cipe, cactus ****
F. buski (intestinal fluke)	MYC		starvation, BWT, MSM, spices, 6 fresh seed recipe
F. buski (intestinal fluke)	Flu	death of parasite host	
F. buski (intestinal fluke)	HIV	benzene	
Onchocerca	JUN		BWT, starvation, levamisole
Plasmodium (malaria)	SV 40-HIV		6 fresh seed recipe, Eucalyp-tus, starvation
Strongyloides	CMV (Cytomegalo -virus)	lauric acid (lard, food oils)	starvation, levamisole
Strongyloides	EBV (Epstein Barre virus)	linolenic and palmitic food oils	
Strongyloides	SRC	lauric acid (food oil)	
yeast (bread)	RAS	asparagine	turmeric, chromium deprivation

Fig. 60 Parasites, their oncoviruses and triggers

** Not parasites, of course, but playing the role of parasites when we eat them. MYC is not killed by ordinary cooking, baking or frying. But 3 hydrochloric acid drops kills it.

*** BWT refers to the whole green Black Walnut tincture recipe, including wormwood and cloves.

143

If we have 10 oncoviruses, should we expect to have about 10 parasites as their sources? Yes. At first, a newly diagnosed cancer patient might only have 5 or 6, but as the disease advances the numbers and varieties go up. The body becomes the host for a teeming population of bacteria, yeast and parasite stages, trading their oncoviruses with each other and adding to their total number.

Meanwhile, the bacteria have changed, too; they are not acting like themselves anymore because of their multiple viruses. Our tumor cells are now full of these infected bacteria besides oncoviruses. They might look glassy, waxy, pink, and rounded, not at all normal. Skin with tumor cells is rough and hard, not smooth and soft. In the past, these places were called "proud flesh" or "cancer" (meaning crab-like). They might grow "roots" or tangles or wrap-around sheaths, not normal cell behavior. The genes inside the tumor cells have been adulterated with those from viruses, bacteria, and even bread yeast. All these must be killed and stopped from multiplying before the tumor can shrink.

Remember, shrinking a tumor requires 3 processes: apoptosis, ordinary digestion, and white blood cell phagocytosis. This means self-digestion, digestion by pancreatic enzymes, and phagocytosis (getting eaten) by CD8 and CD14 white blood cells. First, we will stop its growth by removing SCF and HGH. Then we will start its apoptosis by removing Ascaris and all other parasites bringing us oncoviruses. External digestion will follow and we will supplement it. Then we will remove the remains with CD8 and CD14 white blood cells whose immune power is restored. When all 3 processes are started, it may take only days to see shrinkage visibly or feel it internally.

Growth itself always occurs in 2 parts: the accelerators and decelerators (brakes). The main accelerators are SCF and HGH, but contributors are DNA suppliers, Ribonucleotide Reductase starters, thiourea suppliers, carcinoembryonic

---

**** This is prickly pear cactus, ethnic food in Mexico.

antigen (CEA), human chorionic gonadotropin (HCG), and south pole forces. The decelerators are our longevity-limiter gene, pyruvic aldehyde, and north pole forces. We will soon get to know all of these.

Stopping making SCF and HGH is quite easy by stopping the erosion of the hypothalamus and pituitary glands, namely with diet. By now you may already have done this. Stopping overproduction of DNA, RRase and thiourea is quite easy, too, by killing Clostridium bacteria. Stopping HCG is easy, by killing Fasciolopsis cercaria, along with the rest of F. buski stages. CEA will be removed by killing Yeast. Switching south pole to north pole forces is instantly accomplished by removing nickel, even though it is buried in wheel bearing grease and will return many times before the whole body is degreased.

Cleaning and feeding the WBCs is quite easy. Starting apoptosis depends on killing oncoviruses. Supplying pancreatic enzymes is quite easy. Bringing back the longevity control over tumor cells depends on killing Ascaris. Supplying pyruvic aldehyde is easy with homeographic drops. The pair of substances, thiourea and pyruvic aldehyde, were discussed in the earlier book, *Cure For All Advanced Cancers*. And north pole forces can be brought in, too.

We will be in control of the tumor's growth and shrinkage if we can test with a Syncrometer® for what has already been accomplished. The *Testers' Flow Sheet* shows you your status at any time (see page 273).

The miracle in our lives is that even at this late stage we can still fix this desperate problem. We can get rid of all the unwanted items. But first we must continue with our search for more facts about growth, so we can be efficient later, and do all the essential things together, in the *3-Week Program*.

CHAPTER 7

OUR COSMIC CONNECTIONS

Healing

The body must heal itself regularly to repair the damage done by living. It seems to do this at night. We may go to bed with aches and pains but wake up good as new...at least in childhood. But nighttime is a difficult time to study anything with a Syncrometer® so more details are badly needed.

The body must also heal special places if big traumas occurred, like burning, cutting, smashing. These places get healed day and night. This is the kind of healing I studied for this chapter. It is a subtle, quiet process, as astounding as the study of stars and the cosmos. Maybe we should not be so surprised.

Falling down from the sky, as gently as miniscule feathers, is the cosmic dust. Day and night, night and day, sometimes more, sometimes less, cosmic dust and bits of meteorite land on everything...the grass, the ponds, the fur of animals...everything except human beings. Only we humans have sheltered ourselves from the cosmic dust most of the time, especially in the last century.

It comes down in larger amounts during a rain. Animals lick it off their fur. They drink it from the ponds, rivers and tiny trickles that run through the ground. Even plants drink it up through their roots. Only humans do not. We "purify" our water. First, we filter it, thereby adding aluminum, and then add a very strong oxidizing disinfectant, such as chlorine. We do not eat or drink the tiny flakes of cosmic dust, or at least very little. We have given up a precious natural resource, the cosmic dust, and with it the life-giving element, iridium.

What is Iridium?

A black layer of dust landed on our planet 65 million years ago. Now it is only ¼ inch thick, compacted under all the layers of sediment that have since been added. This thin layer contains large amounts of iridium. It fell to earth with the meteor that landed swiftly and suddenly at that time, digging a huge crater in the soil and raising a dust cloud that circled the earth. Dust loaded with iridium would fall for 100 years afterwards, and then stop, leaving only the gently falling cosmic dust again. What is on a cosmic dust particle?

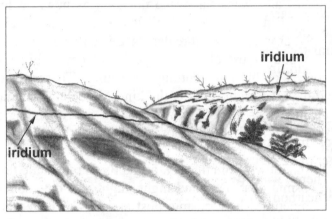

All around our planet a thin (¼ ") line of black sediment is the iridium dust that landed 65 M years ago. It marks the end of the dinosaur age. Read more about this K-T boundary on the Internet.

Fig. 61 Drawing of earth's iridium layer

Catching the Cosmic Dust

If you set out a new zippered plastic bag, unopened, on a dinner plate, you can catch a sample of cosmic dust outside anywhere. Other kinds of plastic might seep and contribute their own elements. (The bag should not test *Positive* for laundry bleach, either, or it will contribute many more elements. You can find a good one with a conductivity indicator, see page 581). Let it stand outside for 10 minutes only. Cut a 2" x 2" square of paper towel, dampen it slightly with tap water and take a swipe across the bag. Hurry indoors to test it by Syncrometer®*. You will find an iridium compound, a cobalt compound, a selenium compound made of selenite, a chromium and a germanium compound, a vanadium compound, a rubidium compound, but most of all, iron. It is magnetic iron, Fe_3O_4, also called magnetite. Remember to test the tap water alone, too, as well as the paper and a part of the plastic bag (bottom side) to serve as "controls", in case these elements come from them (they will not).

Now carry it all indoors. After 20 minutes take another swipe from the same plastic bag and notice that some "chemistry" has happened. What was coming down earlier was **tetra iridium dodecacarbonyl**. Each molecule of this compound is made of 4 atoms (tetra) of iridium surrounded by 12 (dodeca) carbonyl groups. Carbonyls are just carbon and oxygen held together with a double bond (C = O), also called carbon monoxide. Altogether, it is 4 iridium atoms inside a cluster of 12 carbon monoxide molecules.

There was tetra cobalt dodecacarbonyl, and triiron dodecacarbonyl and similar other minerals. But soon these are all gone. In 20 minutes they have become much more oxidized. Now we see some plain iron, plain selenium, plain cobalt and chromium, plain vanadium, plain rubidium, and even some plain iridium powder, like the ¼ inch earth layer.

If the cosmic dust is wet, the minerals oxidize much faster. Fresh raindrops develop these oxidized elements in less than 10 minutes. And if the sun is shining on them (not so common while it's raining) they switch their polarization!

The falling dust is north polarized as long as it contains Fe_3O_4 (magnetite). But in 10 minutes Fe_2O_3 is being formed which is south polarized. Polarized does not mean simply

---

* Place it in a zippered plastic bag for testing; later, test the controls for those things you find in the dust.

having a "pole". It means it shows the <u>influence</u> of such a pole.[*]

All the raindrops and rainwater collected is north polarized when it lands on earth (in Italy, Spain and USA). All living things drink it in this state. Again, only humans waste it. Humans drink municipally supplied water, which has no predictable polarization. All the laundry bleach waters were south polarized! NSF-bleach water was often north polarized.

What is Polarization?

We are familiar with the north and south poles of a magnet. Many kinds of iron, even nails and tin cans of food have a north and south pole in them, showing us the strength of the earth's magnetic field, which produced them. Less than ½ gauss, which is the approximate strength of the earth's field in USA, sounds small but it had the strength to produce these magnetized items! That is not polarization, though. It is **polarity**. All magnets have a south and north pole, called polarity. Often many poles lie like a pile of logs, not neatly aligned, in metal objects. Going around the rim of a tin can with a compass even shows <u>reversals</u> that identify where the pole's axis is switched. Each axis has poles at the ends.

There is never a south pole without a north pole and, actually, all molecules whether made of iron or not have some polarity. To produce a polarity, all that is needed is a moving charge such as moving electrons and these are possessed by all molecules. But sometimes the polarity of a molecule is very strong and sometimes very weak. Strong polarity can reach out to neighboring molecules and align whole blocs of molecules into domains so that the crystal structure of a piece of metal is

---

[*] Testers, use a sample of very pure water, in an amber glass bottle that has been placed on a large ceramic magnet labeled north for 3 to 5 minutes. The large magnet size ensures that you won't be near an edge where some flux lines of the other (south) side might trespass. Label this sample *north*. Also make a *south* water test bottle.

affected by them. Iron molecules are especially capable of this, so iron makes strong magnets.

If you have a rather long magnet, such as a 6 inch nail, the influence of each of the poles can be seen separately. One end is north and the other south. These forces are not the same, or merely in opposite directions. Water is influenced differently by the north and south pole of a magnet. Water is our most important substance. It is part of the very nature of life, present everywhere in our bodies.

When a small bottle of water taken from the kitchen faucet is placed on the north pole of a magnet (actually standing right on it) something happens. It can easily be identified by the Syncrometer® later. After a few minutes the water will resonate with the north pole of a magnet and not with a south pole. A tiny 10 gauss ceramic magnet held 3" above the Syncrometer® plate with the north side down resonates the circuit when the north pole water is placed on the sister plate. Water placed on a south pole magnet will resonate with the south pole of a magnet held above the plate. Notice that the water develops the same polarization as the magnet it is placed on. It resonates with the same magnetic field that created it. This is opposite to the behavior of a metal like iron. If a piece of iron is placed near one pole of a magnet, the opposite pole is produced in the iron. And as surely as one pole is produced in iron, there is another pole produced farther away so that in reality both poles are produced.

Water behaves differently. It has been influenced by the magnet to produce the same pole-like behavior. Living tissue behaves like water. Only the same polarization is produced as the pole that made it. No equal and opposite polarization has ever been measured by Syncrometer®.

When rainwater falls into a plastic bag and is immediately tested with a Syncrometer® it is north polarized. It always contains Fe_3O_4 which acts like a north pole. It is the same for the southern hemisphere. But its chemistry soon changes to more oxidized forms of minerals, and from Fe_3O_4 to Fe_2O_3, from magnetite to ferrite. When this has happened the water switches to south polarized. It now resonates with the south pole end of a real magnet or any sample of water that was placed on a south pole.

Water is called **diamagnetic**, maybe for similar reasons. Water without any iron is unpolarized. Water with both varieties of iron shows bipolarization, both north and south.

Should we be drinking water that is north polarized, namely, bringing minute amounts of Fe_3O_4? Or should we be drinking south polarized, unpolarized, or bipolarized water? The water that induced cancer in all our cancer patients was south polarized. Remember that SCF is attracted to south polarized regions. Cell division only occurs in south polarized places, according to Syncrometer® tests. Asbestos in water makes it south polarized.

Water is never pure in Nature. It has innumerable elements and compounds dissolved in it or floating about in it. Water from your tap has many more chemicals besides. They were added without regard for polarization. I believe it does matter, judging by these Syncrometer® observations.

Food, too, in its natural state is north polarized, except for the seed, which is south. Cell divisions will begin in the seed after water enters. The seed grows in water; all life takes place in water. Is the south pole a villain? Does it represent all that's bad? Not at all! Plant matter and animals are only north polarized by daytime! They switch in the night to south polarized. The switch back comes in the early morning with the first rays of sunlight, and repeats the cycle in the early evening, before sunset. South polarization must have vital importance, too.

Plants reproduce at some location within themselves. These locations are south polarized, just as they are in the human body. And the entire south polarized region, but never north, has stem cell factor present in it.

Back to Stem Cell Factor

Surprisingly, stem cell factor does not come alone when it arrives from the hypothalamus gland at a south polarized organ. It brings a gift to the healing zone. Stem cell factor as it comes in pure form from a manufacturer is just a bit of protein. But in the body it has company. Clustered together with SCF are these unusual substances:

- tetra iridium dodecacarbonyl
- tetra cobalt dodecacarbonyl
- triiron dodecacarbonyl
- Fe_3O_4 (magnetite)
- a selenium compound (not identified)
- tetra ruthenium dodecacarbonyl
- tetra rubidium dodecacarbonyl
- a germanium compound (not identified)
- a chromium compound (not identified)

There was nothing else, though not exhaustively tested.

Are these not surprisingly similar to the cosmic dust particles?

Do these represent elements needed by the body?

Should the sick body have been given rainwater, iridium supplements, cosmic dust, compounds of minerals found in cosmic dust, Fe_3O_4, food that is perfectly fresh? All these questions must wait till more research can be done on them. But rainwater and fresh food need not wait. Fresh vegetables are the preference, in fact, the requirement, for many animals, and rainwater is all they drink. Rainwater is the true elixir of animals and plants. It tastes full-bodied and very good. Collect it after the rain has been coming down for an hour or so, after all smog and industrial chemicals have been washed down out of the sky (this is very important). Test it by Syncrometer® for beryllium (jet fuel), strontium, vanadium, and chromium to be aware of any local pollutants. Do not drink such polluted water. Do not let your rainwater stand in sunlight (it switches polarization). Do not let it stand open. It absorbs so much carbon dioxide from the air it soon tastes "sharp", like carbonation. Do not filter it except through coarse paper like kitchen paper towels that you have boiled 5 minutes and rinsed in your own pure water. Use a double layer, or simply stuff it into a stainless steel or HDPE♲ funnel. You can test this paper-stuffing later to find out what was coming down with the rain in your area. Store the water in the same polyethylene bottles that your distilled water came in to avoid heavy metals leaching from other plastic or glass. Refrigerate it to retard bacteria. Daylight indoors and artificial light do not switch its polarization. But as an optional final measure, set it on the zappicator to restore north polarization. We will discuss zappication later[*].

Catch snow in a stainless steel container or plastic zippered baggie and treat it similarly after melting. It is all north polarized and rich in iridium and the ultra trace minerals of life. There was no lead, aluminum, cadmium, mercury, or other toxic metal, not even nickel, though these were not exhaustively studied, either.

There was a time some decades ago when rainwater or snowmelt was shunned, due to the need for storing it in cisterns. We were taught and knew instinctively that we should not drink <u>standing</u>, namely stagnant, water. It was a cardinal principle, taught in school, to drink only flowing water.

But such common sense gave way to the bottled water industry. We have been drinking "stagnant" water for several decades already. Drink your rainwater fresh, storing only enough to get you to the next rainfall.

Drink it in small amounts, daily, at first. Add nothing to it. It is one of Nature's perfect foods.

Don't expect miracles from this. We must not "judge" it until we know what to judge. The Syncrometer® sees that the body shares this iridium with all the organs that have low levels instead of letting it go first to the most needy organ. To see a result and actually measure effectiveness of rainwater, a homeopathic or immunologic system of measurement could be created. When this is done, the youngest and the healthiest of people are seen to have the highest, most "potentized" levels of

---

[*] Testers, do not zappicate any water to be used for copy-making or drop-making. Its ability to hold the frequency pattern is affected.

iridium substances. All animals have iridium, but very few plants do, that is, in measurable amounts by Syncrometry. The legume family and many herbs do. Water from municipal sources that have no heavy metals from its bleach treatment often does! Spas do, and natural springs do, those known for their health-giving properties.

Later, we will see what iridium actually does; how it combats the power of nickel to change our iron atoms to south pole. We need it to heal our battered, sick bodies.

Research is needed to explore the biosphere's reliance on cosmic dust for life's ultra trace minerals and perhaps even for life itself.

We will be able to heal ourselves again, using iridium from good water and herbs, to bring back our iron enzymes. We will be able to control growth again, when we can take back stem cell factor and HGH from our invaders. We will be able to control DNA and Ribonucleotide Reductase activity. We will take back control over the longevity gene and thiourea. They were much too liberally shared with our invaders. We will take them all back to serve our own purposes as originally intended by Nature. Then we will challenge the invaders themselves who have stolen our strength. First we will challenge the oncoviruses. Who, exactly, are they?

CHAPTER 8

SICKNESS BE GONE

Cancer does not make you <u>feel</u> sick, although you may <u>be</u> sick. Tumors do not make you sick either. Even your parasites and allergies do not make you feel sick. That is why a cancer diagnosis comes as a complete surprise to many victims. There will be no sickness to warn you. Only indigestion of a minor kind!

Sickness comes from very mundane sources...just a handful of bacteria and viruses—the kind that have always made people sick, with or without cancer.

Clostridium does not even make you feel sick, although one of them, C. botulinum makes you depressed and weepy if they overrun you and reach the hypothalamus in your brain. Here their special poisons overpower the hypothalamus's ability to make neurotransmitters for you and joy cannot be felt. You can't even enjoy success when you are told these Clostridiums come from <u>dead</u> liver flukes. Clostridium is easily vanquished.

The most important troublemakers are E. coli and Salmonella typhimurium. Third comes Salmonella enteriditis. Fourth is Streptococcus pneumoniae, causing all your pain. Much less common is Strep G; it can cause high fevers, even extreme fatigue, enough to put you in bed. Mycobacterium avium/cellulare gives you night sweats and some fatigue. Mycoplasma pneumoniae gives you constant coughing. Mycobacterium TB gives you coughing and fatigue. Pseudomonas aeruginosa is very destructive in your lungs. Most of these will be present in lung cancer, but not due to the cancer.

Antibiotics do not help against these bacteria as they would for a non-cancer patient and we will soon see why.

The troublemaker <u>virus</u> is only one, common Flu. Others may be swarming, but you do not feel them.

The troublemaker "sub virus" is called a prion. This will make you feel dizzy, light-headed, and disoriented. It is quite serious…able to cut you off from your own brain by stopping your neurotransmitters.

Again, antibiotics can do nothing against these. We will need to find their weaknesses, where they hide and what their nutritional requirements are. Depriving them of their essential needs will give you a recovery that will last. And if any one does come back you will know immediately what to do to get rid of it again.

We have more than these bacteria and viruses in us, of course, in different organs. But they do not seem to make us sick and miserable. Their contribution is more subtle. Staph, for instance, makes the skin pink, especially the breast in breast cancer. The breast can be hot and sensitive, yet without pain. There is mumps virus, swarming all over the body, unnoticed by sick or well people, except in the telltale sign on the blood test. The neutrophils have come down while the lymphocytes have gone up. It can be drastic, from a normal ratio of 75 to 20, to a ratio of 30 to 60.

And lurking everywhere is yeast, biding its time, it seems. No symptoms are felt to make you sick. But its spread accelerates until it gets enough chromium and nickel plus sugar (your blood sugar!) to simply starve you. But even that does not make you feel sick. Anti fungus and anti yeast medicines do not help. It just keeps spreading.

With these pathogens living on your resources, an entire organ can be gradually destroyed, and then another and another until the whole body is wasted. Why don't medicines work? And why are they not discovered?

The secret is in the gang of oncoviruses and their leader, SV 40. Only in our 2 immunodepression diseases, cancer and HIV, do we see this virus. It has the ability to round up a group of viruses and herd them into our tumor cells. But it can also herd them into our bacteria. This changes them.

Now the oncoviruses give immortality, not just to our tumor cells, but to our worst bacteria, even yeasts and other viruses. Our ordinary bowel and skin bacteria now have a partnership with a gang of oncoviruses. In this way the bacteria have acquired a disguise. They do not behave the same as always. I believe (this is conjecture only) they do not culture the same as uninfected bacteria, or they would have been found long ago. I believe we have not developed immunity against these, and even if we had, the immunodepressed state would not allow it to work. To conquer them we need to know each one's habits and its needs, all the better to pull the rug out from under them. This will enable us to conquer the invincible E. coli, Salmonellas, Staphylococcus and Streptococci that are making you sick.

This mere handful of bacteria, viruses, and prions that are making you sick have been studied in regular research for a few decades. It was a huge help to the Syncrometer® studies. This is what the Syncrometer® found.

The Oncovirus Gang

1. SV 40 is present in every cancer and HIV case I have seen in the past 5 years. This means there was no case without it. People without cancer or HIV/AIDS do not have it, but this conclusion is based on only 2 dozen, or so, case studies. It enters our tumor cells, even our bacteria. It can attach itself to other viruses. It even attaches itself to HIV virus. It appears to be attached to other viruses as if they had been joined one at a time. After a row of 3 or 4 is formed you could call it a little gang. They do not form a cluster. SV 40 is never in the middle of the row. It is always the first in line to touch a cell or a nucleus. The others do not have an order. The gang enters yeast buds, too. The cancer patient's body is full of these oncovirus gangs, though hidden inside bacteria and inside our tumor cells and maybe even in other viruses*. Each of the gang members

---

* Testers, it has not yet been possible to distinguish between in and on viruses.

159

contributes its bit to the changing behavior of their host cell no doubt. Bacteria and yeasts already had immortality before they got invaded. Somehow they benefit even more, with the extra genes of viruses at work inside them.

SV 40 does not appear to combine with all viruses, though. And it is not clear what symptoms it might itself cause, either. But transporting other viruses into our cells to make them sick, unrecognizable, and immortal, is a very important behavior. We can kill it with DMSO, six fresh seeds, turmeric, and wintergreen. Best of all, we can eliminate it by killing its host-parasite, pancreatic fluke. We must certainly never trigger it to multiply with gallic acid. But killing is never as powerful as starving. SV 40 requires **strontium, chromium,** and **gold**!

2.   **RAS** is one of the gang. When RAS is inside our cells, in tumor cells or in bacteria, these now can divide, time after time, without rest. The resting phase between cell divisions is much too short. It may be suitable for yeast, its true home, but not for us. RAS comes from ordinary baker's yeast, which grows in people without cancer, too. In fact it is especially common in fat or overweight people.

It is partly <u>why</u> we are overweight. Yeast steals our chromium, which we need to make use of our insulin. Without insulin, our cells go hungry. We must eat more to gain energy. RAS virus is often widespread in overweight people because they are full of **asparagine**, the trigger for RAS. Asparagine is found wherever decayed food is found. Nearly all the food we eat is partly decayed, be it plant or animal. Our bodies have tiny islands of asparagine everywhere. Fortunately, we can digest our islands of asparagine with a few handfuls of digestive enzymes. Normally, the **asparaginase** enzyme of the pancreas would digest it for us constantly, but it is missing from the pancreatic enzymes of cancer patients. If we ozonate our food to destroy asparagine and don't wait for it to decay again (over 2 days), we can stay clear of it. This does stop RAS from emerging from yeast buds. We should also stop eating <u>live</u> yeast, which brings RAS with it. All the bread in the USA brings us live yeast, because it is under baked. But in foreign cultures, for example, in Mexico, small loaves are baked and always baked crisp; their baked goods never have live yeast left in them[*]. Bake your own bread. All bread maker bread kills its yeast, as it should.

A normal white blood cell can eat all the RAS viruses that are free, having come out of yeast buds. But if the viruses have infected our bacteria, they will be shielded from our white blood cells, while speeding up the bacteria cell divisions. All this is easiest to see in advanced breast cancer. The skin develops redness and a strange roughness where yeast, RAS and staph bacteria have invaded together. Yeast and staph bacteria appear to have an affinity for each other. In reality, they are competing for the chromium supply. The RAS-invaded staph is not killed by antibiotics applied to the skin. It has become invincible like the Yeast. Soon it widens and deepens its territory, racing along like a prairie fire. It enters the blood stream, joining yeast, to consume the blood sugar and starve the patient. Then only weeks remain. But a miracle can still happen. When all chromium metal is removed from water, food, teeth and cookware, Staph and Yeast are starved instead of us. Leftover chromium and asparagine can be taken out with drops and if no mistakes are made, a life is saved. It takes extreme measures at this point, as you can see in the *3-Week Program*.

3. **MYC** is almost always found with mumps, an ordinary virus, as if they were partners. Many people with chronic illness, with or without cancer, have MYC and mumps from head to toe. Yet MYC comes from chickens, and from Fasciolopsis parasites, while mumps comes from Ascaris parasites. They find each other in us. Again, our white blood cells can easily keep up with free MYC viruses, gobbling them even as we eat them alive with chicken eggs and semi-raw chicken meat. But after they form an alliance with mumps they get protection. Our white blood cells refuse to eat them. The

---

[*] Testers, use a packet of dry yeast to search bread stuff for living yeast.

161

trigger for mumps is **casein**, a milk substance. The trigger for MYC is not known yet. But cancer patients have a steady stream of them coming from their multitudes of Fasciolopis stages. Casein often goes undigested when drinking too much milk and accumulates as deposits in our salivary glands, especially the **parotid glands** inside the cheeks. Again, handfuls of digestive enzymes clear them out. After this, no more milk should be drunk till the liver and pancreas can digest better, and then only with digestive enzymes and lactase supplements to help it along. The liver will digest better as soon as the wheel bearing grease, motor oil and heavy metals are out of it. We must be patient. MYC speeds up cell division by supplying essential proteins according to text books. MYC and mumps are eliminated easily with turmeric enemas. The results come quickly on a blood test, showing the ratio of neutrophils to lymphocytes going back up to normal. Its requirements are not yet known.

4. **FOS** is an oncovirus that speeds up growth, according to clinical research. Cells, be they bacteria or tumor cells, with FOS infection cannot die. A link in the apoptosis chain is somehow blocked. FOS comes to us from common heartworm of dogs. We carry the larval stages of heartworm even if we don't own a dog or get the classical disease. Along with this parasite we develop a buildup of **coumarin**. Coumarin is another food phenolic antigen that can give us an allergic effect.

The allergy to coumarin causes bleeding so a little purple patch can be seen, usually on the backs of our hands or arms at first. It is called purpura and could easily happen in the brain where it would be called stroke. If you see these patches, or are already on coumadin-like medicine, stop eating coumarin-containing foods. Kill your Dirofilaria (heartworm) with levamisole. Stop feeding the heartworm larvae with milk. It is the lactose sugar in milk that attracts them because they require it. There will be tiny ponds of lactose all over the body when heartworm larvae are present. We can digest them away with lactase enzymes. Most Dirofilaria infections are not obvious, merely giving you heart diseases of different kinds and starting snarls around themselves and lymph nodes, that turn into free-floating masses. Hodgkin's lymphoma is an example. The FOS oncovirus is triggered out of heartworms by oleic acid, a very common food oil, like olive oil. A weak liver and pancreas cannot digest much oil, so bits of it are left throughout the body, even in the saliva and lymph. When you stop eating olive oil and milk the Dirofilaria leave by themselves, taking FOS with them.

5. **JUN** is a **transcription factor**. This means it can attach itself to our DNA. JUN attaches at a place where normal cell growth is controlled, thereby commandeering this vital control center. It comes from a parasite called *Onchocerca volvulus*, another dog parasite belonging to the same filaria family as heartworm.

Onchocerca prefers to live in the vein valves, which tends to block the veins and gives you varicose veins. It leads to menadione allergy, another phenolic that can give you purple patches on your skin, to tell you the blood is not clotting properly. Distended veins can be in places like the chest, arms, breast, or even unseen in the esophagus. Stopping eating corn reduces their population immediately. They require it. But deposits of corn are everywhere and need huge amounts of lipase and pancreatin to be digested away. Even the tiniest amount of corn, as in cornstarch used to make capsules, must be removed to starve Onchocerca. Onchocerca parasites are easily killed with the Black Walnut-cloves-wormwood recipe and levamisole. JUN, its virus, is triggered by 3 oils: myristic, oleic and palmitic, as in nutmeg, olive oil, and palm oil. It goes away in days, as you stop eating these. But it may have formed an alliance with FOS if heartworm is also present. Then they stick together and survive. Yet, even the combination is easily killed with turmeric enemas, as we will do.

6. **SRC** is a <u>s</u>a<u>rc</u>oma virus, originally found in Rous Sarcoma Virus disease of chickens decades ago. It was found to help combine phosphates with tyrosines, as in orthophosphotyrosine. This will speed up growth of a tumor to

the malignancy level. The Syncrometer® sees it coming from common Strongyloides, parasites in us and many animals.

Potatoes are essential food for these parasites. Stopping eating potatoes and taking digestive enzymes to remove any leftover deposits of them reduces them in days.

SRC will be easy to kill with enemas, too, but we must not trigger it with **lauric acid**, a food oil also found in lard and beef. We must kill our Strongyloides with levamisole, too.

7. **NEU** is also called **ERB**. It may be the most difficult of all to destroy because it comes from our ever present Ascaris parasites—both varieties. Its trigger is linolenic acid, unsaturated food oil, highly prized by nutritionists. NEU is clinically detected in **erythroblastosis**. It is thought to keep turning on the common **epidermal growth factor** as its immortalizing method. But the Syncrometer® suggests that the natural block on endless life is affected. The telomerase inhibitor gene is gone. This is a powerful immortalizing method, too.

Imagine having 4 or 5 of these gang members, RAS, MYC, JUN, FOS, SRC and NEU joined in different combinations to SV 40, all inside a human cell. It would become immortalized, too…in 6 different ways! Together they prod the gene for **bcl-2** to make much, much more bcl-2; bcl-2 turns on cell division. This is to the viruses' advantage. That is how <u>they</u> get reproduced. But, for health, bcl-2 should not outpace the gene for **bax**. In cancer patients the ratio can go to 2:1, then 3:1, then 4:1 and eventually to 15:1! These genes are growth regulators. We count on them during healing to set their pace correctly, which they always do. The impact of the oncoviruses is to skew the ratio extremely in favor of bcl-2.

The bcl-2 gene is somehow linked to Ribonucleotide Reductase (RRase), an enzyme. This is the enzyme that makes DNA out of RNA, absolutely essential for cells to divide. This enzyme has an iron molecule in it. Is it being activated by the southern polarization brought into the tumor zone? DNA levels and RRase levels first double, then triple, then go to 4:1, until they reach 15:1, too! They are clearly acting from a single huge force and on a grand scale. Is SCF the controller? Our tumor cells with oncoviruses inside them show the bcl-2 increase, DNA increase, DNA polymerase increase, Ribonucleotide Reductase increase and thiourea increase in the same proportions.

Thiourea is another cell division stimulant found by Syncrometer® and discussed in the earlier book, *The Cure for All Advanced Cancers*. It normally keeps a 1 to 1 ratio with pyruvic aldehyde, the growth inhibitor. It, too, reaches a 15 to 1 ratio in advanced cancer, but only when Clostridium bacteria are present, producing toxic amines. When Clostridium is gone, the extra DNA, DNA polymerase, and thiourea are gone, too. But Ribonucleotide Reductase remains increased as long as SCF or yeast genes are present.

A less vicious group of oncoviruses, I call Gang II, are CMV, EBV, Adenovirus and Hepatitis B. They do not attach to SV 40 so readily, so they do not enter cells on such a large scale. In fact, they prefer to enter bacteria, yeasts, and tumor cells in the respiratory tract, mainly the lungs. In lung cancer both gangs are at work. Maybe this explains the extra high rate of lung cancer. The lungs are already targeted by many of these viruses before any cancer developed.

We can see that tumor growth is stimulated by potent forces long before OPT has arrived on the scene. It is initiated by SCF and HGH, and later assisted by all these oncoviruses and yeasts.

Cancerous tumors always have SV 40 in them. Most of them have RAS inside; most have MYC; in fact, most of them have 5 or 6 varieties inside, besides immortalized <u>bacteria</u>!

Notice that these oncoviruses are not making you sick. They only immortalize those viruses and bacteria that do! Each oncovirus is triggered out of a parasite.

With so many parasite varieties in existence and present in our animal neighbors, why should immunodepression bring us only certain ones? It could not be chance.

Maybe we should consider a new concept. Our parasites may not enter us in ones and twos, during some accidental contact. Maybe their eggs and other stages enter us <u>every day</u>. But perhaps they only stay with us if the "table is set" for them. Potatoes for some, oats for others. Without their food they leave, forever searching. Our diet seems to be the selective force that decides who will parasitize us. We should stop eating our monodiet.

There are, undoubtedly, other important parasites bringing more oncoviruses, but killing these seems to be enough for success. Ascaris is probably the most important because it is the most prevalent and seems to bring more than its share of oncoviruses. It is a roundworm. Each of our 2 varieties brings with it a remarkable impact on our longevity gene. This gene makes **telomerase**.

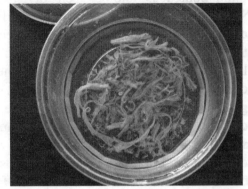

White "strings" with pointed or curled tips identifies Ascaris. At lower left the longest one is about 2", coming apart at the middle. This was retrieved from a colonic treatment.

Fig. 62 Ascaris has pointed ends

Telomerase

Long, very long ago it was "decreed" somehow that humans would not live forever. It had to be decreed because the tendency of living things is to keep on living and reproducing. Our earliest root-origins did keep on living and reproducing. Amoebas and bacteria, for instance, never just die. They do not have a lifespan. They can only be killed. But we, along with other complex beings were given a lifespan and a rather good one, though not knowing just what it was. But our **chromosome ends** do know. Our chromosome ends, the very tips, tell this story. Every time the chromosomes divide to produce a new cell, they get a tiny bit shorter. After 50 or so divisions they are altogether too short to do their job properly and the cell is tagged for apoptosis. The tag is **phosphatidyl serine** (PS). We can search for this with a Syncrometer® to see if a tumor has begun apoptosis, namely, to digest itself. It is a normal event for all our tissues and should be happening in tumor cells, too.

Primitive beings like bacteria and yeasts have a gene, called **telomerase** that keeps adding back that tiny portion of the chromosome tip that gets missed during division. Their lives are not limited. Their cells need not age and die. But we complex beings have a **telomerase inhibitor** that blocks this gene. We are destined to age and die. All our cells have this destiny. Even our tumor cells, with their frantically over-stimulated cell divisions, should reach their limit of 50 (or so) divisions quite soon and then be naturally barred from continuing. But they do not. If Ascaris parasites are nearby, and NEU is being produced, our telomerase inhibitor is gone. This shows that the cancer cells have been given immortality in yet another way. But when both Ascaris varieties are killed our telomerase inhibitor is promptly back again. Just killing Ascaris seems to be enough to rid ourselves of NEU oncoviruses <u>and</u> telomerase. The fastest way to rid ourselves of Ascaris is to starve them, while killing them, as we can do for other parasites.

How each parasite contributes to cancer and illness is given in the table on page 178.

The Secret of Sickness

We have just learned the secret of sickness in cancer patients. There are only a few bacteria and viruses really responsible, and they are even the kind that are easy to recover from. But a cancer patient cannot recover from them. The patient is pronounced terminal instead.

All because no medicine, antibiotic, treatment, or herb has ever been able to clear them up in a cancer patient. It seems to be a special situation. Sickness goes from bad to worse, to hospitalization, to heroic measures, to pumped morphine, to defeat. A half-million cancer deaths go this route each year in USA.

If we could find the weaknesses of each single attacker and use them all together in a very short time, <u>such as one minute</u>, so none could escape, could we not destroy both shelter and sheltered, partnerships and gangs?

We Can Do That

We already know the <u>needs</u> of some oncoviruses and the parasites they come from. Next, we should learn the <u>needs</u> of bacteria. We can even learn the requirements of our regular viruses, as well as our prions and yeast.

Bacterial Lords

Bowel bacteria can leave the bowel when immunity is depressed. They can get right through the walls of the intestine, find their food in some distant place and stay there. Such bacteria "gone wild" make it appear that "new resistant" strains have evolved, and, certainly, new genes received from viruses are at work, but not simply from overuse of antibiotics.

Bacteria make very toxic substances that ruin your appetite, keep you nauseated and fatigued, and disinterested in life—even your own.

They dump their waste product, ammonia (the smell of a diaper pail) in you. Although our bodies can make **urea** out of it, the **urea synthesis cycle** is largely out of commission from the azo dyes in your drinking water. That is why the blood test shows a <u>low</u> BUN (blood urea nitrogen). Check yours.

Bacteria cause pain and fever, chills and sweats, fatigue and apathy, coughing and wheezing, inability to sleep, and much more.

They have made themselves **lords of the land**. Let's identify them, all the better to conquer them.

1. **Escherichia coli** (E. coli)—This is the most common and makes the most sickness in cancer patients. The symptoms can be anything. It comes from the intestines. It invades any organ that provides a south polarization and vanadium,

molybdenum, manganese, chromium, or nickel. This makes it very versatile. If the cancer is in the colon, rectum, stomach or pancreas it makes the cancer marker CAA-GI. It can be invaded by most of the oncoviruses and the others as well, to make it invincible and unrecognizable. Turmeric and fennel are the traditional way to kill the uninvaded ones, but do not conquer the invaded ones without more help. Birch bark and cleavers herb also kill it.

2. **Salmonella typhimurium**—It comes from the intestine, too, and invades any part of the body. It is itself invaded by many oncoviruses as well as regular viruses. When the cancer is in the ovaries, it makes the tumor marker CAA-O. When the cancer is in the breast it makes CAA-B. It needs gold, molybdenum, and ruthenium, which makes it easy to starve. Salmonellas come out of killed F. buski flukes to be part of detox-illness. Diarrhea, constipation, bloating, fatigue and fever are common symptoms. Outright killing with iodine (Lugol's) is fast and sure for uninvaded ones, but not for immortalized ones.

Salmonella paratyphi is next most common and has similar behavior and needs.

Salmonella enteriditis is much more selective about its home. It prefers to live in the pancreas. Here it does the decisive damage to our digestion that allows islands of undigested food to develop in the body of every cancer patient. It requires the same exotic metals.

3. **Shigella dysenteriae**—This is intestinal in origin, too. When the cancer is in the breast, colon, lung, ovary, rectum, or stomach and this Shigella invades, it makes the marker CA72-4. Shigella sonnei is less common and causes depression. It invades the brain when the allergy to caffeic acid is keeping brain cells wide open to invasion. It causes severe nausea and vomiting. Turmeric and fennel, together, is the traditional treatment for uninvaded ones. They require manganese metal.

4. **Staphylococcus aureus**—This is the breast, skin and bone bacterium present on all our skins. It can only invade our

bodies, certainly the skin, when the white blood cells are not able to capture and kill them. And when the skin is inflamed from its allergy to acetaldehyde. Acetaldehyde is made by yeast, which is another reason why yeast and staph are seen together in breast cancer. When the cancer is in the breast or skin over the breast, these bacteria make epidermal growth factor (EGF). Staph causes redness of the skin, but not pain. It is immortalized mainly by oncovirus Gang II, CMV and Adenovirus, but also some of Gang I. It's chief partner is yeast...the bread yeast variety, which supplies RAS to these bacteria, immortalizing them further. No herb that kills staphylococcus (Staph) specifically is known. This Staph requires chromium.

5. **Streptococcus G**—This brings fevers, sweats, fatigue. It brings sore throats, coughing, cold-like symptoms. The bacteria prefer breast, lung, teeth, and respiratory tract. They are immortalized by CMV, Adenovirus, EBV and Hepatitis B, besides Gang I oncoviruses. It is often found with staphylococcus, Streptococcus pneumoniae, and yeast, probably because chromium is available there! They require it.

6. **Mycobacterium avium/cellulare**—This brings much more severe sweats, fever, and diarrhea. It is found anywhere in the body. It comes from Ascaris along with Adenovirus. Both are triggered by myristic acid, a less common food oil. Mycobacterium requires the metals, strontium and vanadium. Strontium is present in all municipal water and all (?) air, and consequently corn. It brings corn allergy.

7. **Mycobacterium tuberculosis**—This brings a low grade fever, chronic cough with sputum, and deep fatigue. It requires strontium.

8. **Mycoplasma**—This lingers long after other coughs and fevers have gone. It hides in the upper trachea, benefiting from a lower body temperature there. Keep your temperature normal with extra clothing worn high on the neck. It requires strontium and induces corn allergy.

9. **Streptococcus pneumoniae**—This is the pain bacterium. It is found wherever there is pain. It is often

accompanied by staphylococcus aureus and other streptococcus bacteria. It colonizes locations with blood and is easiest to kill after bleeding stops. It is mostly immortalized by Gang II but includes some regular Gang I oncoviruses. It requires chromium.

10. **Pseudomonas aeruginosa** is considered especially hardy and difficult to conquer—never cured. It depends on gold and strontium, gradually spreading in lungs till oxygen is too low to survive.

Other bacteria can play an important role in cancer, too. The Progenitor variety, found by Dr. Livingston-Wheeler a few decades ago, is especially inviting for study. Helicobacter is inviting , too, and possibly others found by earlier therapists.

Not everybody has all of these, but a very advanced patient will have 5 or 6. There will be some overlapping requirement for them so it will be quite easy to starve them and stop triggering them.

Virus Villains

Ordinary viruses, not only bacteria, make you sick. They have escaped your white blood cells because your WBCs are powerless. They can easily hide inside bacteria. Some survive by attaching themselves to other viruses and becoming disguised that way. But none, by themselves, is life threatening.

1. **Mumps**—This is a virus we all thought had come and gone in childhood. But very many people, sick or not, with cancer or not, have huge numbers of mumps viruses, circulating everywhere. Antibodies are not wiping them out, although the salivary glands do not get inflamed and swollen. When MYC arrives, these two combine. They are somehow protected by MYC while at the same time sheltering this oncovirus. Mumps does not enter bacteria or tumor cells while MYC always does. Stopping drinking milk till the cancer is cured helps most because mumps is dependent on casein, undigested milk protein. It comes from Ascaris megalocephala. It is also associated with Mycoplasma.

2. **Epstein Barre Virus** (EBV)—This acts like an oncovirus but does not seem to attach to SV 40, making it less vicious. It associates with staphylococcus, streptococcus and yeast, especially in the lungs. It is triggered by linolenic and palmitic food oils. It is dependent on aluminum, which is present in all municipal water. It comes from Strongyloides parasites.

3. **Cytomegalovirus** (CMV)—This acts much like EBV, not riding into cells with SV 40. It prefers to enter staphylococcus, streptococcus and yeast, on its own, leading to chronic lung disease apart from lung cancer. It is triggered by lauric food oil and is dependent on strontium, which is always found in municipal water, the air, and even corn. It too, comes from the parasite Strongyloides.

4. **Adenovirus**—When it is free, Adenovirus gives you the "common cold", with or without extra complications. It always coincides with an Ascaris-boom in the body. This happens for everyone at least once in the Fall, and once in the Spring. At this time the body mobilizes its parasite-killing capability. Such automatic Ascaris killing happens very frequently, even at other times[*]. Catching a cold <u>from somebody</u> who is sneezing or coughing nearby seems to start Ascaris killing too. Research is badly needed into the common cold. It does not ride into cells with SV 40. It prefers to enter staphylococcus, streptococcus and yeast in the respiratory organs. It has special environmental triggers, like smoke, vapors, and foods. It comes from Ascaris and often flees (into you) when you kill Ascaris, giving you a cold if immunity is down.

5. **HIV**—This is seen for short times in many cancer patients and non-cancer patients. Always, there is benzene present where the virus is. When benzene leaves, the virus leaves, too. It first colonizes the genital organs, thymus and bone marrow, but will appear anywhere when a Fasciolopsis

---

[*] Testers, search for A. megalocephala and A. lumbricoides at onset of someone's cold.

buski is nearby and benzene is present. Its contribution to cancer is not known, nor are symptoms obvious, but coming from the same parasite makes it very important. P24, a part of the HIV virus requires gold. Its enzyme, reverse transcriptase, requires strontium. More research is badly needed. It is pulled into cells by SV 40 and even into our blood cells when they are parasitized by Plasmodium, the malaria parasite.

6. **Hepatitis B**—This comes from the human liver fluke and is triggered by **umbelliferone**, from the raw, common carrot. It is in the peel. Oats feed the liver fluke. Hepatitis B associates itself with Gang II viruses. When the liver fluke is killed, Clostridium botulinum appears, to feed on the remains, producing a toxin that blocks a neurotransmitter, **acetyl choline**. This causes sudden weepiness if the bacteria arrive in the hypothalamus, often baffling everybody, when the patient is really doing quite well. Weepy patients should take hypothalamus drops and drink eucalyptus and birch bark teas to kill this clostridium.

7. **Influenza A and B** (Flu)—This makes us quite sick if our white blood cells are not in action yet[**] and you are already killing Fasciolopsis buski parasites. This is popularly called "detoxification-illness". When the Flu seems to be extra vicious, the victims' white blood cells are not only inactive but also don't have any organic germanium, selenite, or vitamin C. Flu comes from Fasciolopsis buski when they are being killed in any manner. The body is quite capable of spontaneously killing parasites, at least at certain stages and at certain times. This leads to Flu attacks, too, often at the same time as colds because Ascaris is included in the body's killing-sweep. The difference between healthy and sick people is the capability of the white blood cells. Many people in hospitals, even

---

[**]Testers, search for Flu in the WBC when a sick person is said to have the flu. If they are empty, search for the immunity destroyers: PCB, benzene, asbestos, mercury, nickel, dyes. If they are full, search for organic germanium, vitamin C and selenite; these will be absent. Flu is often present in WBCs of persons who are not sick. Their WBCs do contain the Flu viruses, but these 3 "foods" are present.

emergency rooms, are there because of undiagnosed flu. Even when other causes are found and treated, it is Flu that silently decides when they are released because that is what is causing illness. If the white blood cells improve in the hospital and begin eating and killing Flu viruses, the person gets better. Regular zapping often clears enough WBCs to stop a Flu attack. Flu becomes chronic easily because HGH can attach itself to this virus, as can SCF. Flu can attach itself to other viruses too, especially NEU, but not to SV 40. Flu requires vanadium.

Detox-illness consists of Flu and Salmonella attacks, occasionally with prion protein as well.

Pesky Prions

Prions come from Salmonella bacteria, but must be triggered. Both require gold, leaving it behind if they get killed. Prions are never seen unless Salmonellas are being killed before the white blood cells have been cleared of their 5 destroyers and fed with organic germanium, selenite and vitamin C. This means there was a big population of Salmonella, coming in turn, from killed F. buski. Nevertheless, prions are not produced unless Salmonella is being killed in an organ that is making PGE2, the allergy-antagonist. This happens frequently in cancer patients and other sick people because the Salmonellas have been growing in the sick organ with allergies, which is making the PGE2. And that, in turn, is due to a growing F. buski population, which often releases its Salmonellas. Suppose you are allergic to muskmelons, which have the antigen that goes to your muscles. The muscles make PGE2 in protest. Your cancer will appear in the muscle; there will be Fasciolopsis buski stages there, too, causing the allergy and contributing to the cancer in several ways. Your body, besides your own therapy, will succeed in killing many of them, releasing the Salmonellas from dying Fasciolopsis stages. If your body kills the escaping Salmonellas too, prions will be triggered in the muscles and escape to the nearest nerves and brain. They will not be triggered if you stopped eating muskmelons. You will not be sick from any of it, nor even notice it if your white blood cells are already free of their 5 destroyers and have enough organic germanium, selenite, and vitamin C. The preventive treatment, of course, is to take large amounts of these, while removing the 5 immunity destroyers from kidney WBCs. This should include gold, molybdenum, rubidium, and ruthenium to starve both prions and Salmonella. The food allergen should be stopped, too.

Prions can be free or still attached to Salmonella bacteria. They can stay free or attach themselves to Flu viruses. They exit with the urine. They enter chromosomes like other viruses but do not associate with Gang I or Gang II. They are exceptionally easy to kill if, but only if, you can get rid of the Salmonella attack and remove any gold. The main symptom of prions is dizziness, disorientation, and lack of emotion; you could even have a pleasant emotion.

Yeast Queens

A yeast "takeover", consuming your body's sugar, happens quite often, even in a non-cancer patient when immunity is lowered. But a cancer patient's low blood sugar cannot feed two. Together with your poor appetite, this could bring you unintentional starvation.

Yeast makes you fatigued from low blood sugar. It also gives you allergic symptoms from acetic acid (vinegar) and acetaldehyde because it constantly produces them.

Vinegar has a tropism for the prostate and colon. Acetaldehyde goes to the skin. Antifungal medication for yeast is not effective, but taking away its RAS virus and its metal, chromium is very effective. Just stopping the RAS trigger, asparagine, is already helpful.

Very many yeasts and viruses live in the intestines. This means we can kill them with several well-chosen enemas. These enemas are used, not to empty the bowels, but to be absorbed and to act locally to kill the oncoviruses, regular viruses, yeasts and bacteria, all together in a massive approach.

You can feel like a new person after 5 days of these special enemas at bedtime. See Help #16, page 263.

You can improve your sickness symptoms in the first week of the program with these herbal enemas, if you have already changed your water and diet. Now you can <u>enjoy</u> the prospect of succeeding in curing the cancer. But you must still be vigilant against detox-illness. Keep up your protective methods on an exact schedule.

Follow your Progress

First make an exhaustive list of your symptoms, leaving nothing out. You might fill 2 pages with 50 or more symptoms.

There are 3 kinds of sickness to follow that you can tell apart if you can test by Syncrometer®. They are pathogen-illness, toxicity-illness and detoxification-illness. (Notice that it does not include cancer-illness.) You might have all of these already or only <u>one</u>, or maybe none. If you can't test, and feel sick, assume you have all.

Detoxification-illness is unique and temporary. It has only 3 ingredients and they are always the same. It is a combination of Flu viruses, salmonella bacteria and prions. Syncrometer® testing tells you in minutes which ones you have. They can be so plentiful that they are all visible in your body fluids, including saliva.

The symptoms they cause are nausea, loss of appetite, blurred vision, even a temperature. You only get this illness if you kill parasites before you have removed wheel bearing grease, heavy metals and dyes from your kidney white blood cells[*]. That is why the program begins with their removal.

It is easy to prevent detox-illness because the *3-Week Program* begins with freeing your white blood cells for action. But sometimes you already have these symptoms, before you begin anything. Plain zapping, taking Flu and bacteria-killing herbs, along with Lugol's iodine can clear it all up in 3 to 4

---

[*] Testers, search for wheel bearing grease, heavy metals and dyes in systemic WBCs first, (place WBCs beside saliva) then in the WBCs of the kidneys (place WBCs beside the kidneys).

days. Delay parasite-killing till you are caught up with detox-illness and have cleared the kidneys for 4 days.

Notice which symptoms on your list are gone after treating detox-illness. It is very important to keep such notes. Later, when it happens again, you will know what is causing your symptoms and how to clear them. Clearing up the detox-illness leaves you with toxicity- and pathogen-caused sickness.

Pathogen-illness includes bloating, gassiness, no appetite, weight loss, headache, insomnia, pain—both mild and acute requiring morphine, constipation, diarrhea, coughing and wheezing, requiring oxygen, hiccups, headache. These are the conditions that make you <u>feel</u> sick. Getting rid of them early in the program will let you enjoy the 3 weeks of cancer curing. These symptoms are due to bacteria and their oncoviruses. It is these we will kill by special enemas, starvation and zapping. It includes E. coli, Staphylococcus and Streptococcus varieties and others. After this, you will still be left with those symptoms due to toxicities.

Toxicity-Illness

These do not make you <u>feel</u> sick, although they cause effusions, edema, anemia, bleeding, jaundice, kidney failure, and liver failure. We will discuss these later.

Notice that these illnesses are much more life-threatening than those that make you <u>feel</u> bad or depressed. But feeling better comes first, so you can be energized to conquer the toxicity variety. Fortunately, all 3 illnesses have overlapping causes so you will be helping the others by clearing each one.

And notice that we did not include cancer-illness, because there is none! The exception is when the tumors cause pressure somewhere, so the blood cannot flow and food or urine or bile cannot pass. These symptoms do not make you <u>feel</u> sick, but, of course, are extremely serious. We have learned, though, that the cancer's growth, which causes the pressure, is due itself to oncoviruses, bacteria, and parasites. These will be our first target. Which parasite and pathogen brings each problem is given in the table below.

Parasites and Their Contribution to Cancer

Parasite	Contribution to Cancer and Illness
Ascaris lumbricoides (pet roundworm)	1. makes tricalcium phosphate "bony" deposits 2. blocks telomerase inhibitor II 3. blocks cathepsin B 4. brings NEU oncovirus
Ascaris megalocephala (pet roundworm)	1. makes tricalcium phosphate "bony" deposits 2. blocks telomerase inhibitor II 3. brings NEU oncovirus
Clonorchis sinensis (human liver fluke)	1. causes erosion of pituitary gland to make tumor nucleus 2. brings Hepatitis B virus
Dirofilaria (dog heartworm)	1. makes abdominal masses 2. makes Hodgkin's tumors 3. brings coumarin allergy to lungs 4. brings FOS oncovirus 5. brings Mycobacterium phlei
Echinoporyphium	1. brings kidney cancer
Eurytrema (pancreatic fluke)	1. causes erosion of pancreas to make tumor nucleus 2. brings SV 40 oncovirus
Fasciolopsis buski (human intestinal fluke)	1. brings Bacillus cereus bacteria 2. brings d-tyramine to the body from Bacillus cereus 3. brings allergies to all parasitized organs by means of d-tyramine 4. makes orthophosphotyrosine together with isopropyl alcohol 5. brings MYC oncovirus 6. cercaria bring Human Chorionic Gonadotropin (HCG) 7. releases Salmonella bacteria when killed, causing PGE2 allergies
Fasciola hepatica (sheep liver fluke)	1. brings fibronectin 2. blocks cathepsin B
Onchocerca	1. brings abdominal masses (lymphomas) 2. blocks ubiquitin 3. blocks cathepsin B 4. blocks telomerase inhibitor II

Parasite	Contribution to Cancer and Illness
	5. brings JUN oncovirus 6. brings carcino embryonic antigen (CEA)
Paragonimus (lung fluke)	1. brings potato ring rot, zearalenone, and benzene locally
Strongyloides	1. brings yeast, Saccharomyces cerevisciae, as in bread, beer 2. causes erosion of hypothalamus to make tumor nucleus 3. brings SRC oncovirus 4. brings CMV virus 5. brings EBV virus (makes CEA)
yeast (S. cerevisciae)	1. blocks caspase 2. blocks telomerase inhibitor II 3. brings RAS 4. makes CEA

Fig. 63 Parasite contributions to cancer and illness

1, 2, 3 Done

We now know a lot about the cancer process. You can separate it into 3 processes: the cancerous growth itself, the sickness that later accompanies it, and the toxicities that spread through your body steadily. The toxicities feed and accelerate the first two.

The cancer process is almost the easiest to stop.

Your new cancer diet that leaves out allergens and foods that feed parasites or trigger oncoviruses will do 2 things:

1. Stop the growth of tumor cells.
2. Allow the natural death of these same tumor cells.

You can do this even before starting the rest of the program.

Your new clean water and food will return your immune power. It will bring quicker relief if you feed your WBCs high quality food without letup: germanium, selenite and vitamin C.

CHAPTER 9

STOPPING METASTASES

Many are Unreal

Seeing hundreds of tumors in the form of lumps under the skin or throughout the lungs or liver may seem daunting when you first look at your CT scan or actually feel them. But it need not be so daunting when you realize they are not true metastases at all. They are merely more of the <u>same</u> kind you already have. You are simply making more and more. If you can get rid of one you can get rid of all. Obviously more and more tumor nuclei are making a successful fusion with the primary organ, be it skin or lung or lymph nodes.

Why are they getting so numerous? The fact that the fusions are occurring in the same organ is your clue. The inflammation in the skin or the lung or lymph nodes is spreading, so the tumor nuclei can fuse with more and more cells. You must ask: Am I still accidentally eating the food antigen for this (the primary) organ? Find the food antigen in the *Cancer Location Table* (page 186); then check the *Food Table* (page 36) to see which foods have this antigen. For the skin the food antigen would be **acetaldehyde**. In the lungs this would be **coumarin** and **SHRIMP** for lymph nodes.

You may feel quite certain that you are not eating the food that has this antigen. Yet your recovery depends on finding it. Try to find a Syncrometer® tester to help you. It is not necessary to be physically present for the tester[*]. The ability to

---

[*]Testers, if you find acetaldehyde in the skin, search next for yeast (any package of dry yeast) which makes acetaldehyde. Then search for asparagine which feeds this yeast. Search for chromium and cobalt deposits which are necessary for yeast to grow. Then search dishes and food for presence of chromium or cobalt. Search in powdered food supplements, herbs.

make a homeopathic or homeographic copy of your saliva sample lets the tester receive it by mail to search for your antigens. The saliva itself is considered a biological waste and hazardous to ship. Instructions are on page 586.

When tiny tumorlets have started everywhere it is because these food allergens have caused "inflammations" everywhere, and that resulted in PGE2 being made everywhere (see page 59). Prostaglandin E2 is a substance made by your tissues when they are irritated by an antigen. If Fasciola stages and Ascaris eggs are everywhere, too, we can expect a lot of gluey threads to be made. Tumor nuclei in large numbers will be detained and fuse here amidst this glue. Wherever they get close enough, long enough, to your organ cells they can fuse with them. As soon as the pancreas end of the tumor nucleus fuses to your skin or lungs or lymph nodes, a tumor growth is started there. And if the pancreas end is bringing the SV 40 virus, it can slip into your skin or lung or lymph node cells through the fusion site. See the diagram, as interpreted from Syncrometer® data.

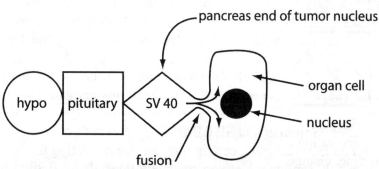

Fig. 64 Diagram of fusion to body cell by tumor nucleus

There are many free-swimming SV 40 viruses too. But they only enter the cells of an inflamed organ that is making PGE2, and at first that is only the primary organ. Sometimes SV 40 is alone, but sometimes it is not. Like an engine pulling a train of freight cars SV 40 pulls its train of other oncoviruses with it. Three or four of these are commonly seen: MYC, RAS,

FOS, JUN, SRC and NEU. It does not so readily pull CMV, Hepatitis B, nor Adenovirus or EBV.

Your organ cells were already being goaded by stem cell factor from the hypothalamus part of the tumor nucleus and by HGH from the pituitary part. A switch in polarization to south had already been made. There was new growth invited to start everywhere. But with the newly arriving SV 40 and its onhangers there is now no apoptosis. The new tumor must enlarge because there is growth without natural cell death. The speed of growth will depend only on how many Fasciolopsis stages arrive to share their OPT-making enzymes and how many Clostridium bacteria arrive to share their DNA-making capability. The fires for malignancy are being built everywhere. Yet, they are very easy to put out at this early stage. Stop drinking the south polarized water, which has laundry bleach and nickel in it. Stop eating the onion family of foods which feeds Fasciolopsis buski. Stop triggering the SV 40 virus with gallic acid. Kill Clostridium bacteria. Kill the oncoviruses, and all the bacteria and yeasts that give them shelter. But most immediately stop eating the food that inflames the organ being targeted.

> Check the *Cancer Location Table*, then check the *Food Table*, then analyze your diet. Eat nothing that isn't listed and found safe. Use no "loopholes".

Suspect the foods you have "always" eaten. Obviously, you are eating a lot of the culprit food. If there are no clues or no time, change it all. Eat nothing that you were eating before. Eat Thai food, Korean food, Chinese food, Japanese food, Mexican food—anything but American if you are American and vice versa.

Such a diet switch can't guarantee that you won't get the same allergen in one of the new foods. But chances are excellent that your switch will work. Learn to do food testing yourself with a Syncrometer® if that is possible. It will give you the freedom to be a connoisseur in spite of deprivations in whatever land you live.

The overriding truth is that you can cure all the hundred lumps I call **pseudometastases** and start them shrinking in days. Lymphomas are an example. Stopping eating SHRIMP puts them on hold immediately. Inflammation and PGE2 go away. No new lymph nodes catch the tumor nucleus to start a new cancer. SHRIMP means seafood and fish, but amazingly, this food substance is in the tops of carrots, too, where the green rings are, easy to avoid. Spreading cancer means the responsible food allergen is spreading and this, in turn, means the allergy is getting worse due to spreading Fasciolopsis buski and Salmonella bacteria. Go on an intensive F. buski and Salmonella-killing program. Find every buski and Salmonella-killing method mentioned in this book and do them all, without delay.

Real Metastases

When a <u>new</u> organ gets involved in your cancer it is a <u>true</u> metastasis. Something new has happened. In reality you have acquired a new allergy of the PGE2 kind.

Why does a new allergy develop? As you eat a certain food, the liver can not digest and detoxify all of the substances in that food. Food is a complex mixture. All food has phenolic substances. They give the food its color, its flavor, its fragrance. You may have put yourself on a diet rich in cabbage, broccoli and other members of the "cabbage-family". These will bring the substance PIT[*]. Or on a diet of carrot juice! This brings **umbelliferone allergy**. The intention to eat much more of these fine natural foods was good, but you can be misled. Your metabolism, the body's quiet chemistry, has been disturbed by interlopers, Fasciolopsis buski, and Salmonella enteriditis. They bring allergies.

---

[*] Testers, purchase phenylisothiocyanate, or improvise with a cabbage leaf, copied, and labeled CABBAGE (RAW).

How did the allergy happen? One small part of your body was turned southerly by the heavy metals in your drinking water, specifically nickel. If that part also acquires a Fasciolopsis stage, its own partner bacteria will be very stimulated to multiply. Its partner bacteria are *Bacillus cereus*, ordinary soil bacteria. But they produce tyramine in a steady stream. Tyramine formed in a southerly region becomes d-tyramine, not the kind your body can work with. Soon its closest relatives, l-tyrosine, l-thyroxine, and l-phenyl alanine will all become d-forms, too, in the neighborhood of Fasciolopsis buski. These cannot be used by your body either. Your ever-alert immune system will notice this immediately because having no useful thyroid hormone (only d-thyroxine) is an emergency. It will start to destroy them. It will destroy any "wrong form" amino acid anywhere in your body and those that you <u>eat</u>, too. Examples are coumarin in the lung, menadione in the blood, d-histidine and any other d-forms at other organs. You may call it a mere allergy when you have symptoms like cramps, rashes, and swelling, but the Syncrometer® detects that your white blood cells are hard at work in an allergic tissue. They are eating and getting rid of these wrong forms. See also page 65.

How Salmonella enteriditis causes allergies is not yet known. Its preferred location is in your pancreas, so your pancreatin enzymes are missing asparaginase. You begin to burp and have discomfort after eating. You get "gassy". Maybe it was the liver's job to change all the wrong d-forms back to their correct l-forms. But that will not be possible if the liver itself has turned southerly in spots or just can't keep up.

As soon as you sense a new allergy or suspect a new lump, rush to do a liver cleanse (see page 563) and do one every 2 weeks till your liver action is much better. Rush to rid yourself of more Fasciolopsises by depriving them of onion-chemicals. Rush to find your source of gold, molybdenum and ruthenium. Rush to find the allergy.

Try to find out which organ really has the new lump. Even very small organs may have a unique antigen. Start removing this organ's metal collection, particularly nickel, which implicates wheel bearing grease. EDTA chelation would always help. Avoid the food antigen for this organ. Kill your parasites, bacteria, and oncoviruses. Do all you can to switch this organ back to north.

In fact, even if you have only a primary tumor, you should do liver cleanses to <u>prevent</u> metastases. A cleaner liver gives you better digestion, fewer parasites, and less allergies.

Cancer Location Table

This list of cancer locations and food antigens is not complete. Many, in italics, need further verification. Testers are encouraged to find more and share results.

Cancer Location	Food Allergen (antigen)
abdominal or chest mass (includes a lymph node)	lactose (milk sugar) and SHRIMP
adrenal gland	mandelonitrile(almonds),*aldosterone*
aorta	menadione (raw greens & grains)
B-cells	*CORN*
bile duct	acetic acid (vinegar)
bladder	cinnamic acid
bone	PIT*, umbelliferone
bone marrow	limonene
brain & spinal cord	caffeic acid
breast	apiol
capillaries	*hippuric acid, pyrrole, benzoic acid*
cardiac (upper) stomach	phenol
cartilage	wheat
cervix	ASA (aspirin)
cochlea (ear)	malvin
colon	acetic acid (vinegar), pyrrole
crista (ear)	malvin
diaphragm	*choline, NGF, hippuric acid*
epiglottis	naringenin
esophagus	menadione
esophagus, upper	menadione, *acetic acid, caffeic acid*
eye	lily family (onion, garlic)

---

* phenylisothiocyanate

Cancer Location	Food Allergen (antigen)
eye, iris	galacturonic acid
Fallopian tube	umbelliferone, *DOPA, aldosterone*
fimbria	*chlorophyll*
gallbladder	acetic acid (vinegar)
heart	tryptophane (amino acid)
Hodgkin's lymphoma	lactose, SHRIMP, *acetaldehyde*
hypothalamus	chlorogenic acid
Islets of Langerhans in	
• head region of pancreas	quercitin
• tail region of pancreas	phloridzin
To find these, touch insulin sample to pancreas sample and add 1 pF or µH for head region, and 2 or more µH for tail region.	
kidney	albumin, casein (dairy food)
liver	umbelliferone
lumbar spine	caffeic acid
lung	coumarin
lung lymph nodes	tryptophane
lymph node	SHRIMP, D-mannitol
lymph vessel valve	lactose
malignant melanoma	phenyl alanine plus mercury
medullated nerve	*apple* (not phloridzin), *caffeic acid*
medulla + 1pF	*galacturonic acid*, allyl methyl sulfide, diallyl sulfide
medulla	*apiol, onion*
medulla, left	*tryptophane, piperine, gallic acid*
megakaryocytes	ASA (aspirin)
non Hodgkin's lymphoma	SHRIMP & CORN
osteomyelitis	umbelliferone (carrot)
ovary	phenyl alanine, apiol
pancreas	gallic acid
peripheral nerve	apiol, *caffeic acid*
pineal gland	*gallic acid*
pituitary	phloridzin
platelets	limonene
prostate	acetic acid (vinegar), naringenin
RBC (red blood cells)	fructose (sugar in honey)
rectum	NGF, D-mannitol
salivary glands	casein
skeletal muscle	melon (not cantaloupe), *lemon*
skin	acetaldehyde, *NGF, apiol*
spleen	*peanut*
thymus	naringenin (oranges)

Cancer Location	Food Allergen (antigen)
thyroid	d-tyramine
tongue, filiform	MSG (monosodium glutamate)
tongue, fungiform	naringenin
trachea	*phenol, phloridzin*
ureter	*beets, avocado*
uterus	phenyl alanine
vagina	acetaldehyde, ASA
veins	*menadione*
vein valves	*CORN*

Food antigens invite the tumor nucleus to the allergic organ.

Fig. 65 Cancer locations and allergens

How Metastases Happen

To make the primary tumor, the tumor nucleus fused itself to one of your organs to make a 4-tissue combination. We can also call it a quad-tumor or just a "quad", perhaps a quad-breast or quad-prostate (see diagram). Quads can be seen floating in your body fluids everywhere. These quads can fuse to another new organ to make a quint-tumor if the new organ is inflamed. This could be a quint-breast-lung or quint-prostate-bone. The quint combination is the first true metastasis. Certain combinations are more likely than others because the organs are nearby and share their parasites. If you have 4 or 5 metastases, you might have very many different combinations of organ cells. For example, you could have octets of hypothalamus, pituitary, pancreas, breast, bone (rib), skin, lung, lymph node (neck location). Or you could have octet-tumors of hypothalamus, pituitary, pancreas, breast, lung, bone (collar bone), lymph node (at collar bone), and bone marrow. There does not seem to be a limit on the number or the order of new organs involved. Only the first three organs and their order stay constant for all cancers.

Organ combinations without the hypothalamus, pituitary, or pancreas exist, but they do not form tumors or cysts.

Combinations of organs with <u>one</u> of these three exist, too, but do not form malignant tumors. Different combinations with pancreas cells exist. These should contain SV 40 if gallic acid is being eaten in the diet. Their behavior has not yet been studied.

Even if you have tumors everywhere, quite uncountable, and the picture looks completely hopeless, these metastases and pseudometastases can be stopped abruptly. The principles are the same as for the primary tumor. Only now it is much more urgent. Put your emphasis on the other parasites, too.

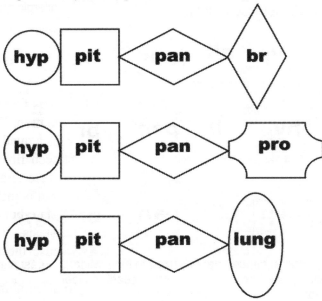

Top: primary breast tumor; Middle: primary prostate tumor; Bottom: primary lung tumor. The 3 organs at the left of each are the tumor nucleus.

Fig. 66 The primary tumor

It is the spread of Fasciola and Ascaris that is making metastases possible with all the gluey fibers being made. Stop eating wheat, the essential food of Fasciola, and the food oils that trigger its viruses. Stop eating the essential foods of the 2 Ascaris varieties we all have, d-carnitine, and quercitin.

Success is swift. In 3 days you can sense the shrinkage of a new lump after starving the parasites and avoiding the food antigen for that lump. Kill more and more Fasciolopsises and Salmonellas since they are responsible for the allergy phenomenon. Remove nickel steadily, namely wheel bearing grease, since it provides the south pole force to make antigens.

What becomes more and more difficult is finding safe food for yourself. Yet, the splendid variety of local and imported foods in our food stores makes it easier than it ever was in the past. Learn to cook new foods! Get help cooking and shopping. You should not lose weight.

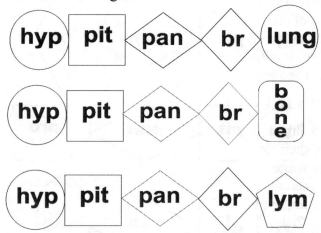

Top: breast cancer metastasized to lung; Middle: breast cancer metastasized to bone; Bottom: breast cancer spreading to lymph nodes.

Fig. 67 Quint tumors become the first metastases

You have already stopped the primary tumor's growth and now you have stopped your metastases, too. You are even preventing metastases from forming with liver cleanses to make you less allergic. You can relax and focus again on clearing up accumulations inside the tumors. But instead of using the brute strength of massive amounts of detoxifying supplements, we will first reactivate the immune system. We need the immune system, namely your WBCs, as our ally because it avoids "detoxification" symptoms that we can get with other ways. The immune system knows better than our reasoning minds how to attack parasites and remove your tumors. Together, the immune system <u>and</u> supplements will remove the accumulations fastest, followed by the tumor tissue itself.

Kidneys and Bowel Come First

It would do no good to scrub, sweep and dust your whole house if you couldn't get the collected trash <u>out</u> of the house in the end. And no kitchen could get its work done without a system of removing the garbage.

It could be a sink and sewer system or even just buckets, but that is what keeps the whole household running. Your kidneys and bowels are your body's garbage removal system.

What's In Urine?

Healthy kidneys have a northerly polarization by day. This means their tiny cell channels for accepting food and pushing out its wastes will be open and working. Throughout the day, the Syncrometer® detects mercury, thallium, copper, cobalt, vanadium, dyes, PCBs, even asbestos and malonic acid in the urine. That is what we have been eating! At night healthy kidneys turn southerly. They make very little urine and put very few toxins into the urine. Only spent iridium, a quota of iron, the bleach in your drinking water, undigested oil, yeast and its oncovirus, RAS, stem cell factor and HGH are regularly seen past midnight. The kidneys need their "sleep" no doubt. See the table of urine contents for a healthy person by daytime and nighttime.

Nighttime Urine

Syncrometer® Urine Test in health		
N=*Negative* (means it is not there)	NIGHT	DAY
P=*Positive* (means it is there)	3:00 am	9:00 am
north polarized	*Neg*	*Pos*
south polarized	*Pos*	*Neg*
ferrite, Fe_2O_3 (oxidized) form of iron	*Pos*	*Pos*
magnetite, Fe_3O_4	*Neg*	*Pos*
cortisone	*Neg*	*Pos*
PGE2 (universal reactant to allergies)	*Neg*	*Pos*
hypochlorite (bleach from water)	*Pos*	*Pos*
mercury	*Neg*	*Pos*
thallium	*Neg*	*Pos*
copper oxidized	*Neg*	*Pos*
cobalt oxidized	*Neg*	*Pos*
vanadium oxidized	*Neg*	*Pos*
germanium oxidized	*Neg*	*Pos*
selenium oxidized	*Neg*	*Pos*
chromium oxidized	*Neg*	*Pos*
manganese oxidized	*Neg*	*Pos*
nickel oxidized	*Neg*	*Pos*
iridium, oxidized	*Pos*	*Pos*
aluminum oxidized	*Neg*	*Pos*
thulium oxidized	*Neg*	*Pos*
MYC (oncovirus)	*Neg*	*Neg*
JUN (oncovirus)	*Neg*	*Pos*
SCF (stem cell factor)	*Pos*	*Pos*
FOS (oncovirus)	*Neg*	*Neg*
RAS (oncovirus)	*Pos*	*Pos*
HGH (growth hormone)	*Pos*	*Pos*
PS (phosphatidylserine)	*Neg*	*Pos*
oleic acid (undigested oil)	*Pos*	*Pos*
yeast	*Pos*	*Pos*

Fig. 68 Nighttime compared to daytime urine contents

In cancer patients the kidneys have turned southerly by daytime, quite unsuitable. Asbestos and the oxidized forms of iron besides nickel are stuck in them, trapped by thick sticky wheel bearing grease that cannot leave. Being southerly signals them that it's time to sleep. Very few toxins show up in the urine now, even though it is daytime and even though the kidneys are full of copper, cobalt, vanadium and other toxins waiting to be excreted. It is no wonder that these metals and toxins go elsewhere to accumulate. See the table of urine contents compared with kidney contents for a cancer patient.

Kidneys Asleep in Cancer

Syncrometer® Urine and Kidney Test in Cancer		
DAYTIME	**Urine**	**Kidneys**
malonic acid family (5 M's)	*Neg*	—
aluminum	*Neg*	—
cadmium	*Neg*	—
CEA	*Neg*	—
chromium	*Neg*	—
cobalt	*Neg*	*Pos*
copper	*Neg*	*Pos*
dyes	*Neg*	*Pos*
Fe_2O_3	*Neg*	*Pos*
Fe_3O_4	*Neg*	*Neg*
HCG	*Neg*	—
Human Growth Hormone	*Neg*	*Pos*
iridium	*Pos*	*Pos*
iridium 4 dodecacarbonyl	*Neg*	*Neg*
lead	*Neg*	—
mercury	*Neg*	—
nickel	*Neg*	*Pos*
north	*Neg*	*Neg*
Ribonucleotide Reductase	*Neg*	—
SCF	*Neg*	*Pos*
south	*Pos*	*Pos*
strontium	*Neg*	—
thallium	*Neg*	—
thiourea	*Neg*	—
vanadium	*Neg*	—
yeast	*Neg*	—

Fig. 69 Kidneys clogged but urine empty in cancer

In cancer patients the kidneys switch to northerly at night, which is wrong again, but at least they should be able to work. Only now other organs are not cooperating with them because they are "sleeping". White blood cells work day and night. They are constantly switching between northerly and southerly, picking up debris while north, releasing it while south. But releasing requires 3 supplements and if they are missing even one of these, the release is stalled. The white blood cells are stalled in their south state. They are waiting. Waiting for organic germanium, organic selenium and organic vitamin C. These 3 supplements feed the white blood cells so they can release their toxic cargo into the bladder and go back for more. We will use hydrangea root, sodium selenite and rose hips to supply them, though they are less than perfect. We will also use manufactured vitamin C and Germanium-132 as well as various nuts to increase dosages. See page 76.

Getting strong excretion by the kidneys is a pressing problem for the cancer patient. Unless our detoxifying program is accepted by the kidneys, we can't be successful. The elimination system, our bowels, can come to the rescue, to some extent. Other alternative therapists have made the most of this, too. They may rely on enemas, several a day, to get toxins out of the body. We will do this also, even using enemas as a vehicle to deliver herbal treatments.

The Syncrometer® shows that the liver, too, has regions that become south polarized in cancer patients. So it cannot detoxify enough harmful chemicals during daytime. It cannot fill its bile full of toxins and bacteria and pour it into the intestine, as it should, thereby moving the bowels. Constipation is common.

At night, when the sick liver regions finally become northerly (wrong again), they do not get the cooperation of the healthy organs that it serves, because now they are "asleep"; so it does not make bile flow and move the bowels then, either (nighttime).

Other alternative therapists have discovered that a stimulant like coffee could be used by enema to activate the liver, forcing it to make bile and release it into the intestine. Coffee enemas are a standard part of other programs. They would certainly be useful for us, too, if it were not for the asbestos and processing solvents in coffee. Even though asbestos can be filtered out, its iron is set free and left behind as Fe_2O_3, the south pole kind, altogether too risky. Still we must activate and cleanse the liver somehow. We will use herbs.

Removing accumulated ferrite iron (Fe_2O_3) and asbestos (which supplies such iron) will come first in our body clean up, together with nickel from automotive greases and mercury from amalgam. This will give kidneys and liver their northerly polarization back by day in order to do serious detoxification and excretion.

Vitamin C dissolves some iron deposits but does not attack asbestos. You need it in large amounts, so it will also have a diuretic effect. Be sure to use regular l-ascorbic acid, not a neutralized variety. Instead, take your calcium, magnesium and potassium supplements along with it. Find how much you tolerate before the bowels get too loose. It could be 10 or 20 grams (2 or 4 tsp.). Of course, a loose bowel is just what is needed to speed up elimination, but not beyond endurance.

Intravenous vitamin C can give you up to 100 grams a day, when used by a skilled therapist who gives enough calcium and magnesium in the same IV to keep it all neutral. It gives a diuretic effect at the same time as removing iron deposits.

Rose hips are a source of organic vitamin C, quite a bit more potent that the pure synthetic form. In nature it comes with extra factors that help with its action. A great deal of manufactured vitamin C in the market place is contaminated with thulium, a lanthanide! This kind of supplement would be much more harmful than helpful. Lanthanides were discussed in earlier books. Thulium, in particular, is very harmful (testers should search for this toxin). Supplements of vitamin C are often contaminated with laundry bleach. Avoid this kind. Rose hips, coarse ground, including seeds are best.

Drinking northerly-polarized water helps immensely to switch back the kidneys and liver to their correct polarization. Drink one pint in the morning, when thirst is greatest. Putting herbal teas and rainwater on the zappicator to make them north polarized helps, too. How this combats wrong polarization is not clear. But the kidneys will get right to work excreting toxins for a short time. Do not drink it after 8 p.m. since toxins would not be normally excreted in the night. The good effect of north polarized water is temporary, so keep it up till you are cured and beyond.

Wearing north pole magnets of low strength (10 gauss) over the kidneys helps them become north polarized, too. Be extra careful to put the correct pole touching your skin; always test your own with a compass. Do it yourself because confusion is everywhere. Wear them by daytime only.

Sitting on a stronger magnet of several thousand gauss is helpful, too. A 4" x 5" coated ceramic magnet of 3000 to 5000 gauss switches the kidneys to north after 5 minutes. BE SURE YOU ARE SEATED ON THE NORTH POLE SIDE. If you can't be sure, don't use it. Use any small compass to check, twice. Then get off it for 25 minutes and repeat the cycle throughout the day. The northerly polarization lasts about 20 minutes each time. The force reaches through your clothing and upward through your body to the kidneys.

Zapping the kidneys changes the polarization to north for 20 minute periods. Taking kidney drops also does this. In fact the urge to empty the bladder is often felt right afterwards.

With all these ways to repolarize the kidneys, we might think it should be easy and permanent. It is not—for a special reason. With every load of ferrite iron and asbestos brought from the tumor zone and now passing through the kidneys, they tend to get stuck in a south state again. Only after the tumors and body are cleared will the kidneys stay north polarized without help. It could take three weeks. But you do not have to wait to get this done before starting to detoxify. As long as the white blood cells are being fed, their immunity destroyers being removed, and 2 quarts (liters) of urine being excreted, it will be enough. As long as the bowels are moving every day, either naturally or by enema, it will be enough to get started.

Angiogenesis

If tumor cells had no oxygen, no food, and no way to get rid of their wastes, they would be forced to die in spite of their extra longevity from oncoviruses. This is exactly what happens to large tumors because they need more of everything to do their metabolism than do small tumors. The middle of a large tumor suffers the most, being furthest from the bathing lymph, which supplies the foods and oxygen. So at the middle it turns into a decaying, putrid mass called a "necrotic center". That is sometimes how a biopsy tells the difference between normal tissue and malignant tissue.

The shortage of oxygen, together with decaying tissue, makes it possible for an anaerobic bacterium like Clostridium to start its colonies there (anaerobic means 'requiring the absence of oxygen').

Necrotic tissue and Clostridium toxins are very, very toxic. Your body tries to remedy this by, at least, wrapping up the whole mess in a tough coat to protect you. Your body also tries to remedy the fundamental problem of oxygen lack by growing new blood vessels into the tumor so it will be better fed, get more oxygen and get regular cleaning by the lymph. Remember, the body is nurturing the tumor like an embryo because of it's HCG (Human Chorionic Gonadotropin) hormone (see page 5). The free-floating hypothalamus cells were actually commandeered to make this HCG by the Fasciolopsis cercaria stages. In fact, the Syncrometer® sees that the hypothalamus cells are actually stuck to the cercaria.

New blood vessels can sprout from old ones if they are needed. It is called **angiogenesis**. Our normal laminin is reported to start angiogenesis for normal body needs. But when massive amounts of laminin surround the tumor, because of increasing Ascaris parasites, angiogenesis gets an abnormal boost.

Hurry to kill Fasciolas and Ascaris, not just to prevent metastases, but to prevent angiogenesis, too.

Copper is needed in large amounts for angiogenesis. We can, of course, chelate this out or remove it with homeography. Much of it is stuck in blobs of wheel bearing grease in the brain, spine, and bone marrow. Degreasing is still most important. Replace copper water pipes and take tooth metal out of the mouth. Removing it from the body does no good, if it keeps steadily coming from water pipes and dental amalgam or seeping cookware.

Yeast buds, viruses and all pathogens can get into or out of the tumor much faster after angiogenesis has brought the circulation into tumors. These mark the terminal decline of health. We must hurry.

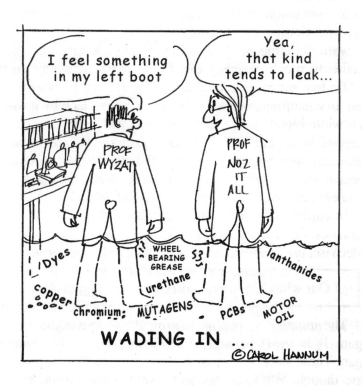

CHAPTER 10

GETTING BACK IMMUNITY

Setting free our white blood cells first, before anything else, will reward us with earlier success and less detox-illness. They can then join us in clearing away the accumulations in our tumors. Otherwise, we would have to take "mountains" of supplements to remove the flotsam and jetsam, like nail polish, shampoo, toothpaste, Freon, felt marker ink, soap, car wax, motor oil, ice cream flavoring, rust remover and wheel bearing grease from our tumors and it would take much too long. After the white blood cells have eaten and removed all this "trash" we want them to start eating the tumor cells themselves, together with their bacteria, viruses, and oncoviruses.

To free our white blood cells from their 5 destroyers we must first stop eating and drinking them. We must think of each white blood cell as a tiny miracle and not burden it with indigestible food or food antigens or frivolous things like cosmetics, toothpaste, or metal jewelry. You came into the world without a single one of these and now your immune system needs its vacation.

In earlier books many recipes were given to replace your cosmetics, dyes, and jewelry if you have a very demanding job. Otherwise, use NOTHING.

Our white blood cells **are** our immune system.

The immune system in each organ takes care of its own organ. It is made of special "soldier" cells that guard this organ. These white blood cells call this organ their home. They may, though, leave this organ to visit ("communicate") with others in other organs. Most of this is done in your lymph nodes, their communication centers. It reminds us of beehives with their elaborate communication systems, all meant to keep the hive unified and thriving. Our white blood cells have the same purpose and for this reason they have special powers.

They can "sense" an enemy of ours from far away, for example, lead molecules or SV 40 viruses. For this they need their "skins". Their outer membranes are their skins. Special sensors are imbedded in them. The rest of the membrane is made of a double-layered "fence" of fat molecules that keep out intruders and toxic molecules.

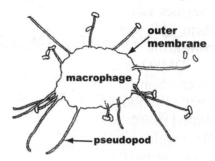

Fig. 70 Macrophage eating salmonellas

The white blood cells can tell the difference between friends and enemies from a long way off. When a macrophage senses an enemy it moves toward it. Its big clumsy feet are called pseudopods but they can make long thin pseudopods, too. It reminds us of an armored tank when we watch it move in a live blood sample. White blood cells have a number of ways they can attack our enemies. Large enemies must be attacked and killed before they can be nibbled away. Smaller enemies like bacteria and viruses can be eaten whole just by engulfing them and then killed after they are inside. They are easily picked up with long thin pseudopods sent after them. Even prions are eaten.

White blood cells can make powerful chemicals called cytokines and leukokines. They include interleukins and interferons.

The Syncrometer® has

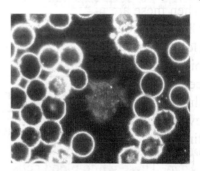

A macrophage, CD14, is at the center. The rest are RBCs.

Fig. 71 Live blood analysis

200

detected many more such chemicals, also in very minute amounts. I have called them _weapons_ (see page 109). Weapons are used to destroy the larger parasites so our digestive enzymes can digest them and our white blood cells can eat them. All available weapons are used in times of heavy parasitism.

DMSO is one such weapon. It destroys **allyl sulfide**, an onion-chemical needed by Fasciolopsis buski cercaria. MSM (methyl sulfonyl methane), another weapon we make, destroys **diallyl sulfide** and **allyl methyl sulfide**, more onion-chemicals. Benzoquinone, in very minute amounts, destroys dozens of toxins as well as one of the Ascaris varieties (lumbricoides). Rhodizonic acid destroys Ascaris megalocephala.

Complement is another very important part of the immune system. It is a family of molecules used as spears! It is a way of spearing our tiny enemies so the white blood cells can eat them.

Different white blood cells are given different jobs to do. They are very organized in their one real task—to protect you.

Using the Syncrometer®, I have distinguished ten kinds of white blood cells. They are CD4 and CD8 lymphocytes, CD37 B cells, CD14 macrophages, and six more varieties that eat dyes and motor oil. The CD4s eat and kill viruses. The CD8s include our _natural killers_. They are even seen killing CD4s when these are not able to kill the viruses they have eaten. The CD14s eat everything, except _you._ Both CD8s and CD14s are flesh eaters; _only these_ can eat tumor cells and large parasite pieces. We can also distinguish, electronically, the red blood cells (RBCs), platelets, eosinophils and megakaryocytes, all of them floating in the blood. Platelets are just tiny chips, not even cells, too small to hold a nucleus. Their job is to fill in the tiny tears and holes that are always developing in the long "pipelines" we call arteries and veins. This job is called blood clotting. Eosinophils are white blood cells that can spit histamine at enemies; they increase as Ascaris increases.

During the accumulating period of a tumor, which I call the middle phase, thousands of things are brought into the organ that has the tumor. They should have been brought to the liver or kidneys but, instead, they were deposited at the tumor site. Why didn't the white blood cells kill or remove all of these undesirables and bits of trash? That was their job. Why couldn't they keep up? They, too, along with the tumor cells and kidneys, became south polarized by the cargo they had to carry. Several kinds of PCBs, benzene, asbestos, dozens of heavy metals, malonic acid, motor oil, and hundreds of dyes as well as wheel bearing grease that had many of these imbedded in it, all arrived together from the drinking water to keep them south polarized constantly. They could not cycle from north to south and back again to do their work. They were meant to pick up a southerly cargo, which temporarily turns them south, process it, expel it, and turn themselves back to north again for the next cargo. Northerly is their normal state for making a pick-up. But it takes work and vital energy to process the cargo and turn itself back to northerly. This system of cycling can fail when the white blood cells are overwhelmed with too much ferrite iron or nickel and other heavy metals that are south. (A small magnet can be overwhelmed by a large magnet to change its polarity.) We will help them catch up with this task first, and then get them into action for us.

First of all, stop all sources of immunity destroyers.

The 5 Immunity Destroyers

PCBs

PCBs and benzene are toxins that get trapped in your white blood cells' membranes. Since the membranes are made of fat, and these solvents dissolve in fat, it is understandable why PCBs and benzene accumulate there and why the white cells then lose their special powers. That is where their sensors are located.

The main source of PCBs is the laundry bleach added to about half the population's drinking water. Since food manufacturers use this water and bleach, the second biggest source for USA citizens is processed food. Since all the produce in the market has been washed several times, and moved from different water zones, over half of it brings us PCBs, again.

Recalling the statistic that <u>all</u> cancer patients who passed through our clinic halls in the last 5 years had been receiving laundry bleach disinfected water; you can assume that your water contains it too.

Recall the second statistic—that all patients who went to a residence with clean water after leaving the clinic succeeded in getting well.

The third statistic was that all patients who deteriorated after leaving the clinic had gone to a residence with laundry bleached drinking water again.

This means that if you got significant alternative treatment, to the point where you were considered well enough to go home, you would have stayed well if you had recuperated in clean water. If you did not stay well you were again using laundry bleached water.

<u>It probably means that the usual clinical treatment would work well, too</u>, if you returned to a home with clean water. Of course, over-radiation, too much chemotherapy, or removing part of the face would still be a handicap. But the usual 5-year "life-allowance" given clinically might now be stretchable to 10 or 15 years, a significant improvement.

Saying that a cancer patient cannot be cured if they return to laundry bleached water is like saying you cannot stay dry by walking back into the rain. Since cancer is an immunodepression disease, you must avoid future immunodepression to stay well. This should apply to clinically treated patients as well as others.

The statistics might also mean that how you were treated for cancer is less significant than where you lived afterwards.

If you have just been diagnosed with cancer, your first question should be, "Am I getting PCBs and the other immunity destroyers from my municipal water? And did I inadvertently and mindlessly put them in my water myself?"

Details on finding the answers are given in the *Help* section of the *3-Week Program*. If you are only preventing cancer for your family, this should be the first question asked when buying a home. And if anyone in your family develops a serious illness, how your water is disinfected should be the first question asked.

Although PCBs are on your food, from spraying and washing in PCB-water, the 2 hot water soaks described in the *Recipe* section can remove it.

After getting away from your PCB source, you can begin to remove it from inside your body with the *3-Week Program*.

Many more facts about PCBs can be found in earlier books and on the Internet. Learn all you can.

Benzene Everywhere

Benzene is another immune system destroyer.

Our agencies, FDA and EPA, have been vigilant over benzene in air, household chemicals and even gasoline but were never in a position to test food or water correctly. Using antiquated tests that can only find benzene in parts per billion (ppb) would never protect American citizens. Although the legal limit set by our agencies was 5 ppb, I never detected such huge amounts. Our immunodepression comes from much smaller amounts. We must be protected from parts per trillion (ppt) amounts, a thousand-fold smaller. The entry of benzene into the food chain was not noticed because of this technical problem. Now it is in and on our food in such large amounts, most private testing labs can detect it.

Benzene has become a huge food problem, due to pollution of food with food spray and laundry bleach water. It comes right from your favorite supermarket and organic food store. You must stop using or eating everything that has benzene.

The body does not have a "safe amount" of benzene. But, as more and more benzene gets discovered in food, the public agencies will shift their focus to higher "safe" amounts. Beware of such a shift and a shift in wording, such as "no significant risk level". This is a deception. It leads to complacency over a very important problem. It will raise our cancer and AIDS incidence still higher. The focus should stay on <u>zero</u> amounts as it presently is.

You must clean all your fruits and vegetables a special way to remove the food spray and bleach-water residues that bring benzene. It is described in the *Recipes* chapter. It does not <u>all</u> come this way, though.

Benzene also enters our food with flavors, colors and fragrance. It enters with pills, whether they are over the counter drugs, food supplements, or prescriptions. Flavors and colors were extracted and manufactured with solvents that came from the petroleum industry, including benzene. It was falsely believed that you could easily evaporate it off. And certainly, enough came off to come under the "limit" of detection for the measuring device. But it only gave us false security.

There are more ways that petroleum products come in contact with food. For example, the grain[*] stored in elevators that will make your bread is doused with "mineral oil" to keep the dust down. It all has traces of benzene. And wherever petroleum grease is used—like in baking pans under cookies and breads—benzene rides along. It may be surprising to find benzene in so many places where the temperature was raised above its boiling point; that is no safeguard. It was evidently trapped or it recondensed.

The attitude of manufacturers and producers is: "You can <u>expect</u> benzene to be everywhere. It's even in the air and the blacktop in your driveway. It's negligible. As long as we meet FDA & EPA requirements, where's the problem?" This reminds me of an event in history, about 350 years ago.

In 1665, the worst year of the bubonic plague in England, the grain that made peoples' bread was contaminated with rat feces and rat urine. It was everywhere in small amounts. You could not smell it or see it because the grain was ground finely into flour. It was not suspected to bring the bubonic disease

---

[*] Search "Grain Dust Explosions" on Internet.

since the sick and the healthy people all ate it. From this terrible tragedy we should have learned one lesson: When widespread illness comes to people we should examine our staple foods first, our bread and water, milk and meat. Bacteria and viruses certainly play their roles, but the vermin bringing them and toxins supporting them should be searched for in food before air and driveways.

Benzene has been known to cause cancer for decades, especially the leukemias. That is why our agencies were given the important task of monitoring it. Yet they have failed to protect us, setting and raising legal levels instead. We have more leukemia than ever before. Why should benzene be legally permitted in beer when half the men are getting cancer? Regulations should not be based on tests done solely on the food later on, when the concentration will, of course, be less, making it all the more difficult to detect, but rather on knowledge of "what goes in".

In a desperate England in 1665, rats were so numerous they crawled the streets openly. How could tiny bits of rat filth in the bread matter? It was everywhere. Besides, bread was baked, that should make it safe. The same "logic" was used then as now. We see people with and without cancer all around us drinking the same water. And it is all chlorinated, that should make it safe. The concepts are flawed. Eventually, instead of killing rats, dogs and cats were removed in England, precisely those animals that could reduce disease, an easy mistake to make when you're just guessing. We should not be guessing. We have scientists. We should be using them. We are only using medical professionals now. We need physiologists, biologists, parasitologists, cytologists, ecologists, when studying a difficult problem. Instead, physiology departments at universities were closed in the 1960's. In the present day USA we are increasing and emphasizing the chlorination of water…the very treatment that is inadvertently doing the most harm.

We should be testing our food and water with the best equipment, of research quality. But we can't expect industry to create high standards for itself. Society must create them independently. Besides, we should not trust corporate testing nor agency testing when their personnel frequently "trade jobs". We must solve the problem of conflicts of interest. We must put renewed energy into parents' and society's responsibility to provide safe food and water for our children— safe from benzene and PCBs at least. Children are most affected by leukemia.

Our white blood cells stop eating anything after they get benzene onto their membranes. The membranes are made of fat, a double layer of it. One of benzene's actions is to let viruses into our genome. A special enzyme called **viral integrase** allows this whenever benzene is present. Oncoviruses lurk everywhere, even in our daily bread (RAS), but would not be allowed in if this integrase were not made for them with the permission of benzene.

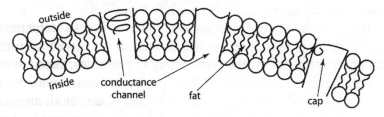

Fig. 72 Diagram of cell membrane structure

Your body has a moderate ability to get rid of benzene without help. Benzene leads to pain and bleeding. Learn how to prevent this in Chapter 15, on page 351.

Asbestos in our Food and Water

We have been so focused on asbestos in walls and ceilings that we missed the most obvious places, food and water. Not being able to detect the smaller fibers (under 10 μm), while these are actually the most harmful and numerous, made the agencies' regulations almost useless. A microscope should have been used and developed into an automated technique.

207

When the tiniest bit of asbestos is put in water, all the water around it becomes southerly-polarized. When a tiny bit gets stuck in your tissue, the surrounding fluid, blood, and tissue become southerly. This is the trigger felt by the hypothalamus in the brain, telling it to release its stem cell factor. The message received could be imagined as "*Iron has been oxidized to south pole; this organ is surely traumatized and open to air, it will be in need of growth to repair the trauma*". Your body cannot be expected to know this is a false alarm. We did not evolve with asbestos in our food or water to make it wary.

But at the same time, your white blood cells sense the truth: "there is a strange intruder; something needs to be eaten; it is not a mere trauma", and begin to eat the flood of asbestos that is arriving. It is followed by drastically unhappy results! Asbestos is made of tiny spears, each with built-in iron! When these tiny spears are eaten by a white blood cell, a lot of iron, of the south pole kind, has entered the white cells. A gene is now triggered to produce **ferritin** because ferritin is the storage molecule for iron. It is the body's way to safely store such iron. Soon an excessive amount of ferritin is produced; so much, it oozes out of the white blood cells and coats their outside membrane. This ferritin coating acts like an oil slick over the immune cells and stops them immediately from eating more asbestos or anything else. They can't see. They can't sense.

Fortunately, we can wash the asbestos off our food if we use the same special hot washes described for PCBs and benzene in the *Recipes* chapter. After this we can use a special chemical, **levamisole**, to remove the ferritin coating from the white blood cells. But cleaning our drinking water would require filtering.

The asbestos in water has not gone undetected. Water is said to have asbestos in it from old clay pipes used to bring it from the water reservoir. Read the pamphlet you get from your water department about asbestos. This could make anyone despair. But the Syncrometer® shows it never comes from the reservoir, even with these old clay pipes. It comes from the same pumping station where the wrongful bleach is added! The bleach itself had it. Perhaps gaskets from the pumps there had it, too. However, bleach of the correct kind (NSF-stamped) does not have asbestos. Nor does water that is treated with NSF-bleach.

There are huge amounts of asbestos on our food, both fruits and vegetables. Being sprayed with bleach-water (laundry bleach) is a common practice to guarantee safety from bacteria. This brings asbestos with it and also wets the food as it rolls along conveyor belts. Conveyor belts are made with asbestos. Old frayed belts add huge amounts to the food, all to be tightly stuck as the produce dries under hot-air blowers. That is why 2 hot washes are needed to remove it.

When asbestos has left your organs, along with nickel and wheel bearing grease, they become north polarized again.

Remember that south polarization is not to be demonized. It is reserved for the nervous system by day and the body's growing and healing points at all times. The blood, though, swings from northerly to southerly and back again, minute by minute.

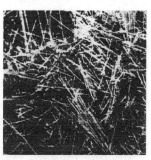

Fig. 73 Asbestos spears magnified

Work is being done here that is still quite mysterious. It is an exchange of iron status, using iridium. And the white blood cells cycle from northerly to southerly and back again, too, with every toxic load they process and shed. You will get back these normal rhythms, and get back to a normal life when the polarizations are correct.

Dyes Stick Fast

Why are young children eating colored candy, colored drinks, colored cakes, and colored pieces of ornamental sugar on their food?

209

Even the most primitive cook knows, and has always known, that food is off limits to tampering. Food is not a frivolous part of life. And paint may go <u>on</u> the body, temporarily, for dances, but not <u>in</u> the body. Such instincts are especially applied to children. Parents, throughout the ages, have seen to it that young children got <u>no</u> tampering.

Why have our instincts gone astray? Did we all feel safe in the care of our government agencies the way children feel safe with their parents while they take risks? Did we believe that enough scientific experiments would have been done and long-term tests required, preventing any catastrophe from ever happening? As food dyes, one by one, were removed from the food market in the 1960s, after a big increase in the cancer rate, we should have become suspicious of other dyes taking their place and of agencies in general. But as a nation of eager consumers, we did not.

Agencies are not all the same. Cautious agents who put the people's health first can be followed by agents who put other motives first. It will take <u>people's groups</u>, who are made up of real parents, not government agencies, to take back control over food and water safety. Agencies have too many conflicting interests. When any piece of meat, chicken or fish has azo dyes, and even the <u>colored</u> produce is dyed, food tampering is at an extreme. It is no wonder that every tumor tested showed the presence of a multitude of dyes. The implication is quite grim…that we have hundreds and more dyes accumulated in all of us. One dye is always present in cancer patients—Fast Green #3 (also called Food Green)[*]. The Syncrometer® detects that it lengthens the life of cells that absorb it, although they become nonfunctional. Life is extended up to 15 times! It is acting just like the gang of oncoviruses! Cancer cells that would have, at least, died at their usual time, are now not able to turn on their own apoptosis. We have already seen oncoviruses doing exactly that. The

---

[*] This is Fast Green FCF with color index (CI)-42053. Search Fast Green, FCF on Internet.

longevity gene, bcl-2, is much too active. This gene is a major controller of apoptosis.

Normal Longevity

Two genes, bcl-2 and bax, have a big role in deciding how long each one of our cells may live. They keep a balance between living too long or too short. The longevity gene is bcl-2, while bax shortens life by triggering apoptosis. A mutation could easily affect these genes, to tip the results in favor of one or the other. We could have suspected dyes since they were found to cause mutations in the past and cancer is always associated with mutations. Why haven't these dye-caused mutations been found in regular research? Research choices are partly economically and partly politically made. Parents would make different choices. The Syncrometer® sees Fast Green dye concentrated in our CD8 natural killer cells. The cells remain quite alive after this, in increased numbers, but not able to kill anything. Food Green is another name for Fast Green #3. It has accumulated in every USA cancer patient I tested. In the *3-Week Program* we will get the dye out with homeography after the dye sources have been removed.

Laundry bleach water contains large amounts of many dyes, although they are invisible. Hundreds of dyes are contained in sprays and essentially all food is sprayed. It is even on our undyed food because laundry bleach disinfectant is used in washing it. It is even on freshly caught fish if the knives and cutting boards are disinfected with laundry bleach. I recently visited a fisherman's booth near a beach in Mexico. The freshly caught fish were whole and laid on ice. We saw the fisherman take his knife from a bucket of "water" and swish his table with a jug of "water". In a corner, on the floor, was a gallon of laundry bleach. I bought a filleted fish and an unrinsed whole fish off the ice. I tested each. The fillets were full of dyes and hypochlorite (the telltale sign of chlorination). A piece of washed fish, not filleted, was full of dyes, too. Only the unwashed whole fish was safe to eat. There is evidently no safe fish in the market place. The Syncrometer® showed that canned fish, frozen fish and fresh fish were all processed with laundry bleach. This food cannot be cleaned up.

Wherever there is organic matter, dyes are absorbed deeply, the same way as in your tumor cells. They were invented to do exactly that—to persist (not fade).

Dyes do very damaging things. DAB is 4-dimethylaminoazobenzene. This dye raises the **alkaline phosphatase** level. Check yours on your blood test results. DAB has filled the white blood cells. When it is too low, threatening organ failure, it is due to Fast Garnet and Sudan Black, together with cobalt. When dyes are in your B-lymphocytes the globulin level is disturbed. Sudan Black B and Fast green can raise your LDH. Check yours. It will be in the red blood cells, stuck there sometimes with vanadium. High LDH and alk phos are drastic events in terminal cancer patients. When LDH and alkaline phosphatase levels have gone over 500 or even 1000 it has been speculated about in clinical science but no true cause found or pursued. The Syncrometer® shows only these dyes and heavy metals are responsible for these high numbers. When they are removed by homeography, both blood tests come down to normal in days. There is a lot of dye stowed away in these cells. Fast Red and Fast Red Violet cause edema and effusates to develop in the lungs or brain or abdomen. This is a common cause of death for these cancers! Fast Red Violet blocks the body's ability to detoxify **maleic anhydride**. It has been known for decades that this substance causes "leakage and effusions" (see The Merck Index, 10 edition). The maleic anhydride comes from the malonic acid in food sprays, in cooking oils, and tooth fillings, and from plastic seepage from your dishes, but mostly from your laundry bleached water. The body has a route for detoxifying it, but not if a dye blocks this (see page 367).

I have studied only seven of many dyes in our food. They need to be studied in all our diseases. The cancer patient must carefully remove all dyes from fruits and vegetables although they are invisible. It is done the same way as removing PCBs, benzene and asbestos—with hot washes. It will be described in

Recipes. Every molecule of dye matters because it prevents recovery of the immune system!

The extent of pollution with dyes is almost unimaginable. Here is a real example. Recently a one-mile stretch of ocean beach was being prepared for a beach festival in California. Regular ocean water samples were taken and found to have some E. coli bacteria, not uncommon in these waters. The Navy forces were called in to make the beach safe. Soon the ocean was pink! The Syncrometer® detected common laundry bleach and many dyes in it. Apparently the Navy poured in bleach, but also added red dye to mark the area that was treated—we tested the pink water. It looked intensely pink for about ½ mile offshore, and lasted for about one week. The public was informed that it was due to "red tide", certain algae! All the azo dyes in my test kit (18) were in the water, including Fast Green, no doubt a pollutant of the red dye and in the laundry bleach. The dye did not go away; it sank to the bottom of the ocean and could be seen for 2 years afterwards in shallow areas. It will bring immunodepression and growth of tumors to fish, sea mammals and shore birds (see page 369 for the eventual outcome).

Modern enamel cookware seeps huge amounts of dyes. Your toothbrush seeps copious dyes. Your plastic glasses and wristwatch seep. Your plastic teeth seep dyes. That is why the extremely advanced cancer patient is told to use NOTHING, wear NOTHING, apply NOTHING, unless tested by Syncrometer®. The plastic teeth will be hardened.

After stopping eating them and absorbing them we can begin to pull the dyes out of your tumors. We will use 2 supplements (vitamin B_2 and coenzyme Q10), round after round of zapping, and finally homeography. But the fear is that the dyes will get stuck again in your kidneys or liver along the exit path. Be sure to keep the bowels moving and the bladder emptying. Be sure to keep taking homeographic drops that protect the kidneys. We must find the dyes in the urine before we know we are succeeding.

213

Heavy Metals in Water and Food

Metals are the fifth and last category of toxins that disable your immune system. This means destroying the ability of your white blood cells to find, pursue, eat and kill your oncoviruses, bacteria, yeasts and even tumor cells. They have a huge task.

Nowhere in animal bodies do we see shiny metals taking part in the growth of an organ or even just being present. Nowhere in the vegetable world, either, do we see bare metal becoming part of a plant. Yet these same shiny metals can be changed by chemistry to another form, called **organic**. Atoms of the metal can be tightly held by special proteins to make **enzymes**. Now they are called **minerals**, not metals, although the elements are the same. Some metals are never changed into minerals: uranium, palladium, and the lanthanides, for example. Find these in the Periodic Table. Lead, antimony, cadmium, aluminum are further examples. The lanthanides were called "rare earths" until recently. There are 15 of them in

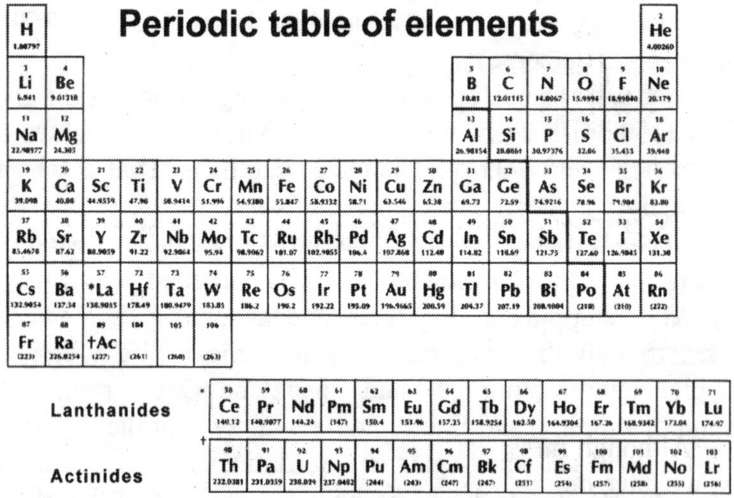

Fig. 74 Periodic table of elements

a group specially marked on the chemical table. They are more magnetic than other metals, though not as strong as iron. They always occur together and can hardly be separated, even with

214

strong chemistry. Thulium, gadolinium and lanthanum are all lanthanides. There must be some very important reason for Mother Nature to keep certain metals and the lanthanides out of our bodies. Are they too oxidizing? Would they compete with other minerals? Would they disturb our magnetic polarization? The real reasons will not be known till biologists have uncovered many more secrets of life, including electronic and magnetic phenomena. Till then, Mother Nature gave us instinct. Metal does not taste good or feel good; the implication is that we should not eat it or wear it on our skin even though we don't drop dead when we do. Nature's rules have millions of years of wisdom behind them. But she could not anticipate "civilization", which should perhaps be labeled "regression", quite often. Metal did <u>look</u> good, with its sparkle and its shine. We fell in love with them, too.

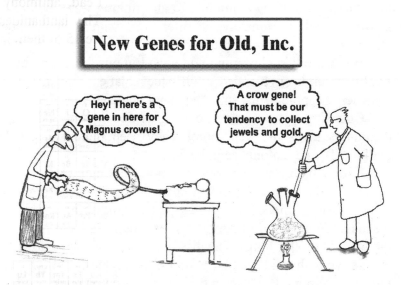

Although metals are safe deep in the earth, far away from us, we have dug them up, thrown them in the air just for thrills (firecrackers on the 4th of July in the USA fill the air with strontium). We have puffed them into the air as car exhaust, wrapped them around ourselves to wear, stuck them inside ourselves as rings, cooked in them and, finally, put them right in our food. We wallow in metal. Aluminum, an unthinkable metal, found nowhere in living things, was actually dumped into our food in the 1880s and has been there ever since. The "invention", called baking powder, was none other than adding aluminum to a liquid; it

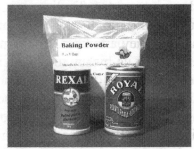

Fig. 75 Aluminum-free baking powder

bubbled! That is how non-yeast-rising breads were born. Now that Alzheimer's disease is rampant with its accumulation of aluminum in the brain, and Herpes and EBV (chronic fatigue) very common, this practice should be re-examined as well as the practice of adding aluminum to all drinking water before it is disinfected. Fortunately, it filters out with a homemade charcoal filter or charcoal pitcher filter.

We wallow in chromium and nickel in our food. Anything finely ground or blended with steel blades that get hot (powdered supplements, smooth peanut butter) brings them.

Choosing plastic, ceramic or glass cookware and food containers gives us even more! They seep mercury, nickel, thallium(!), and malonic acid, besides.

Teflon and glass seep copious amounts of thallium.

Yet, what could be worse than eating metals from our plastic dishes, and copper water pipes? One thing! Sucking metals straight, like lollipops, in your mouth day and night in the form of tooth fillings. The dissolved metal sweeps into your tonsils, your thyroid gland, parathyroids, thymus, and directly into your tumors. If we see a child sucking on pennies or other change we quickly snatch it away…we instinctively know it is harmful. There are about 50 metals in each such tooth-lollipop (see page 328). How could we blunder so badly as adults? Your body is barely able to keep up with the heavy metals left behind by its own enzymes, let alone added ones from tooth fillings. Those from enzymes of all sorts are copper, cobalt, chromium, vanadium, gold, germanium, molybdenum, ruthenium, rubidium, selenium, manganese, zinc, iron and nickel. They are not necessarily from our own enzymes. They are left in us by fungus and bacteria. This will give us some astonishing insights. These metals steal our youth, our health, and our destiny (longevity) as they slowly accumulate with age. If they accumulate suddenly, we are in a crisis—a disease like cancer. If they accumulate slowly, we believe we are aging and accept it meekly. They are our "natural" heavy metals, coming from living matter (living in us!). Obviously, we should not eat more of them to hasten our end.

Copper from water pipes often brings lead, too, from the solder joints. If lead and copper are detected by a Syncrometer® tester or even a water lab, change your pipes to PVC or have them epoxy coated on the inside (see *Sources*).

Natural Heavy Metals

How could a heavy metal be natural? Is it not always toxic? It comes from our worn out enzymes. Each enzyme has a mineral inside itself. When the enzyme has lived its lifespan, it gets digested. First it is tagged with a substance called **ubiquitin** so your own digestive enzymes make no mistakes. But the mineral itself is not digestible; it is left behind in a little deposit, like we leave bones and peelings on our dinner plate. It can't be used again, at least not by us. It must now be called a metal, quite toxic, although it is formed naturally, just by living, right in our own bodies. We dispose of them through the intestine and with the urine, but fungus and bacteria could find them first!

Some minerals, like iron, are partly salvaged by our **reducing** chemistry and seemingly, by iridium.

Nickel, vanadium, gold and ruthenium have a different history. They do not belong to our bodies. They belong to primitive life forms, like yeast, bacteria, fungus and parasites that use them in their enzymes, but live in us. Nickel is built into their **urease** enzyme.

Primitive life is necessary to keep <u>our</u> lives possible. We must not undervalue them. They eat filth, such as ammonia (the vapor of urine). Ammonia is toxic to more recent life forms like us. Yet we make it, too, as a byproduct of our own life processes. We and other mammals have a set of enzymes with the special job of changing all ammonia quickly to **urea**, which is not toxic. Two ammonia molecules are turned into one urea molecule when the **urea synthesis cycle** is at work. The liver and kidneys make most of it. Our eliminations and excretions then get rid of the urea. And there is always a bit left in the blood, called BUN on the blood test. For bacteria and fungus to "clean up", namely feed on, animal excretions in Nature, in the fields and streams, their urease enzyme must go to work to break these urea molecules apart again, back to ammonia. This gives it all a stench and we sense its presence so we can stay away from it. But the ammonia provides valuable nitrogen for them, making their life possible. The element nickel is present in each urease molecule. It is their key to survival.

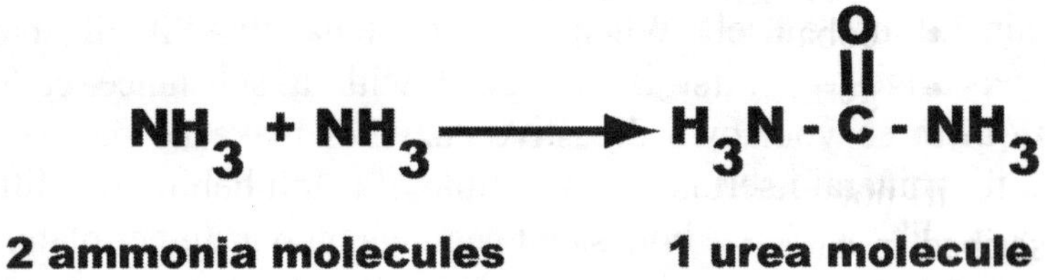

$$NH_3 + NH_3 \longrightarrow H_3N - \overset{\displaystyle O}{\overset{\displaystyle \|}{C}} - NH_3$$

2 ammonia molecules   **1 urea molecule**

Fig. 76 Making urea

Our intestines are always full of bacteria, dead and alive, good and bad, feeding on the leftovers of our digestion. As they die, nickel is left behind, to be picked up by their successors. Gold, in the case of Salmonellas, is recycled the same way. Competitors can snatch away metals left by others. Prions and the HIV virus snatch their daily requirement of gold away from Salmonella this way.

So just by the very act of harboring other creatures in us, we become a repository of all their natural metals. The harm that is done by nickel alone, besides inviting infection, is major. It consumes our <u>iridium</u> and it turns us southerly! Iridium levels fall very low wherever nickel deposits are seen. A tumor, due to its stockpile of nickel, cannot salvage its iron deposits and make it usable again. There is an iridium shortage. Yet, the iron ferrite, Fe_2O_3, deposits must be cleared away somehow to get the tumor zone back to a northerly polarization.

> Nickel turns us southerly.

Healing cannot go forward because of low usable iridium levels. A very low level of 29 is reached (in homeopathic units of 1 in 5 dilution) for iridium near a tumor. Levels in the 80's are normal, and a level of 120 is seen in young children.

Each of us, whether sick or healthy, is full of heavy metals by the time we are old. But it is not a random assortment of heavy metals. It is always these:

- chromium
- copper
- cobalt
- germanium
- nickel
- selenium
- vanadium

Is it not astonishing that these are the same metals described in earlier books to be the common denominators of tumors?

The body's metals in cancer, in disease, and in aging are the same ones, having become oxidized, left behind by dead enzymes of our own and from our invaders. The tumor cells are unable to reverse the process to make organic minerals again and reclaim them. Nor can healthy bodies do this as we age. We just can't keep up with this part of our housekeeping (body maintenance) chores. Copper turns us brown in spots, cobalt gives us heart disease, vanadium and germanium give us mutations, chromium gives us blood sugar problems, gold gives us ovary disease and obesity, nickel brings us immune depression with more and more infection, gray hair, baldness, and allergies. Yet, none of this seems necessary! It should be avoidable!

Metals are required by our parasites, bacteria, and even viruses and prions. They fuel our diseases.

> Illness, including cancer, is metal disease. We should fall out of love with metals.

It makes sense, now, that a few people got cancer as long ago as prehistoric times. It does not <u>require</u> civilization with its <u>novel</u> toxins. It is the <u>same</u> toxins as we always had, but which we failed to respect and now inundate us. We failed to respect them when making our cookware, food containers, jewelry and dentalware. Nor did we develop good body-housekeeping habits. We should be routinely removing these throughout life.

It seems even more astonishing that this set of natural metals includes the same elements that sift down on us day and night from outer space. With one difference! From space they already are in a novel reduced "organic" form. Missing are nickel, gold, aluminum, lead, mercury, thallium, thulium, rhodium...the nonhuman ones. Space minerals seem ready for <u>us</u>. And already packaged in assortments easily attached to our stem cell factor! Are we somehow missing a cosmic connection to our very lives? Which one of the space items brings them? Or is it all simply bacterial matter from earth...dust mixed with organic matter, like carbon monoxide? Bacteria would have brought nickel. Dust would have brought aluminum. Only more research can answer this.

Back in Time

A few thousand years ago there was an occasional case of cancer. How could that happen if laundry bleach is an essential part of the causation now? We should look at the ingredients of this bleach to see which of these could have been in the environment of a few people long ago.

PCBs seem most unlikely. Asbestos seems very unlikely, too. But benzene can come from natural sources—the parasite

220

Paragonimus is followed by a fungus that uses vanadium and makes zearalenone (Chaetomium). Zearalenone is changed to benzene on its detoxification route, according to the Syncrometer®, and described in earlier books. That could provide one of the 5 immunity destroyers.

Could dyes have been an immunodepressant thousands of years ago? The dye industry was thriving in the Middle East in biblical times.

In the past, heavy metals, especially ferrite iron (Fe_2O_3) could have entered the water in some places bringing south polarization to it. Uranium could have been in the water naturally in some places. With two or three of the 5 immunity destroyers available to ancient society, occasional cancers could be expected.

Immunodepression results from any <u>one</u> of the 5 kinds of toxins. These specifically block some part of our white blood cells' protective behavior. Protection from parasitism is a major part.

We must hurry, and we must stay focused on the 5 immunity destroyers as top priority in our health goal for society. It means our chief goal is clean water, tested for these five by Syncrometry, as soon as this technology is automated. It should be tested as it <u>leaves</u> the pump house <u>every day</u>.

Present day dentalware puts a large stockpile of unnatural heavy metals, like cerium, titanium, uranium, mercury, into your mouth besides the natural ones. They are sucked on constantly as fillings, retainers, bridges and crowns. While you are young and strong the dissolved metal will be taken to the kidneys and liver to be removed. But later it gets left in little deposits along the way. It gets left in your brain, your eyes, your nerves, your lungs, bones, colon, kidneys, prostate and any organ you are able to test! I have estimated about 1000 deposits of mercury alone that can be readily demonstrated by Syncrometer®.

Check your Metal Damage

Copper takes part in angiogenesis, the making of extra blood vessels. Copper is needed and is constantly recycled by Penicillium fungus that grows in us if we supply it. Together with Aspergillus, which needs cobalt, chromium and nickel, they are quick to take over a dead Fasciolopsis buski or Fasciola fluke. This is why we use so many digestive enzymes in our *3-Week Program*—to digest the dead flukes <u>before</u> they can grow this fungus. Both kinds of fungus make aflatoxins. In the liver aflatoxins block detoxification of hemoglobin so the bilirubin goes up (check your blood test). The Syncrometer® sees that the **bilirubin oxidase** enzyme is missing. This is how we get **jaundice**, a frequent cause of death for cancer patients. The cancer is not involved in your jaundice. Hurry to chelate out the copper, cobalt, chromium and nickel, or take each one out homeographically. Of course, getting chelation hardly makes sense when you have copper water pipes and metal teeth. Change pipes to PVC and have metal in teeth removed. Changing to plastic water pipes will get rid of lead, too, another big help for the liver.

Cobalt is especially attracted to tumors which motivated the development of Cobalt 60 radiation decades ago. Cobalt inhibits our basic metabolism, the glycolysis part, just what was found by scientists to start tumors 70 years ago! A <u>low</u> LDH or a <u>low</u> alkaline phosphatase in your blood test reflects on your slow metabolism, due to cobalt toxicity. It may be in the liver, RBCs, platelets, WBCs (CD4s, CD14s). Check yours. Cobalt affects red blood cells so they can't carry much oxygen. This could be why it is the main heart toxin, too.

Vanadium causes p53 gene mutations and lost regulation over albumin and globulin production. Check your blood test. Vanadium raises the RBC, the B-cells (so they make too much globulin), and the CD8s. It is required by E. coli, our worst enemy in cancer illness. It is also needed by Flu viruses.

Germanium, the metal, removes a block on mutations that organic germanium had put in place to protect us. Now the effects of vanadium are greater. The metal form accumulates in the spleen.

Chromium, along with nickel, has been rated as a top metallic carcinogen (cancer-causer) for decades. Its deposits accumulate in the intestine wall to feed the yeasts there. It feeds staphylococcus and streptococcus bacteria, besides yeast. Possibly for this reason staph, streps and yeast are often seen together in tumors, especially in breast cancer. In "well" people it causes overweight and high blood sugar. Check yours.

Nickel supplies bacteria and fungus with their needed element to make the urease enzyme. It accumulates in the prostate and in the scalp at the hair roots! The prostate and scalp get infected and inflamed. The scalp goes bald and the prostate enlarges from chronic inflammation. The prostate invites parasites from the nearby colon and cancer has its opportunity.

Not much is known about the specific actions of unnatural metals.

Mercury , like dyes, gets stuck in the WBCs. Then they are immediately prevented from killing anything even though they manage to eat them. CD4s, your virus eaters are especially vulnerable to mercury and thallium. CD8s often eat these disabled CD4s. Then they get stuck with the mercury, themselves, Soon invaders gain the upper hand in your body due to widespread immunodepression from mercury.

Tungsten, platinum, palladium and the remainder are not yet studied. Cadmium is easily found in the kidneys of every high blood pressure victim. Aluminum is found in abdominal and Hodgkin's tumors, by Syncrometer®, and in lymph in EBV illness, besides in Alzheimer's disease.

The lanthanide elements are especially toxic. They have only been in commerce since World War II and are already deposited in us. They are **paramagnetic** and have the effect of changing DNA timing in our bodies. Much is already known about the lanthanides (see the book pictured). DNA timing is discussed in the *Syncrometer® Science Laboratory Manual*.

Gold accumulates in ovarian cysts, the hypothalamus (in obesity) and pancreas. Gold feeds our Salmonella bacteria (S. typhimurium and S. enteriditis). It even supplies our prions! How do they use it? Prions are on the upswing and will lead to BSE and CJD (Bovine Spongiform Encephalopathy and Creutzfeldt-Jakob disease), if not controlled by us. We should stay far away from gold, in or on our bodies.

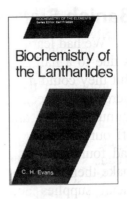

ISBN-0-306-43176-9

Fig. 77 Lanthanides disrupt fundamental biological processes

Strontium, a most unsuspected metal appears to be used by a number of our hardiest invaders: Streptococcus pneumoniae, our pain causer, Cytomegalovirus (CMV), Mycobacterium avium/cellulare, even SV 40 and HIV (in reverse transcriptase enzyme). Strontium has become ubiquitous in our environment. Why? It is in all bodies of water. Why? It is in air. Why? It is even in 2 natural foods, corn and honey. These foods also bring beryllium, another air pollutant, perhaps from airplane fuel. Sick people should not eat these.

Ruthenium, another unsuspected metal, feeds our Salmonella bacteria, the scourge of both AIDS and cancer patients. It comes attached to activated charcoal and is in distilled water. That is why carbon filters, even though disinfected with NSF bleach, must be boiled 5 minutes and cleaned regularly.

We have gained an arsenal of knowledge that can be put to use to defeat illnesses that are due to metal toxicities. We can go back to stopping sickness again. And we will stop it by depriving the bacteria and viruses of their essential food (metals). Their essential foods are our toxicities! How fortunate for us.

Banish Sickness Again

We had learned that feeling sick is not due to the cancer. It is due to a half dozen well known bacteria and their viruses. But they could not be identified or killed the usual way. They were given special rights by their own viruses, to evade our immune system and invade our organ cells. Their genes turn off our apoptosis and make our cells multiply faster. But we had found their vulnerability...they still need their metals to make their enzymes! It will be a simple matter to cut off their metal supplies and get relief from sweats, fever, coughs, bloating, organ failures, deep pain, and plain sickness in less than a week. Here are their daily requirements. Items in italics need further confirmation.

Pathogen's Daily Requirements

(items in italics need confirmation)	
Adenovirus	
Aspergillus (fungus)	cobalt, chromium, nickel
Chaetomium (fungus)	strontium
Clostridium	nickel, *cobalt*
Cytomegalovirus(CMV)	strontium
E. coli	vanadium, molybdenum, manganese, chromium, nickel
Epstein Barre Virus (EBV)	aluminum
Flu (Influenza A & B)	vanadium
Herpes I & II	lead
HIV	gold (attached to core) strontium (attached to reverse transcriptase)
Mumps	manganese, copper, zinc
Mycobacterium avium/cellulare	strontium, vanadium
Mycobacterium tuberculosis	strontium
Mycoplasma	strontium
Norcardia (Parkinson's)	titanium, *tantalum*
Penicillium (fungus)	copper
Pneumocystis (coccidia)	strontium
Prions	gold, *ruthenium*
Pseudomonas aeruginosa	strontium, gold

Salmonella enteriditis	gold, ruthenium, molybdenum
Salmonella typhimurium	gold, ruthenium, molybdenum
Salmonella paratyphi	gold, ruthenium, molybdenum, rubidium
Staphylococcus aureus	chromium
Streptococcus G	chromium, vanadium, nickel
Streptococcus pneumoniae	chromium, strontium
SV 40	chromium, strontium, gold
Yeast (bread and alcohol)	chromium, nickel, cobalt

Fig. 78 Our pathogens' daily requirements

We had learned that cancer, feeling sick, and toxicity-disease are 3 separate illnesses. If you have been sent to Hospice and can hardly endure living, a loved one can still rescue you. You may have all the symptoms mentioned in *Sickness Be Gone* (page 157). But you can banish them all in this simple way:

Eat no metals, drink no metals, wear no metals.

This means, move to an NSF-bleach water zone. Find a local distilled water in a 1 gallon bottle that tests zero with a conductivity indicator. Filter this distilled water twice through a filter pitcher that you harden yourself and has charcoal that you boiled for 5 minutes in tap water. Make sure it delivers water with none of the metals given in the pathogens' requirements table (page 225). If possible, test by Syncrometer®. Beware of simple human errors like wearing earrings, a necklace or watch. Drink this chlorine-free water and cook with it. Improvements begin in 2 days.

As soon as you get relief from illness, although some pain persists, get all metal removed from your mouth by extraction. Harden the plastic in your mouth to stop metal seepage, using a toothbrush zappicator. Eat or store food in non seeping plastic.

Then start DMSO in tiny doses ($\frac{1}{8}$ to ¼ tsp.) to excrete wheel bearing grease and all its trapped metals. The lower dose is for the most extreme illness. It should have been tested for thallium. If not available, start the kidney cleanse (page 561).

Keep removing metals with homeographic drops for the kidneys and lymph.

Early success could bring you new hope and soon a goodbye forever to Hospice. They did their best. They are to be commended on carrying on <u>without</u> hope. But your life beckons as you prepare to start the program.

Magnetic Healing

There is much more that is wrong with metals. But form and magnetic properties are everything. In organic mineral form, or with correct magnetic property, a very toxic element can be quite healing.

The commonest metal of all, plain iron, displays this feature the most obviously. It may be the most important actor in our metabolism and also the most important disruptor of metabolism in cancer and many diseases. In illness it has become the victim of other metals' oxidizing actions.

As a mineral, iron is essential. It is in your hemoglobin, for instance. But after it is oxidized (to the ferric form, or to ferrite, Fe_2O_3) it is quite harmful if it accumulates in the wrong place. I believe this is partly because it is so easily magnetized. Any little bit of metallic iron can become strongly magnetized, even if it seems not to be magnetic, like a tack or paper clip. Take the cans on your food shelf for example. They are easily magnetized because they contain iron.

Even the tiniest pin would not stick to a can of food, though, because the can's magnetism is not strong enough. Still, you may be surprised to detect the force yourself with a small compass. Choose a can of food that has sat on the shelf a long time (weeks) with the same end up. Measure it at the top—your compass might find it is actually north pole. Measure it at the bottom, it will be south pole. You may find two places north, side by side, or a north and south pole on the sides, across the can. For every north pole there is a south pole somewhere. Numerous poles are possible, even side by side and upside down. Nearly anything is possible with iron, a

227

situation that the body could never allow for its iron and survive.

The earth's magnetic field magnetized the tin can and does this rather quickly. You can turn the can upside down and a few days later find the poles are reversing! The same thing could happen to iron deposits in you if they were allowed to develop. Your body is not shielded from earth's magnetic field; in fact your body depends on it. Small deposits that are free to turn would behave like compasses. The earth's magnetic field, about ½ gauss, is actually very powerful.

The total amount of iron in the body is quite small (about the size of a pea), probably for this reason…it must be so carefully controlled! Some varieties of iron are obviously magnetic. Others are not. Simple oxidation or reduction, done in a second by your body, can make it non-magnetic or switch its poles, a drastic change. Iron supplies almost half our enzymes and all the hemoglobin in our red blood cells and myoglobin in our muscles. The cytochrome enzymes in every cell and P450 detoxifying enzymes are iron-enzymes. Even the very enzyme that makes DNA from RNA, called **ribonucleotide reductase**, contains iron. Maybe this is the critical iron atom that senses the magnetic field. It's traveling electron has an extra long path to take as it shuttles back and forth to make DNA, long enough to be the sensor, perhaps. Such iron could not be allowed to turn into oxidized form and change its polarity, uncontrolled. Perhaps this is why we have evolved such a good salvaging method for used-up iron. After red blood cells die and abandon their iron or when your enzymes need replacement and abandon theirs, it is quickly salvaged. Special white blood cells shuttle it all into a little ball of protein called ferritin (see also page 208). Inside the ball, it forms a tiny clump of thousands of molecules. Perhaps it can't be magnetized inside this cage. Perhaps the cage is a magnetic shield. The Syncrometer® finds the iron going into this cage to be south polarized but no magnetic field or polarization can be detected from ferritin afterwards. It also finds iridium molecules, the oxidized kind, inside ferritin. Are they sheltered together? Is the iridium reducing the iron back to usable form? Read more about ferritin on the Internet.

When iron is deposited <u>outside</u> of this little living cage it becomes magnetized into a strong south pole. A north pole may be presumed to be present somewhere, but has never been found by Syncrometer®.

The same thing could happen inside your body as happens inside the tin can. The food near the north part of the can will be north polarized. And the food just inside the south part will become south polarized. You cannot see this with a compass or even a magnetometer, but a Syncrometer® finds it easily. It is an <u>effect</u> of the north or south pole force nearby. The molecules have turned in one direction under the influence of the north pole and the other direction under the influence of the south pole. The Syncrometer® distinguishes them. They coincide with the letters d- and l- given to sugars and proteins.

l-molecules of amino acids have north polarization; d-molecules of these same amino acids have south polarization. Sugar molecules seem to have the opposite rule but are much less studied. A mixture of d- and l-, such as in citric acid made in a laboratory has no polarization.

The water surrounding a deposit of iron is given the same magnetic property as the deposit. I called such water north polarized or south polarized earlier (see page 150).

The Syncrometer® finds that an organ with iron deposits becomes south polarized when it should be north polarized. The white blood cells there do the same. When the iron is safely inside ferritin, it does not polarize the region around it, the organ stays north polarized when it should, daytime.

Certain organs are naturally south polarized by day, the whole brain, spinal cord and nerves, for example. The eggs inside the ovary and sperm inside the testis are also south by day.

Organs that are south polarized are capable of experiencing a powerful growing force, as if the ribonucleotide reductase enzyme had been turned on explosively. In the body, growing yeast can turn this enzyme on. When a manufactured

South Pole magnet is used for this, all the doorways into the cells, called channels, are opened allowing them to feed constantly, see page 207. These cells are treated like queen bees or sumo wrestlers.

When nature is in control, the small molecule called stem cell factor arrives at these locations, presumably to stimulate the stem cells into growth and to feed them with all the essential minerals at the same time.

The true nature of the growing force streaming from south pole magnets through water and living matter to produce south polarization is still not clear. Is it simply the opening of all feeding conductance channels? Is it the simultaneous turning on of DNA-manufacture? Is it the arrival of stem cell factor? Is it the bending of light to the right? A study of this force may reveal a fascinating story of how non-chemical life forces are transmitted and maintained.

The body will excrete the iron that was abandoned by cells and didn't get salvaged promptly, even using the nighttime to do this (see nighttime urine, page 192). It evidently is urgent to the body. But if there is an overwhelming amount of south pole iron it can get stuck in the kidneys on its way out. Then the kidneys becomes south polarized. <u>This is the critical damage done to a cancer patient</u>. All cancer patients have disabled kidneys even when nothing appears to be wrong with them.

It could be fixed, though, by removing nickel and supplying iridium. Your job will be to unload the nickel and to convert as much oxidized iron as possible to reduced forms. When this is done your cancer will turn around, bringing back your health and youth.

You now have a map that shows you the scientific path we will take to reach the goal. The goal is a scan or x-ray with the tumor missing, the illness gone, and the toxicity diseases gone. It is a more demanding goal than we had in the advanced cancer book. We were satisfied then with the tumor missing. Notice how many patients were completely surprised even by this. Yet, it should come as no surprise now because it is rational and can be monitored with a Syncrometer®. The various apoptotic steps fall in place and the white blood cells can be seen eating the leftovers.

You are now ready to start the *3-Week Program*, knowing why you are doing everything. And why it has to succeed.

Syncrometer® testers can follow the *Testers Flow Sheet* to help avoid mistakes and speed up the cure.

Summary:

1. The immune system is a vast network of guardian cells, called white blood cells. They have special powers, like traveling wherever they wish, mobilizing other white blood cells to help them, going to conferences at different lymph nodes, and listening to the beat of a different drummer that understands our lives much better than we do…perhaps a magnetic force.

2. In cancer patients many of these white blood cells cannot see, hear or taste; some cannot fight, some cannot travel nor capture trespassers, our invaders. They are disabled. Others are clogged. They had to eat so much motor oil, wheel bearing grease, dyes, and plain rust, they cannot disgorge it all for want of enough organic selenite, vitamin C, germanium and iridium. They are completely loaded, but stuck.

3. Their payloads are south pole materials on delivery to the urine for dumping. Unless they get fed with supplements of organic germanium, selenite and vitamin C, we cannot succeed. They will have to set their cargo free. Although iridium is plentiful in rainwater, and can be drunk there, it is not advisable to take iridium chemicals as supplements. Only Nature, as in rainwater, could be trusted.

4. After feeding our WBCs, we can come to their rescue by removing 5 things, the immunity destroyers. All of these came from the laundry bleached water but also came from other sources. If clean, NSF-bleached water can be found quickly, the chance of recovery is excellent. Otherwise, no matter how good a cure or a clinical remission it is, it will soon

fail again. Moving away from your "Cancer House" is by far the best advice, landing in a good water zone.

5. The *3-Week Program* starts by removing all 5 together, trapped as they are in our wheel bearing grease deposits in the kidneys. Soon the kidneys and their WBCs are able to help clear the rest of the body of its wheel bearing grease and other toxins.

6. Getting the white blood cells to unload the accumulations inside tumors is much faster than relying on huge amounts of supplements.

7. Metals can be divided into natural and unnatural varieties. Natural metals are those used by living things.

8. Metals and minerals are one and the same element, but in different form. When they are used in an enzyme or by a living being they are in organic or mineral form. They are sensitive to strong oxidizers, or high heat cooking, losing their structure, so the element gets oxidized to metal again. Metal forms are toxic to organic forms.

9. We can destroy all our invading bacteria and some viruses by taking away the metals they need to survive. We do not need antibiotics to rid ourselves of pathogens. Starving bacteria and viruses is faster than using medicines or herbs although they should not be condemned. This can deal the final blow to your symptoms of sickness.

10. Removing metals can cure some toxicity diseases, too, like anemia and emphysema. But other toxins, malonic acid and dyes, for example, are responsible for effusions.

11. Healing is not understood but a small beginning has been made. We need our stem cell factor to be devoted to us alone, not cut loose from its master in the brain. We need the correct magnetic polarization. We need iridium and perhaps even a cosmic force. Fortunately, it all happens without our understanding.

CHAPTER 11

3-WEEK CANCER CURING PROGRAM

Seeing the Big Picture

We all carry some of the same parasites that cancer victims have. But they are held in check by our immune system, our white blood cells. <u>You</u> got cancer because your immune system was destroyed by laundry bleach that was added to your drinking water for years. This allowed <u>excess</u> parasitism to develop. It is your highest priority problem to solve. This *3-Week Program* will not work unless you find clean water. The main cancer parasite, Fasciolopsis buski, is only one of a dozen or so that once were rare but now are prevalent. They bring us new bacteria and viruses, their own. We are exposed to the cancer-causing parasites and viruses from the animals around us because they have them. To stop this route of contagion we only need to be more caring. We should protect <u>them</u> from parasitism in order to protect ourselves. We are very thoughtless now.

Even with a moderate degree of parasitism we would not get cancer unless we drink laundry bleached water. Consuming 2 quarts of water a day in your food and beverages would give you 10 ng PCB and 10 ugm benzene daily, if the water had 5 ppt PCB and 5ppb benzene, the legally allowed amounts. It is far too much for nonbiodegradables and xenobiotics.

Having rather large bodies it takes us some time to reach our limit in detoxifying ability and storage capability. Eventually our bodies are teeming with lower life forms that have managed to gain a foothold. Some seem new to us like the parasites but some are old "acquaintances" like E. coli and Salmonella. These are intestinal bacteria, which explains our indigestion, burping, weight gain and loss of energy. It is telling us that they are escaping into our bodies, implying that our immune surveillance has deteriorated. It also implies that they are getting enough of their own essential food factors to thrive, even away from the intestinal tract. We are drinking and eating enough chromium, vanadium, ruthenium, molybdenum and manganese metals and even absorbing enough gold to give them all opportunity to thrive and expand their territory. We cannot guess...because we consider it unthinkable, that our food, water, even dishes are bringing serious toxins like all of these, and even mercury, thallium, motor oil, wheel bearing grease and malonic acid. Now it is understandable that immunity fails; we are poisoning it. Unknowingly, we swallow all toxins blithely, like a dog lapping water from a ditch behind a gas station. For any symptoms we take remedies like antibiotics, antacids, sleep potions, stomach soothers, pain medicine and laxatives. We limp along, doing our best, between stimulants and sedatives. Finally our invaders are so numerous they can form partnerships, exchange DNA and make new hybrids, giving them new characteristics. They bewilder us, leading us to believe they have come from distant lands, or from scheming terrorists, or have evolved from overuse of medicines. But there is no evidence for that. There is evidence for immunity lowering, in Africa and in our cancer explosion. We have allowed ourselves to become an immunodepressed society. That is a public concern, not one to be hushed up or politicized. Average WBC counts have steadily dropped in the last few decades. Labs change their ranges to accommodate to this! The Syncrometer® shows we have burgeoning populations of parasites, bacteria and viruses and ever rising levels of toxicities that nurture them. Altogether they lead to new diseases, based on both infections and toxicities. Their paths become linked.

We must hurry to repair our immunodepressed state. It may not merely have short term effects like cancer, AIDS, and new diseases; it could have long term consequences that can be passed to our babies, to be born with parasitism and toxicities already started. Then it would appear to be genetic and lead us down yet more blind alleys.

You as an individual cancer victim can do nothing to undo society's immunodepression. But you can take yourself out of its trap and rescue yourself. Then you can help your family and friends.

If you have early cancer it will be quite easy to succeed and when the cancer marker or doctor says you are "in remission" you might think you cured it. But you did not. Not unless you reversed your immunodepression. The marker and tumors may be gone, but the new varieties of bacteria and viruses together with your toxicities will stay on. Getting rid of the tumor is not the same as curing the disease. A new round of cancer must follow.

If you have very advanced and terminal cancer you will need to do everything, not missing a step: cure the cancer, kill the bacteria and viruses and get rid of your toxicities.

It is these most advanced and terminal victims that I have challenged with this 3 week program. If you have been given your hospice "ticket" but can still eat and expel, this program is for you. It is compatible with any clinical treatment and other health program if you are creative about diet and lifestyle. Listen to the voices of love and life around you. Then do your best to stay with them.

Doing the Program

If you do each step of this program with precision you can expect <u>more</u> than a 95% success rate. This is almost equivalent to a guarantee. But the more advanced you are the less forgiving the program will be. You cannot skip steps or swallow even one bleach-polluted supplement a day without destroying the guarantee. You cannot <u>wash</u> yourself or your food or clothing in PCB-polluted water or drink even one cup. Then you would also have to be lucky instead of certain. Substitutions, additions and subtractions from the program do lower the success rate. Asking a therapist to administer the program for you lowers the success rate. Your life is worth your own, personal investment of time. Time would be minimized if you could be plunked into a safe environment with safe food, free of your antigens. I encourage such enterprises.

As you proceed with this program don't get caught in the realm of unrealistic dreams. Wake yourself up before it is too late. You should be improving with this program. If you are feeling worse, be sure to rescue yourself first from simple mistakes. Actively treat your detox-illness, or bloating and bowel bacteria, or pain, or water holding and swelling of feet. Do not assume "it is your cancer spreading" when it is actually your bacteria spreading. They belong to the infections and toxicities, not the cancer. You can eliminate them. And pay much more attention to <u>preventing</u> detox-illness and bad digestion than you had thought necessary. If you are not seeing any improvements, choose a different path. Do more. Improve your compliance. It would be wiser to give up a body part in surgery than your life, even if you will miss it later. Never punish yourself for making such a decision.

Cancer is your newest challenge. If you choose only the clinical path, what is your life expectancy? Will you be caught in another unrealistic dream? Read statistics. Discuss them with your doctor if you can. Read all the books you can get your hands on. Discuss these, too, if you can, remembering they appear as competitors to your doctors. Discuss them with others who already <u>have</u> experience. Do more than you need to. Don't be satisfied with luck. Ask for help through rough spots. Don't cut any corners. Be very patient with friends and family. They do mean well. But your life is your own and you must fight for it. Finally, go at a pace you can tolerate, even enjoy!

To keep yourself in good compliance draw a table for yourself with the necessary items listed down a column on the left side. Make another column for each day. Then make a check mark for each item taken or done. Ask your friend or loved one to pull you through when your motivation weakens. Promise your caregiver to say <u>yes</u> nine times out of ten when asked to sip, swallow or chew. Reward your caregiver with announcements that you feel improvements when you really do. Don't spare the praise. Look at the birds outside your window. They seem so carefree. But is cancer and extinction waiting for them, too? You must <u>cure yourself</u> to help the birds, the flowers, the butterflies escape such a plight. Toxicity and disease will surely reach them. Only a cure has true value for the biosphere. There is so much work to do and you are needed so much. Laugh a lot—especially at yourself, and anything you can find to laugh at. Even find the humor in your tumor.

The Program

The First 5 Days

This program is designed for the extremely advanced cancer patient who must do **everything**: clear the cancer, clear up infections, and stop toxicities. If you are also in clinical care, try to get the cooperation of your doctor in:

a) **not** using isopropyl alcohol on your skin; bring an unopened high strength ethyl (drinking) alcohol

b) **not** giving contrast injections with your scans because they fill the body with lanthanide metals or dyes; request ultrasound or dye-free scans in spite of less detailed views

c) **not** doing a bone scan or whole body scan <u>without evidence of bone or whole body disease</u>; getting radiated till the whole skeleton or body glows is too invasive just to satisfy curiosity

d) **not** using plastic IV bags; to avoid the PVC, the diallyl phthalates and other plastic derivatives, use glass

e) **not** doing a biopsy when chemo is not a choice anyway and when a history of cancer makes malignancy the most probable description; avoid this new trauma and the spread of cancer cells out of its enclosure

f) **requesting** allergy testing so you can minimize PGE2 formation. The RAST food test is most helpful. If you have corn allergy, request saline instead of dextrose in your IV.

g) **recommending** alternative therapy to you when hope for survival fades, or as an adjunct

There are about 50 things to do in this program. The speed is up to you. Going too fast is likely to give you unnecessary detox-illness. Find a helper to get you through detox-illness and help you prevent it.

Items you will need to purchase are underlined.

Try to get started on every item by the fifth day so you have a full 3 weeks of treatment behind you before scheduling a retest. But you can go slower and retest later. Each item is discussed further at the end of the program, page 250, to help you with details. Use the *Testers' Flow Sheet* on page 273 if you have a Syncrometer® tester to help you. You may test yourself. Test 3 times a week, at least, to know your status.

1. Find safe water for drinking, cooking, washing and laundry. Move to this good-water zone. It will be identifiable by a Syncrometer® tester given a single sample from the cold or hot kitchen faucet. Sending a sample from 5 or 6 gas stations in a chosen area would be quickest. Repeat the test later for the good water locations. The presence of only National Standards Foundation (NSF) bleach in the water sample and the absence of *water softener salts* means it is good water. The presence of local laundry bleach or softener salts identifies the bad water. Also identify the bleach yourself with a 2-month home test (see page 579). Three common NSF-bleaches that you can buy at pool and spa stores are Desert Star, Sani Clor, and Water Guard, though, of course, you are not at liberty to choose the bleach for your water. For drinking, in addition to being in a good water zone, buy distilled water in polyethylene 1 gallon jugs. Test several brands with a conductivity indicator to find one that reads **zero** and has no chlorination (see page 581). Filter this slowly through a filter pitcher whose activated carbon was boiled for 5 minutes (see page 589) in tap water. The pitcher and plastic filter unit themselves must be hardened, see page 587. The pitcher filter removes the strontium, ruthenium, rhodium and aluminum still left in the distilled water. The boiling removes ruthenium from the charcoal. If you are extremely ill, filter twice, through a second pitcher, treated the same way. Reboil your charcoal every 2 weeks. For

cooking use the same pure, distilled-filtered water. Dechlorinating your whole body this way is a huge help.

Read the alternatives in the *Help* section on page 250.

2. Request these blood tests:
   - CBC
   - Urinalysis
   - Blood chemistry (called SMAC) of about 24 items
   - A cancer "marker" test, but only if your oncologist used one; we will use orthophosphotyrosine, HCG and CEA.
   - Blood clotting tests
   - Serum iron

Other tests are seldom necessary and create needless cost. The test results will give you a starting point to compare with new tests to be done after the *3-Week Program*. Use *Blood Test Results* on page 311 to understand your test results and to know what to do about each one.

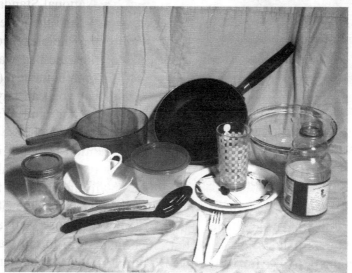

Glassware, canning jars, Teflon, toothbrushes, paper plates, plastic ware, and "good" china seep heavy metals, malonic acid and thallium! Ceramic and enamelware also seep.

Fig. 79 Kitchenware that seeps

3. Stop using <u>all</u> commercial cosmetics, body products such as soap and shampoo, herbs, teas or supplements, unless they are tested by Syncrometer® for laundry bleach, azo dyes, isopropyl alcohol and PCBs. This applies to prescription drugs, as well as over the counter varieties. A single bad one taken daily will hurt you. Find unpolluted, uncolored varieties before going off your own. Stop using metal jewelry; harden all plastic items in sonicator (20 min.) or in steaming (not boiling) hot water for ½ hour.

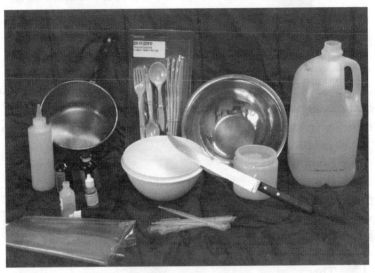

Stainless steel, high density polyethylene ♻, zippered plastic bags (at front left), and the white Tupperware bowl do not seep.

Fig. 80 Cookware, cutlery and containers that do not seep

4. Cut a place setting from HDPE♻ water bottles such as your distilled water jug. Purchase cookware, cutlery, and containers that do not seep. Eat, cook, and store food only in containers tested for heavy metal seeping. Test them yourself with a conductivity indicator (see *Sources*).

5. <u>Hydrangea root</u> powder, ½ tsp. 4 times daily and <u>Germanium -132</u>, (150 mg), one, 4 times daily. You may use both. But if you have a chronic cough or cold, eat Hazel nuts

instead of both (four, 4 times daily). When cough lifts, add Ge-132. If cough stays away, also add hydrangea powder.

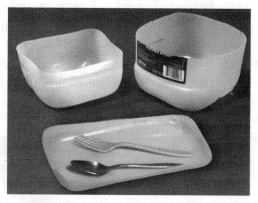

Homemade dishes, bowls, plates and cups can be cut from HDPE♲ water bottles. Use these while testing others with a conductivity indicator.

Fig. 81 Temporary place setting

6. <u>Sodium selenite,</u> (200 mcg), take one 4 times daily.

7 . <u>Rose hips powder,</u> (2 capsules), 4 times daily, coarse ground with seeds. You may take additional <u>vitamin C</u> if tested for thulium by Syncrometer®, (1000 mg), 2 capsules 4 times daily.

These 3 items, #5, #6, and #7 <u>feed</u> your white blood cells. You can never miss a dose without slowing down the whole program or getting detox symptoms. All 3 are destroyed by microwave cooking. Use stovetop or hotplate.

8. Start taking homeographic drops, according to the homeography schedule on page 116. First, take <u>pyruvic aldehyde</u> drops to stop excessive cell division. Then take <u>kidney protective set</u> and <u>lymph</u>. Take all these 6 times a day, putting 6 drops under the tongue for each dose. Reduce to 3 times a day after 2 days and keep this up for the whole 3 weeks. Also take <u>wheel bearing grease-out-of kidney set</u> and <u>lymph</u>, <u>dyes-out-of kidney set</u> and <u>lymph</u>, <u>heavy metals-out-of-</u>

kidney set and lymph. Take all these 6 times a day for 2 days, then 3 times a day for 2 days, then once a day till you are completely well, beyond 3 weeks. Leave at least 1 minute between drops to prevent mixing them. Swallow before taking new drops. You may start all these together. Continue with schedule on page 116.

9. Extract all teeth that once had metal in them. Then start the *Dental Aftercare* without delay (see page 335). One week later, zappicate all natural and plastic teeth and empty spaces 3 times, see page 344. Partial dentures must be "hardened" <u>by you</u> before you may wear them even one hour. See denture hardening recipe on page 572.

10. Eat only the cancer-diet menu because it has been chosen to avoid the main cancer allergens. Your diet should have no chlorogenic acid, phloridzin, gallic acid, nor the onion-garlic family, nor oats, potatoes, dairy foods (except butter and heavy whipping cream), eggs, lemons, and all cooking oils, including olive oil. Eat only free-range, organic beef, turkey and lamb or buffalo because these do not have linolenic acid deposits, nor d-carnitine or asparagine deposits. Choose nitrogen packed grains as cereals (see *Sources*). Store them in the freezer. Bake your own breads or use a bread maker. If you have lung disease or lung cancer, avoid corn also. If you have multiple chemical sensitivities (numerous allergies), avoid wheat and all beef, too. See the *Food Table* that lists the allergens in foods.

Foods with phloridzin are:

- apples, except Red Delicious and Golden Delicious, very ripe
- pork, ham and derivatives
- soy products including oil, sauce, beans, sprouts, etc.

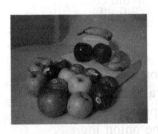

Fig. 82 Pick apples carefully

242

- unripe fruits of any kind
- bananas (freezing destroys the allergen and makes them safe)

Foods with chlorogenic acid are:

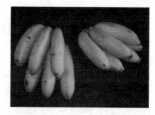

Midget varieties, as well as Machos, Burros, and purple have no phloridzin.

Fig. 83 Safe bananas

- potatoes (cooking very well done destroys this allergen, <u>not frying</u>; no chips or fries are safe)
- cow's milk and all dairy products including butter (boiling for 1 minute destroys this allergen)
- peppers of all kinds, unless cooked very well done
- unripe fruits
- watermelon

Foods with gallic acid are:

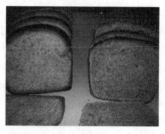

- commercially baked goods and bread (bake your own)
- cereal grains (cooking the cereal very thoroughly destroys this allergen); avoid cold cereal.
- cooking oils

Unbleached flour avoids bromine; baked in bread maker kills all live yeast.

Fig. 84 Safe bread

Also, stay off foods belonging to the **lily** family, besides onion and garlic. They are: **leeks, chives, asparagus,** and **aloe vera**. Also avoid cilantro, beans, roasted peanuts, and canned or processed foods. Store bought spices nearly always have some onion ingredient. Buy pure spices from an herb supplier (see *Sources*).

243

What's Left to Eat?

All the foods you were not eating! That brings home this point: you get allergic to, meaning not able to completely digest, those foods you eat most! That is what the liver, pancreas and stomach can no longer digest and detoxify. But as "buski's" and salmonellas are killed and nickel is drained from your body, you will lose these allergies. Pulling the wheel bearing grease out of your body with DMSO takes the nickel with it, but the whole procedure could take ½ year. Liver cleanses eliminate some automotive greases and speed this up.

11. Check the *Cancer Location Table* for the food allergy responsible for your cancer and metastases. Find the corresponding foods in the *Food Table*. Stay off these foods.

You have now stopped making the tumor nucleus and are starving the parasites responsible for it all.

12. Ozonate all your food and beverages, but not your supplements, for 7 minutes. Place foods in a plastic shopping bag, closed with a twist tie where the ozonator hose enters the bag. After 7 minutes turn off the ozonator, close containers and refrigerate. Let stand for 15 minutes more before eating to let the ozonation process complete itself. Place on zappicator for 10 minutes. These treatments give them sanitation and north polarization. Use a 1 kHz zapper to power the zappicator, connecting only the *Positive* terminals.

13. Five minutes before each meal take 2 vitamin B$_2$ (300 mg), 2 magnesium oxide (300 mg), and 1 iron capsule (10 mg ferrous gluconate). Also take 4 kinds of digestive enzymes at the end of meals: straight pepsin, multiple digestive enzymes, lipase-pancreatin, and bromelain, one capsule of each with each meal. For meat meals take 5 lipase-pancreatin capsules at the beginning and end of the meal in addition. Sterilize them with 1 drop of Lugol's iodine stirred into a beverage, see #16.

14. Put 15 drops hydrochloric acid (5%, food-grade) on your food in each meal, distributing them and stirring with a non-seeping plastic fork. Do not put HCl straight in your mouth, it will dissolve your teeth; it stains stainless steel.

15. <u>Betaine hydrochloride</u> (500 mg), take 3 with each meal (9 daily) to destroy Clostridium bacteria in the intestine. Start counting the days after dental work is completed and continue for 3 days.

16. At the end of each meal (at least 4 times a day) take 6 drops <u>Lugol's iodine</u> in ¼ to ½ cup water. <u>Immediately</u> (within a minute) afterward take 6 capsules <u>turmeric</u> and 6 capsules fennel. This is followed by digestive enzymes. Sonicate the enzymes 10 minutes to sterilize, or use Lugol's iodine.

17. <u>Vitamin D₃</u>, 50,000 units daily. (Don't use a rubber dropper to dispense, the rubber contributes laundry bleach). Don't use a diluted form of vitamin D, containing vegetable oil; this brings malonic acid and benzene pollutants. Use the straight concentrate from a polyethylene self-dropper bottle or do without to avoid risk. Improving your kidneys and sunbathing will supply some.

18. Once daily put 10 drops <u>oregano oil</u> in a capsule and swallow quickly, followed by bread, to destroy Clostridium in your tumors. Make strong <u>Eucalyptus</u> tea, 2 cups a day to destroy the remainder. Also make Birch bark tea, 1 to 3 cups daily.

19. Take 15 digestive enzyme capsules, <u>lipase-pancreatin</u> variety, twice daily between meals (in addition to any taken with meals). Taking more helps. Find the strongest variety available by comparing the units per capsule. Test for bacteria or sonicate them 10 minutes. Also take <u>lactase</u> enzyme, one between meals and one with meals.

20. Take <u>thyroid</u> (one grain) in morning upon rising each day. It must be tested by Syncrometer® for laundry bleach pollution. Test for prions if you are concerned about eating prions from natural gland pills. Sonication for 5 minutes destroys them as well as bacteria. Your body temperature should reach 99.0°F. Use a thermometer placed under the tongue for 5 minutes in the morning before rising. Be alert to the possibility of allergic reactions to some brands of thyroid.

In the next 3 instructions you will begin killing parasites. Wait till you have completed 4 days of homeographic drops

245

that help kidneys and their WBCs before killing parasites. This is to prevent detox-illness.

21. Zap every day for 6 to 8 hours with fresh batteries. Use a plate-zapper box and a ¼ volt *Positive* offset zapper putting out 30 kHz. Use the Zapping Schedule on page 94.

22. Decaris (levamisole) (50 mg), take 2 tablets before each meal, totaling 6 daily. It removes ferritin and kills roundworms.

23. Take 2 tsp. green Black Walnut hull tincture (Extra-Strength) daily from a new, 2 ounce bottle. It should be green. Store opened bottles in freezer to keep their green color. If you are advanced and tolerate more, drink the whole 2 oz. bottle on the next day in sips over a 5 minute period. You may mix with syrup, fruit juice, or water, or heavy whipping cream. Also take 10 wormwood capsules during this 5 minute period, plus 10 clove capsules. Stay seated for half an hour afterwards. Take while zapping if possible. Repeat daily as long as you are not ill with detox-symptoms. If you have brain or spinal cord cancer, take 10 capsules wormwood 3 times daily instead of once.

The next day expect a Flu and Salmonella attack (detox) unless you have been taking flu-preventing teas and salmonella-killing Lugol's. In any case take a single dose of Oscillococcinum at bedtime when beginning to zap and kill parasites, as well as the following teas.

The following teas prevent Flu and colds while you are killing parasites.

24. Drink 1 cup of Eucalyptus tea, (c/s)[*] daily, organic, strongly brewed, sweetened to taste. Drink Elder leaf tea, (c/s), ½ cup, once daily. Drink Boneset tea, (c/s), 1 cup daily. Brew in stainless steel pan. Take these twice daily on zapping days. The extra amounts will help your urine volume to come up to the 2½ quarts (liters) that is recommended when killing parasites.

---

[*] c/s stands for cut and sifted grade. A finer grind, such as powders, regularly has nickel or chromium pollution from the hot blades.

25. <u>Oscillococcinum</u>, homeopathic remedy for Flu. Take one dose at bedtime on zapping days. If you develop a cold or other symptoms take it immediately, at onset, and at bedtime.

To treat more severe detox symptoms take round after round (at least 4) of Lugol's iodine, followed by the herb teas, and Oscillococcinum at bedtime. Include <u>birch bark tea</u> or <u>Reischi mushroom</u> to speed recovery. Have all these handy. Buy birch bark, c/s, tested for thallium and laundry bleach. Also Reischi mushroom (Ganoderma), 1 tsp. 3 times daily, not made into tea.

26. Apply one <u>10 gauss magnet</u> over the middle of spine at back of neck. Apply two over each kidney region (see picture). Use clear packaging tape or masking tape <u>only</u>. Wear by day time. The north side touches skin. Red (south) side faces up. Check each magnet with a <u>compass</u> first (see page 502). Store in their own bag away from homeographic bottles. Soak off in shower.

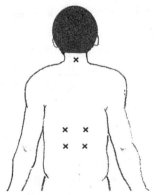

Fig. 85 Kidney and neck magnets are 10 gauss

27. Cook <u>L-G</u> and <u>L-A</u> using recipe. Take 1 tsp. of each liquid 3 times a day. Take separately.

28. Make raw, grated <u>horseradish</u> at mealtime, 1 tsp. a day. Mix with food. Do not store. Do not ozonate. Make raw, grated, <u>red beet</u> at another meal, again as a condiment. Take 1 tsp. daily. Eat straight or in a salad. Do not ozonate or store.

29. <u>6 fresh seeds</u> rolled in a zippered plastic bag to crumble them. Grinding will bring nickel and chromium from the blades. Eat immediately. Choose apricot if possible, if not, use peach, or nectarine seeds. Sweeten or eat plain once daily for 5 days; then take 5 days off; then 5 days on again and repeat till you are well. Do not purchase seeds (they do not work). Do not crack pits ahead of time (they are soon worthless).

NOTE: Apricot seeds have had this warning label to let you know they were once deemed toxic (LOW QUANTITIES MAY CAUSE REACTION. NOT SUITABLE FOR FOOD USE WITHOUT FURTHER PROCESSING–SECTION 10786 TITLE 17, CALIFORNIA ADMIN. CODE). Six fresh seeds has not resulted in stomach aches, headaches, diarrhea, or even fatigue. Their cancer curing magic is easy to monitor by Syncrometer®. Read more on Internet.

30. Make 1 glass north pole water each morning, using food zappicator.

31. Also, drink 1 glass ozonated water daily. Ozonate 5 minutes by immersing the hose in water.

32. Take glutathione (500 mg), 1 capsule, 3 times daily.

33. Take vitamin A (100,000 units) daily. Expect red, itching, peeling skin. If this happens take 5 days off, then resume the vitamin.

You have now taken 3 cell-differentiators: vitamin D_3, l-thyroid, and vitamin A. This will give tumor cells their normal stimulation to recover.

34. Take l-cysteine (500 mg), 2 capsules with each meal (not while driving). Watch for minor side-effects like fatigue. Rest till they are gone. This helps liver and kidneys while killing Ascaris and providing reducing power.

35. Do a Lugol's-turmeric enema daily to kill oncoviruses (see page 269). Do a Lugol's-turmeric-fennel enema daily if you have bloating and gas. Separate these items carefully as instructed in the recipe.

After The Fifth Day

36. After dental extractions floss your remaining teeth once a day with homemade strips of plastic shopping bags, cut ¼" x 4" and placed in steaming hot water ½ hr. Then rub teeth with oregano oil tooth powder, homemade, consisting of baking soda and oregano oil only, both tested for laundry bleach; see *Recipes*. Harden your toothbrush in steaming hot water for ½ hour, done twice. It is permanent.

37. Reduce betaine to 3 capsules once a day.

38. Start <u>calcium</u> (500 mg), 1 capsule daily, with a meal.

39. Start <u>sodium/potassium, "balanced bicarbonate"</u>, ¼ tsp. 2 times daily upon rising and bedtime. If not available, you may substitute plain baking soda tested for laundry bleach. Also check urine pH (using <u>pH strips</u>) upon rising. Reduce to once a day at bedtime when pH is up to 6. Stop when pH is 6.5.

40. Measure how much urine you make in 24 hours. Use an empty gallon jug, a funnel, and container. Apply tape to jug and write time on it after pouring in the first batch. Pour all batches into jug, ending at the same time next day. Guess at the amount made and discard. The goal is 2¼ to 2½ quarts. Repeat once a week.

After 2 More Days

41. Make the <u>Kidney Cleanse recipe</u>, increasing ginger to 2 capsules three times daily and uva ursa to 2, three times daily. See page 561.

42. Reduce vitamin D_3 to 25,000 units daily.

43. Go off vitamin A if you are getting serious skin symptoms; then continue after they subside. Continue as long as possible.

44. Do a liver cleanse on the next weekend unless ill or having diarrhea. Lift suspected parasites into a plastic cup or zippered bag using a plastic fork or spoon. Add a few drops of Lugol's iodine to each for temporary sterilization. For permanent storage add an equal amount of 10% formaldehyde to parasites in small amount of water to keep safely as a specimen. Try to identify yours (see page 100).

45. <u>IP6</u> (inositol hexaphosphate), 20 drops in a glass of water, one to three times daily to help dissolve tricalcium phosphate, the hard part of tumors. Also take <u>inositol</u>, straight, 1 tsp. with each dose of IP6.

46. Take MSM (methyl sulfonyl methane), 650 mg., 1 capsule with or between meals, to destroy leftover ONION chemicals.

Help with Each Item

Help #1. Water, water everywhere, but...

Your water must be free of PCBs, benzene, asbestos, assorted heavy metals, dyes, motor oil and grease, water softener salts, and malonic acid. Even traces of these are no longer being detoxified by your body. Most of these toxins occur together, like a fingerprint, after the wrong bleach is added at your water department's pump house. The telltale marker for all of them is the bleach variety itself, found with a Syncrometer®, or finding a single toxin yourself, like motor oil, which you can see visually (see page 580).

What's in Laundry Bleach?

Because getting clean water is the most important step of this curing program, I will give as much help as possible with this.

Water from your reservoir, river, or wells, before it is treated does not have these pollutants. Water that is only chlorinated with chlorine gas does not have those pollutants either. Water that leaves the pump house where the free chlorine level was tested and boosted with non-NSF-grade liquid bleach does have them. There have been no exceptions in over a thousand tests. This means that asbestos in your drinking water is not coming in detectable amounts from asbestos-cement pipes. It is coming from the bleach added. It means that PCBs are not coming from aquifers or natural reservoirs. Nor is the motor oil and engine grease, although boats may be running there. PCBs and the other toxins found in laundry bleach are added at the pump station, too. Our public water sources are much cleaner than we thought. Pollution comes from willful or accidental additions made to them on the way to your home and the home of your pets and domestic animals.

250

Laundry bleach contents found by Syncrometer®

Laundry bleach Varieties	Cobalt	Motor Oil & Wheel Bearing Grease	Strontium	Uranium	Asbestos	Aluminum	PCBs	Benzene	Azo Dyes	Heavy Metals
#1		N	N	N	N	P	P	P	P	P
#2		P	P	P	N	P	P	P	P	P
#3	P	P	P	P	N	P	P	P	P	P
#4		P	*P	P	P	P	P	P	P	P
#5		P	P	P	N	P	P	P	P	P
#6		P	P	P	N	P	P	P	P	P
#7		P	P	*P	*P	*P	P	P	P	P
#8		P	P	P	N	P	P	P	P	P
#9		P	P	P	P	P	P	P	P	P
#10		P	P	P	P	P	P	P	P	P
#11	P	P	P	P	N	P	P	P	P	P
#12		P	P	P	N	P	P	P	P	P
#13		P	*P	P	P	*P	P	P	P	P
#14		P	P	P	P	P	P	P	P	P
#15	*P		P	N	N	P				
#16	N	N	N	N	N	N	N	N	N	N
#17	N	N	N	N	N	N	N	N	N	N

#1 to #15 are laundry bleach varieties taken off the shelves in supermarkets in USA. #16 and #17 are NSF-rated bleaches available at pool stores. The motor oil and wheel bearing grease samples for testing came from regular cans available at any automotive store. Heavy metals and azo dyes are mixtures. Omitted from the test was malonic acid though it regularly appears. The names of the laundry bleaches #1-#15 are withheld for fear of reprisal. Asterisks reflect extra high levels.

Fig. 86 Laundry bleach contents

Water softener salts do not get added at the chlorine booster station. They get added in your home by running the hot water through a container that holds the salt or in other and newer ways. The salt itself is usually disinfected with laundry bleach. But it isn't just salt either. It invariably has PCBs, benzene, uranium and strontium as its own major pollutants. 'But', you might say, 'it only goes into the hot faucet. I never, never cook with that, or drink it'. Any single lever faucet mixes the hot and cold, even when it is pushed to extreme left or right. Even 2 separate faucets do not prevent spreading of PCBs to the whole house! Samples from the cold side <u>always</u> show water softener if it is being used in the hot side. Water softeners, even with good NSF-bleached water in your home is not acceptable.

…Not a Drop to Drink

All of our cancer patients (100%) had the laundry bleach "frequency-print" in their tap water <u>and in their saliva, blood, lymph and tumors</u>. Very many of them had the water softener "frequency-print", too.

Yet 2 out of 3 water samples sent by friends and family members of patients were not polluted with laundry bleach, at least not before they had installed a filter themselves. Their water departments were using only NSF-bleach, as the regulation requires. About one out of 3 (33%) water samples contained laundry bleach instead of NSF-rated bleach and did not contain both, suggesting that laundry bleach use was a policy, not an occasional choice.

This means, if you have cancer or anyone in your household develops cancer you have a 100% chance of having laundry bleach water arriving at your kitchen faucet. The only question is: Did you bring it in yourself, or not?

Because there is automotive grease in laundry bleached water, you will be able to detect it yourself without help from a lab or Syncrometer® tester. But the grease rises slowly; it could take two to three months. Nevertheless, if your friends and family do the same test, you will be able to find a clean water source by yourself, visually. A non-visual method could be developed using other methods described on pages 581 and 583, but is not ready for accurate determination now.

Two errors can creep into your decision-making. One comes from water softeners. All (100%) water softener salts tested had PCB-pollution, high strontium levels, uranium and, of course, high aluminum since it is intentionally present. Such "softened" water would be making your water toxicity much worse than it already was. If you test your incoming water before it enters your house (for example, at the garden hose) and it does not show grease rising to the surface, you could conclude you are getting clean water from your city. Quickly remove the water softener tank, hot water heater, and hot water pipes. If your municipal water is clean as it arrives, you merely need to replace these items with new ones. You cannot "clean up" PCB-containing grease; it sticks to metal, plastic, and glass surfaces. Be careful not to buy a water heater with a built-in softener.

The other error comes from having installed water distillers, water filters and extra pumps yourself. If even one is in your system, sample your incoming water at the garden hose to decide if the municipal water is clean and you don't have to move.

Cool Clear Water

If your <u>incoming</u> water is grease-contaminated, the only solution is to move, as before. If it is <u>not</u> contaminated, you could simply replace all your pipes and heater. Remove any distiller or filter or pump. This is also the time to change pipes to PVC if you had metal. You cannot clean pipes once grease has traveled through them bringing PCBs. Get new fixtures as well, but not plastic valves because these have hidden "permanent" grease fittings; again PCBs hide there. Metal faucets and valves do not contribute detectable amounts of metal.

All this testing delays your start with the *3-Week Program*. You might think that switching to bottled water would be a solution. It is not. But a temporary solution, while you are spending 2 or 3 weeks searching for a good water zone, is to make your own metal-free water, starting with a distilled water that has very little heavy metal pollution. Use a conductivity indicator to find good distilled water. It is almost as sensitive as a Syncrometer®. You can filter such zero-conductivity distilled water through your own pitcher filter to remove residual aluminum, strontium, ruthenium, rhodium and others. These are ultra important to your illness, besides the cancer. But you must boil your activated carbon first. Boiling does not clean up charcoal that contains laundry bleach due to its own disinfection. Buy clean charcoal first (see *Sources*). Test the water again after filtering. See instructions on page 589.

The only storage container that does not seep is the same polyethylene jug you purchased with the distilled water. Save these.

You might think a good filter would be a solution for your home water supply. It is not. The filters now on the market actually <u>bring</u> these pollutants because laundry bleach was used during manufacturing to disinfect them! Even the activated charcoal is disinfected this way. That is why replacement charcoal for your filter must be a tested variety and must even be boiled to remove its strontium and ruthenium.

You might think that a distiller would be a solution; would it not boil off the solvents and leave behind the heavy metals to give you pure water? It does none of these things. The solvents, heavy metals and dyes in laundry bleach water all carry over with the steam. And any attached filter adds its own laundry bleach to otherwise clean water.

You might think that a reverse osmosis system would be a solution. It uses a membrane that should keep out all toxins. It does not. The membrane itself is made of heavy metals, the very worst ones, such as lanthanides (thulium, yttrium, ytterbium). It is accepted in FDA regulations for such filters. The agency personnel are probably ignorant about lanthanides.

You might think that bringing buckets and bottles or tanks of good water to your kitchen would be a solution. It is the very worst. Many former cancer patients, in fact all who had a later recurrence, had fallen into this "logical" loophole and became a casualty. <u>All the water running from faucets in your home should be free of laundry bleach</u>.

Do not start to detoxify or kill parasites until you are living in a clean water zone. It will all be wasted. Merely getting clean drinking water for drinking and cooking still leaves you with PCB-water (from laundry bleach) for washing. This will not be satisfactory. There will be hardly any progress, even in 6 weeks.

Well Water...

...is a very good water!

One solution is by far the easiest: moving to a home with a well. Now you are in charge. But I must hasten to warn you; some patients who chose this easier path, this sure road to success, still lost their cure because they again had the wrong bleach in their well water! They had allowed someone else to do it by giving them the task of routine disinfection. Once added it could not be removed. The pipes had become contaminated, as well as the pressure tank. Any filter added to your well water would create the same problem as before.

Do not leave any water "chores" to anyone but yourself. Get NSF-stamped bleach ahead of time at your pool store; explain it to your workmen as they drill, clean or repair. Provide it free of charge. But do not give them the responsibility; be present yourself and add it in your presence. Explain to the supervisor that if his workmen accidentally use "store bleach", *you won't be able to use it nor pay for the work. You will have the water analyzed on their last day, to be certain.* Leave nothing to chance. You must provide the NSF-bleach and be sure no other bleach is on the work premises when well digging or servicing is going on. Of course, well diggers don't like to be supervised or watched. But getting free disinfectant is always appreciated. Make sure you get their partly used bottles in exchange. **Calcium hypochlorite** is a good choice for underground repairs and general servicing. It is not polluted and is also available at pool stores.

To disinfect the water if coliform bacteria are found, ozonate your own well water. Any chlorination has other serious disadvantages for a cancer patient. Chlorine is an over-oxidizing toxin and your body already is over-oxidized. The chlorination compounds made by the chlorine are carcinogenic. It makes no sense to chlorinate water and drink extra carcinogens in a society where already about ½ of all men and women are getting cancer and you are already diagnosed!

But do not install a commercial size ozonator. The pumps, filter, valves and fixtures attached to it would surely foil you again. Check into small units without a single filter added or build your own filter.

Well water has special healing minerals, such as iridium, and is the most delicious of waters. Ozonate with a small unit that runs ozone into the holding tank on a schedule. Or ozonate at point of use and only if necessary. Learn to use a coliform test you can find at a pool supply store. Keep yourself safe with a minimum of ozonation.

You may pump water from a well straight into a holding tank that you place high enough to let gravity feed to your plumbing. If you get sediment the well pipe is too deeply placed. You could use a stainless steel mesh strainer. The pump should not be the older submersible[*] variety because the oil contained inside will eventually leak (called pump failure) and let out PCBs again! A warranty of a mere 10 years already tells you this. Even if it didn't fail for 15 years, the result is PCBs in the well water and they don't go away. You have ruined the well. Get a surface pump. A <u>surface</u> pump needs periodic oiling and greasing. Make sure no automotive greases are used for this when repairing the lift-cup in the shaft, use lard. Do it yourself!

Filtering or distilling well water would lose the very important advantage of getting minerals from such water. The heart thrives on "hard" well water minerals. Adding minerals back after taking them out would be a hoax very similar to adding enrichment vitamins back to white bread.

Only a high iron level is reason enough to filter your well water. And only with a homemade filter so you can choose safe activated carbon for it and can recharge it yourself by boiling without having to constantly buy, test, and treat new filters.

---

[*] A newer submersible variety using water lubrication only is available. See *Sources*.

On the other hand, water should not have nitrates, or pesticide. If it does, it is unfit for you. Drilling deeper may lead to better water without these surface "runoffs".

Rainwater

In my opinion this is the best water, but it should be tested for strontium, beryllium, vanadium and chromium first. These can be filtered out with a filter pitcher. It needs no pumping or disinfecting which add risk to it. How to build a cistern, coating it and using a plastic liner have all been described in magazines devoted to simpler living. Find them on the Internet. Water samples I tested from such a source have proven safe, because the plastic liner was hard enough not to seep. If you are sick, bedridden or very advanced, collect your own for personal use (see page 114). This does not replace the need for safe water to come into your kitchen through the faucets, though.

Other Solutions

Another solution is to rent or lease a large, new, uncolored plastic tank on wheels, holding about 300 to 600 gallons. Purchase your NSF chlorinated water from a source you have tested yourself. Connect it to your water line with a metal valve. Fill it regularly. Purchase a water-lubricated pump (see *Sources*). Test it first in a bucket of clean water by sampling the outflow and testing for laundry bleach. Keep extra pumps and tanks to a minimum and test your water again as it arrives in the kitchen.

The house water pipes and water heater should be changed at the same time since the new good water will not clean them.

Yet another solution is to rent an RV and connect it to an RV park water line after you have tested their water. The cost will be low since you are not driving anywhere. Pipe the water in through a new flexible hose to your plumbing system, bypassing your pipes. Buy a new storage tank, water heater and fixtures. Or put an RV on a family member's property where the water is good.

Flee First, Fix Later

Don't wait for all this if you have a cancer diagnosis. Flee from your water immediately. You have a 100% chance of failure at home. Moving anywhere else, to a different water district would give you a better chance of success (at least 50%).

Flee to a motel, apartment, or RV site in a different water district immediately. Make sure that no water softener or "extra bleach" is used by their own installation. It is a common practice in "rentals" to add more bleach personally through an extra dispenser. Water softeners are attached to water heaters, too, usually near laundry rooms. Choose a room furthest from the laundry room that gets a different water heater. Unfortunately, there is no test by a commercial lab that can tell you which kind of bleach is being added to the water. Only a Syncrometer® tester could do this in a very short time.

Test their water first. The water sample may be taken from the outside faucet or a neighboring gas station rest room, as long as it represents the same water district as the motel or apartment you have chosen. Find the motel or apartment first so you can ask the manager if there is a water softener or any water treatment in the plumbing system.

Since the use of laundry bleach in drinking water is a partly personal and partly haphazard decision by the water department, there is no guarantee that "good" water will stay "good". The personality and policy of the department overseers make the difference between choosing laundry or NSF-bleach varieties. But "bad" water is not likely to change to "good" after the habit has begun. Reminders of legalities do not work either. The best decision is to relocate to a good municipal water supply, at least temporarily. This way you have time to make the changes in your own plumbing for your return later, if you were so fortunate as to have a good city supply. If you have friends or family that will do this for you while you are away, you have blessings beyond counting.

The rest of this *3-Week Program* will bring you success with unprecedented certainty, but only if you have moved to a clean water source.

Thousands of people have cured their own cancers. They moved away from their "Cancer Houses". You can join them and plan for a normal life.

Help #2. Use the *Blood Test Results* on page 311.

Help #3. You cannot put PCBs on your face (face powder), on your tongue (mouthwash), on your tonsils (toothpaste), on your eyebrows (eyebrow pencil), on your lips (lip gloss and lipstick), on your scalp (shampoo and conditioner), or on your hands (moisturizer, soap and lotions) and expect not to absorb it. These are very absorptive zones. And all the traces in these products add up to a lot when you are not excreting any. Use only the homemade recipes given in the *Recipes* chapter. Many more are given in earlier books. Be creative. Do not buy "homemade" products unless you have them Syncrometer®-tested. The body is a giant sponge. It miraculously wrings itself clean through the kidneys many times a day. But an overload blocks it. All the supplements you will use should have been tested by Syncrometer® for laundry bleach pollutants. You can expect 90% of all drugs, supplements, herbs and health foods in the market place to have such pollution. This is because the same laundry bleach was used for disinfecting health foods and supplements as regular foods and drugs. The variety of bleach used by a manufacturer is easily identified by Syncrometer®.

Help #4. While plastic, glass and ceramics have been getting worse over the years, that is, softer, leaching every imaginable toxin (even thallium), stainless steel has been getting better, that is, harder. They should still be tested, though. Small plastic items, like toothbrushes or cutlery can be dropped into steaming hot water for ½ hour, as you do for dentures to harden them. Large plastic items would require a large pot or be filled with steaming hot water. Others cannot be hardened.

259

Fortunately, thin unstretchable plastic film as in zippered baggies is already hardened, as is some high-impact plastic and high density polyethylene HDPE♲ used for water and milk. Use such empty water jugs to store water and take with you on travels. A few hard glass items do exist, too.

Most fortunate is that stainless steel pots, bowls, and even utensils and cutlery seep nothing (except titanium and tantalum from some).

But you cannot take all this for granted. Test every food container yourself using a conductivity indicator. See instructions on page 581.

Throw away all "seep ware"; even one will harm you if you are advanced or sick. The seeped metals feed your bacteria with the metals they need while giving you kidney failure, anemia, liver failure, bone marrow failure, etc. A conductivity indicator will not detect malonic acid, motor oil, or wheel bearing grease, nor very low levels of thallium and other metals. But detecting heavy metals with good sensitivity is still very useful. You could then test these by Syncrometer®. Distilled water that sits open to air for many hours absorbs carbon dioxide and the acidity is conductive. Cover open containers when doing kitchenware tests.

Help #5. #6. & #7. These 3 items are required by your white blood cells to be able to kill and detoxify the things they have captured and are going to be eating very soon. Hydrangea root supplies organic germanium but has linolenic acid (oil). Nuts supply germanium, too, but have an antigen that affects skin (except Hazel nuts). The supplement Ge-132 can be used in addition, but has other disadvantages so rotation of all these is best to avoid getting allergic to Hazel nuts. If you have a cough or develop a cough, go off all nuts. The viruses responsible for the cough are triggered by the nut oils. Sodium selenite is a compromise between organic and inorganic selenium since so much is needed. In fact, none of these amounts is enough. Even 10 times as much germanium, selenite and vitamin C is not enough. Your WBCs are so eager to work for you, they always take on more than they can complete and get stuck. For this reason stop microwaving and high temperature cooking. It conserves all three. Nuts also contain selenite. Rose hips supply natural vitamin C in a more effective form than the synthetically made variety. Finely ground herb powders of any kind pose a much higher risk for nickel and chromium from the grinder blades than coarsely ground. When the white blood cells get back to work it is like slipping your car into gear. Everything is in motion and in need of much more fuel. For this reason, do not miss any doses of these three. Mixing them is fine. Sweetening them is fine. Putting in or out of capsules is fine. Making a cocktail is fine. Adding a capsule of ginger or other safe herb is fine, too, but always paying attention to your own special needs and eating them promptly.

Help #8. A copy of pyruvic aldehyde (methyl glyoxal) is easily made as well as a homeopathic form of molybdenum. Pyruvic aldehyde instantly slows down abnormal cell division. Molybdic acid instantly reduces allergic reactions, especially in the lungs. Results can be seen in about 2 days. Getting the kidneys to work well again is first in importance and comes before killing parasites. Use the homeography instructions on page 112 and complete the whole schedule.

Help #9. If you salvage infected teeth with a filling of any kind it could destroy the certainty of success. This method is too new to have statistics for it. In earlier books only extractions were recommended. If you nevertheless choose this risk, the plastic should be hardened with a toothbrush zappicator as a final treatment, see page 344. Porcelain should never be chosen because of its uranium content. Hidden cavitations should be treated later, after you are well, to reduce risk of more infection. They might be gone later, too, so a new evaluation should be done beforehand. Finally, a complete mouth zappication should be done to chase away the mercury still smeared over all the soft tissues. Always harden your dentures again after visiting a dentist.

Help #10. The first three antigens are responsible for making the tumor nucleus. Lemon feeds pancreatic flukes and lung flukes. The onion-garlic family feeds the main parasite, F. buski, bringing its essential food factors, **allyl sulfides**. Oats feed the human liver fluke. Potatoes feed Strongyloides. It is not surprising that our main parasites are dependent on our main (staple) foods. Practice cooking other-culture foods and those of your childhood to get away from your allergies. It's amazing how much food is still left to eat, a tribute to our Agriculture Department. Avoiding corn is important in chronic lung disease including lung cancer and emphysema, and may be important in many other diseases, too. Corn has incorporated beryllium and strontium in large amounts in its grains. Vanadium and chromium are present in lesser amounts. These are major air pollutants in food form that supply our worst bacteria and viruses, all converging on your lungs. For food hints, see *Recipes*, page 507.

Help #11. All food has antigens (allergens) in the form of colors, flavors, and fragrances. To be less allergic means you are more able to detoxify phenolic-type antigens. Molybdic acid 4 x helps greatly. Not eating the allergenic food helps most. When taking Molybdic acid drops while avoiding the food, you may recover from allergic lung symptoms in days. Fasciolopsis, Fasciola, and Salmonella bacteria are most responsible for becoming allergic, but the mechanisms are not clear.

Help #12. You don't need to put the ozonator hose into the food itself. The plastic bag builds up a small ozone pressure that can penetrate to the bottom of a quart of liquid and right through meat and butter. You must <u>open</u> the quart container and any packaged food, though. Ozonate longer to detoxify more difficult items. Ozonating 15 minutes clears hypochlorite (chlorine) and estrogens from dairy products. You may zappicate while waiting after ozonating. Do not accidentally use the *Negative* zappicator terminals. This would send the pulses to ground instead of the food.

Help #13. Vitamin B$_2$, magnesium and iron taken together stimulates pepsin and HCl formation by the stomach. The 4 kinds of digestive enzymes will get the food through the stomach in record time, to prevent bloating, indigestion, and more food deposits in your tissues. But eating meat demands stronger enzyme action. Learn to cook foods on your menu in creative ways from old cookbooks. There will be dozens of entrées and recipes that you have long forgotten but are suitable now. Do not use the microwave oven. It oxidizes natural minerals to the heavy metal form, destroying organic germanium and selenite. Use the stovetop. Make yourself a food warmer in minutes that is almost as quick and very little clean up, also suitable for a hotplate. Any animal tissue could have bacteria. Either sonicate your enzymes or empty them into water and add 1 drop of Lugol's to sterilize.

Help #14. The HCl should be food-grade. It helps sterilize food while improving digestion; 2 drops added to pepsin powder in water sterilizes it. It kills MYC in eggs (3 drops each). Count the drops; do not squirt. It can make spots on your stainless steel sink. Use only 5%.

Help #15. Betaine hydrochloride is not meant to be a source of hydrochloric acid. Its amazing ability to remove Clostridium from the intestinal tract removes the source of reinfection of tumors. If it brings any discomfort, space them through the meal.

Help #16. Lugol's kills parasite stages, yeast, all bacteria and even viruses if it can come in close enough contact with them. But it cannot reach the sheltered oncoviruses <u>inside</u> bacteria and tumor cells. Turmeric kills SV 40 viruses that are free. To kill those SV 40 viruses that are sheltered inside yeast buds or in bacteria you must first kill these (with Lugol's) then kill the escaping SV 40 viruses, all in 1 minute. This same combination (Lugol's followed by turmeric) can kill many bacteria filled with other oncoviruses, too. Your tumor cells are filled with viruses and bacteria that have SV 40, the "ringleader" in them. This turmeric-Lugol's treatment can destroy them all if used by mouth and by enema together. Take one of your daily doses while you are doing the enema. You must not <u>mix</u> the Lugol's drops <u>with</u> herbs or supplements because their essential ingredients will be destroyed. A ½ minute interval after Lugol's prevents that. Don't put Lugol's in **anything** except water.

Help #17. Tumors have vitamin D_2 instead of D_3. This is due to an influence from nearby Ascaris parasites that changes your body chemistry. Along with vitamin D_2, the body produces hard deposits of tricalcium phosphate in solid tumors but not true bone. Making deposits is possible when bacteria are growing there, producing a very alkaline pH that results in precipitation of calcium phosphate salts. Giving vitamin D_3 helps remove these deposits by "mobilizing" the calcium in them. But the pH must be corrected too, for this method to succeed. Killing the bacteria by acidifying with IP6 works best. If the calcium level in the blood is over 10 for any reason, wait till it falls to 9.9 before giving this supplement. Get all-polyethylene pipettes or pour the supplement into a polyethylene dropper bottle. Use very tiny drops to go down to 25,000 units.

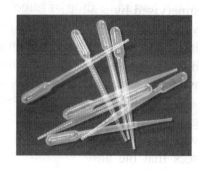

Fig. 87 Polyethylene pipettes or droppers do not seep

Help #18. Oregano oil is fierce if it accidentally touches the mouth. Keep bread handy to swallow in case this happens. If it flows over the capsule rinse it off. Do not dispense it from a rubber dropper because the rubber seeps laundry bleach. Pour yours into a polyethylene dropper bottle or use a polyethylene pipette, used for only this purpose. Not many herbs can kill Clostridium bacteria. Eucalyptus and Birch Bark can.

Help #19. Digestive enzymes taken between meals can roam the body but are not effective in the presence of Ascaris. Ascaris blocks trypsin enzymes. Enzymes let the tumors open for further digestion and for our white blood cells to enter and help with the clean up. They also digest asparagine, which otherwise triggers RAS in yeast, and digest casein, which triggers mumps virus. They digest deposits of food oil, but not lactose, only lactase enzyme can digest milk sugar.

Help #20. Chronic low thyroid levels are typical for cancer patients, as well as very low body temperature. This favors the viruses. The Syncrometer® finds the hormone thyroxine to be changed to d-thyroxine at tumor sites, quite useless as a differentiator and metabolism booster. A blood test would not distinguish between d- and l- hormones, so you would not know you were thyroid-deficient. It is wise of the body to treat it as an allergen. Earlier therapists gave much more than 1 grain, perhaps for this reason, but you should be supervised by a physician if you want to take more. They said you could "burn up" a tumor, especially breast cancer with large doses, together with natural wintergreen, watching for too high a pulse (over 120) as a precaution. Do not take wintergreen for long time periods because it is an aspirin.

The adrenal glands have been especially stressed by the glandular tissue bits of tumor nucleus landing there for years with their inappropriate hormonal impact. The Syncrometer® sees that the adrenal glands produce hardly any cortisone in cancer patients. At the same time they overproduce estradiol, estriole, and estrone. These 3 estrogens circulate everywhere, in men as well as women, over stimulating ovaries and the breast, even in men. Perhaps it is this high-estrogen state that lowers thyroid levels. At any rate, giving a low dose of thyroid will not shut down this gland and will provide much needed stimulation of metabolism besides a rise in temperature.

One grain is $^1/_5$ of your daily requirement. Take enough to raise your temperature to normal. But allergy to thyroid pills is common. Switch varieties if you feel bad an hour after taking them. You could test for prions if you wished, but it does not seem important to me. I believe we all carry prions in our Salmonella bacteria anyway. What is important is not triggering them with PGE2, (any allergies), nor supplying them with gold.

Help #21. Purchase slides (digestive set and anatomy set, at least). Learn to use a battery charger, rechargeable batteries and voltmeter. Purchase 4 inductor-capacitor (I-C) sets of 1 pF and 1 µH each. Start zapping the blood, lymph, WBCs, cerebrospinal fluid, lymph vessels and nerves and veins, called "L", and arteries, more nerves and more veins, called "A". Start zapping early in the day and end at sunset to minimize the burden on kidneys at night. Purchase or build a copy-maker plate. Purchase ½ oz. amber bottles of polyethylene and glass. These do not seep. For drop-making, get polyethylene bottles with built in drop dispenser. Use rainwater or distilled home-filtered water, stored only in HDPE♲ containers for drop-making. Complete the whole zapping schedule. Before you are done, you will have had several bouts of detox-illness. Go to #16, #25, and #26 to be sure you know how to prevent and stop any illness before it worsens.

Help #22.   Levamisole kills Ascaris, Strongyloides, and dog heartworm, Dirofilaria. It also removes ferritin from your white blood cells, so they can sense and pursue your enemies again. Ferritin coating of our white blood cells is caused by asbestos in your food and water. It only takes a week to remove ferritin, but the second week helps against parasites. Go off after 3 weeks.

Help #23.   While capsules of freeze-dried green Black Walnut hull have great value, you cannot expect them to replace the fresh green tincture from a newly opened bottle. Potency is important when you are sick or advanced. Stay seated while taking this potion. Preferably take it while zapping. Many parasite eggs are stuck in your wheel bearing grease and disappear as it is removed. Patient daily removal plus extermination is best.

Help #24.   Do not microwave since it destroys organic germanium, selenite and other minerals. Purchase cut and sifted (c/s) herbs to maximize potency and avoid nickel and chromium pollution from grinder blades. Make teas fresh daily. Purchase organic grade if possible; others often have thallium and laundry bleach.

Help #25.   If you neglect symptoms, Salmonella bacteria increase and soon release prions. This is probably the true source of prions (BSE) for animals, too. Prions cause dizziness and disorientation, even psychosis. But your white cells eat them quickly and kill them if they themselves are not disabled by dyes or nickel. Prions are triggered, like any virus, but this time by PGE2. This means any food antigen at the location you are killing a F. buski parasite could trigger prion release from the Salmonella that is escaping. Watch your diet carefully to stop all PGE2 from forming (avoid your food allergies). Prions have a requirement for gold, but Salmonella does too and must release it when it is killed. Then prions can snatch it. Your gold level goes down about a week after removing every bit of it from your body. If you have a tendency toward dizziness, be sure all gold is out of your dentalware, eyeglass stems, chains, rings. Regular zapping is best for detox symptoms.

Help #26. Medical tape varieties, as well as band-aids test *Positive* for mercury and thallium. Do not pull tape off skin—let it loosen in shower. Dropping them or heating them could change their polarity. Test polarity next day. Treat them gently. An alternative to these small skin magnets is sitting on a large magnet of several thousand gauss. A 4" x 5" ceramic magnet of 4000 to 5000 gauss reaches the kidney white blood cells. Sit on it for 5 minutes, then get off for 25 minutes. Repeat as often as possible throughout the day. Handle any large magnet with great care. Always store on the floor with north side up, in a double plastic shopping bag. The patient should not touch, pick up, or get near the south side.

Help #27. Do not mix them because their chemistry changes as they react together. They will remove heavy metals for you. One removes mercury and <u>unnatural</u> metals. The other removes nickel and the remaining <u>natural</u> metals. Bring to a boil every other morning to sterilize. Add ¼ cup water and reboil if a white precipitate forms. They both have a tropism for the thymus, which is beneficial.

Help #28. Horseradish kills Ascaris and thereby removes an important longevity factor for tumor cells. It also provides peroxidase, an oxidizing enzyme. Raw beet helps the liver greatly with digestion. Less phenol (and food antigen) is produced. Use a stainless steel grater, not plastic.

Help #29. These seeds can kill the tumor nucleus and SV 40 virus! Even other oncoviruses, when they are sheltered inside yeast buds, can be killed quickly with this. It even destroys some food antigens. This is not the same as laetrile. Seeds, once removed from their pits lose potency in an hour. Refrigeration does not help.

Help #30. This immediately stimulates the immune cells to go to work. It also adds to northerly polarization needed by body tissues. If you start with rainwater, the effect is stronger and lasts longer. Just standing the water on the north side of a large magnet has some effectiveness, too.

Help #31. For this, drop the ozonator hose into the water, seeing that the diffuser produces many tiny bubbles. Ozonated water brings an oxidizing action that can kill many invaders. It can oxidize metals[*] and PCBs, making them more soluble in water so they can be removed more easily.

Help #32. Glutathione can combine with many heavy metals, making them easier to remove. It is particularly valuable for lungs and liver.

Help #33. Itching and flaking of skin, especially in groin, often lets you rub off small warts and blemishes. Be patient with its healing action for a few days before taking a break.

Help #34. Cysteine helps kill Ascaris. It helps both liver and kidneys to heal and renew themselves with new tissue. It can heal cystic kidneys if malonic acid is stopped. You can see this after 3 weeks on an x-ray. Sometimes a dose produces a detox-symptom; stay seated. Do not drive a vehicle.

Help #35. The purpose of the enemas is not to empty the bowels. It is to kill the oncoviruses and even the sheltered ones in colon bacteria. It needs to reach quite high up to reach them in the rest of the body. It cannot reach the head and eyes or

---

[*] Testers, note that oxidizing metals can make them "disappear". To find them again you would need to test for the metal oxide (magnesium oxide, for example) or metal hydroxide.

268

neck. That is why you should take these combinations by mouth at the same time.

Doing the Enema

Purchase 2 kinds of enema equipment, the popular Fleet bottle and the bucket from *Sources*. You will need to do pre-enemas to clear the colon first. Buy a Fleet bottle (set of 2), at a pharmacy; throw away the contents, wipe and wash away the grease on the nozzle with very hot water. Throw away the nozzle cap; it cannot be cleaned. This will be used for the pre-enemas to clear the colon enough to allow the plastic tube of the enema bucket to reach high up on the left side later. Fit the plastic tube on the bucket spigot. Push stop valve onto the closed position. Practice this.

If the Fleet bottle is not available, you can improvise with a 1 pint or 1 quart plastic bottle used for bottled water. Attach a nozzle meant for other enema equipment. Make a pinhole in the bottom of the bottle, leaving the pin in place. After inserting, pull out the pin and control the flow with your thumb. Another improvised quick enema is with a 50 or 60 ml syringe. Attach rubber tube.

The 2 pre-enemas take only 5 or 10 minutes each. Fill the Fleet bottle with very warm water; then add 6 drops of Lugol's to the top. Apply homemade soap to nozzle for best lubricant and to anal area to prevent hemorrhoids. After washing, disinfect your hand immediately in Lugol's water (1 drop per cup of water, made fresh). Insert nozzle while bending over near the toilet, aiming nozzle toward navel. Bear down, with a pushing force, to make insertion painless. After removing, sit on top of closed toilet seat at least 5 minutes for best results. Keep a magazine handy to occupy yourself while waiting. Then empty bowels. Repeat, being sure to lubricate well again. This time hold it 10 minutes before emptying. After that you are ready for the real enema using the bucket. Do it right away, to be near the Lugol's timing. Prepare it ahead of time.

Have ready 6 capsules turmeric already emptied in the bucket; close valve and add 1 cup very warm water. Run it in slowly to avoid expelling it. None of this super enema is to be expelled at all. That is why so little water is used. Do not pull out the tube yet. Sit on it or lean back to reduce pressure. After 20 to 30 minutes put 6 fennel capsules in the bucket, add ½ to 1 cup water and run it in very slowly. Do not pull out the tube yet. After another 20 minutes, open 2 coenzyme Q10 capsules into hot water, they will cool en route. Keep these in for 15 minutes. Then add a final ½ tsp. of Lugol's to top of tube. After running each one in, lie down, read or watch entertainment till all urgency to expel is gone. Leaning back helps, too.

If you did need to expel, reduce the water volume next time.

This "super" enema, given correctly, has the most powerful effect on how sick you feel. Even if you feel immediately better though, these bacteria and viruses will all come back unless you complete the whole program. Do not premix Lugol's or other items with each other. Wash the bottle, nozzle, bucket and hose using Lugol's in water until color is visible, it kills everything it contacts. For more help, read earlier books by this author.

Help #36. Oregano oil stings; do not get it onto mouth or any other open surfaces. You can make your own oregano oil toothpowder, see page 573. Test your supplies first for laundry bleach. To apply it after dentalwork, wrap a strip of paper towel around your finger. Dampen in clean water and dip into powder. Rub each tooth, inside and outside surfaces.

Help #37. Begin counting the betaine-days right after dental work is complete. You need 3 days of 3 capsules, 3 times a day from the end of dental work.

Help #38. Do not take more because locations where bacteria are growing are much too alkaline and would precipitate calcium deposits, as has already happened in the tumor.

Help #39. Cancer patients are much too acid where phenolic substances or formic acid or malonic acid have accumulated. Lactic acid (LDH) levels might be much too high, too. All these acids reduce the kidneys' ability to excrete its daily toxins—a serious handicap. Neutralizing the acids with bicarbonates like baking soda or the balanced variety that includes potassium is an efficient way to get them all excreted. It could take a week to get rid of formic acid and stop internal bleeding, but even hemorrhage can be stopped with the help of bicarbonates, as long as the source of acids has been stopped. Do not take more than this because of a possible effect on hemoglobin. Purchase urinary pH paper at a pharmacy. Tests are only valid if done upon rising, before eating.

Help #40. You should make a minimum of 2¼ quarts (liters) urine a day (24 hours). Test daily till you get that much. Then test once a week. Drink your teas before supper time to reduce nighttime urination. Do not try to make more than 3 quarts.

Help #41. Ginger and uva ursi remove methyl malonate from kidneys. This is the main kidney toxin, causing both kidney failure and cystic kidneys besides blockage. You can expect a sudden increase of urine lasting a week. If it doesn't happen you are still getting malonic acid.

Help #42. To reduce your dose, dispense a much smaller drop. It does not have to be precise.

Help #43. Do not put any lotion or oil or salve on your skin, nor soap of any kind. Use only borax solution, minimally. You may use butter.

Help #44. See Liver Cleanse on page 563. Use olive oil for this purpose only. Do not use grapefruit if you have brain or spinal cancer; it contains caffeic acid, the antigen for brain. Use citric acid dissolved in apple juice to make a tart but pleasant substitute. The next day use double the lipase-pancreatin in the program to get rid of the oil deposits again. No other oil seems to be able to replace olive oil for the liver cleanse. Lugol's for such use does not need to be pure. Ask a pharmacist to make 10% formaldehyde for you. Or dilute 37% formaldehyde with an equal amount of water. This gives 18½ %. Dilute this again with an equal amount of water to give 9%. This is close enough.

271

Help #45. IP6 is organic phosphate and extremely sour. It alone can dissolve the hard calcium deposits in tumors. Tricalcium phosphate deposits form easily but dissolve very, very slowly, because the pH is so alkaline all around it from bacteria nearby. IP6 is helped by inositol and vitamin D_3 but the whole program is necessary to remove them. It requires that the CD8 and CD14 WBCs (your immune system) actually eat the tricalcium phosphate and deliver it to the urine.

Help #46. Read about MSM on the Internet. In scientific tests much more was given than we are using. Feel free to use more, but only if tested by Syncrometer®.

CHAPTER 12

SYNCROMETER® TESTER'S FLOW SHEET

For the 3-Week Cancer Curing Program

This flow sheet gives you a path that leads to success with certainty. Follow each number to its counterpart in the set with asterisks(*) on page 278. Complete each instruction given in the asterisk set. From there, go to the underlined set that tells you what changes to make. And from there, go to the bracketed set with instructions on how to clear your body of the unwanted items. Copy the flow sheet for a convenient report form.

The flow sheet uses 4 levels of body cleansing (detoxifying): saliva, lymph, organ with the tumor, and the tumor itself. The saliva represents the systemic (system wide) level where major problems would make themselves evident and testable. Things recently eaten or of major significance can be detected here. As soon as a major problem begins to subside, it is no longer detectable in the saliva, but could still be detected in the lymph. As it subsides further, it is only detectable in the organ that has been accumulating it and finally, only in the tumor. Each level should be cleared, but often you can skip a level or go right to the tumor. Write results in the blank columns.

Purchase or make your own test substances, organ samples, parasite, pathogen and metabolite samples (see *Sources*, also *Syncrometer® Science Laboratory Manual*).

Syncrometer® Test Flow-Sheet

Test substance	should be	at saliva	at lymph	at organ with tumor	at tumor
		RESULTS			
1. laundry bleach	Neg				
2. water softener salts	Neg				
3. motor oil	Neg				
4. wheel bearing grease	Neg				
5. asbestos	Neg				
6. mixed heavy metals	Neg				
7. mixed azo dyes	Neg				
8. malonic acid set*	Neg				
These eight are accumulations from your drinking water.					
9. north pole	Pos				
10. south pole	Neg				
These are magnetic polarizations, see text.					
The following metals are tests using atomic absorption standards, namely, inorganic.					
11. mercury, thallium	Neg				
12. gold	Neg				
13. uranium	Neg				
14. copper	Neg				
15. cobalt	Neg				
16. chromium III & VI	Neg				
17. germanium, strontium	Neg				
18. vanadium	Neg				
19. selenium	Neg				
20. nickel	Neg				
21. aluminum	Neg				
22. lead	Neg				
23. bromine	Neg				
24. cadmium	Neg				
25. thulium	Neg				
26. formaldehyde	Neg				
27. arsenic, ruthenium	Neg				
28. methanol	Neg				
29. benzene	Neg				

---

* malonic acid, methyl malonate, maleic acid, maleic anhydride, D-malic acid

274

Test substance	should be	at saliva	at lymph	at organ with tumor	at tumor
	RESULTS				
30. PCBs	Neg				
31. hypochlorite	Neg				
32. ferritin	Neg				
33. Flu (influenza) virus	Neg				
34. prion protein	Neg				
35. mumps virus	Neg				
36. S.* enteriditis	Neg				
37. S. paratyphi	Neg				
38. S. typhimurium	Neg				
39. Shigella dysenteriae	Neg				
40. Shigella sonnei	Neg				
41. Staphylococcus aureus	Neg				
42. Streptococcus pneumoniae	Neg				
43. Streptococcus G	Neg				
44. Aspergillus fungus	Neg				
45. Penicillium fungus	Neg				
46. aflatoxin	Neg				
47. Escherichia coli	Neg				
48. formic acid	Neg				
The next 8 are oncoviruses (oncogenes).					
49. MYC	Neg				
50. SRC	Neg				
51. JUN	Neg				
52. FOS	Neg				
53. FOS/JUN	Neg				
54. NEU	Neg				
55. RAS	Neg				
56. SV 40	Neg				
57. CMV	Neg				
58. EBV	Neg				
59. Hepatitis B	Neg				
60. Adenovirus	Neg				
Next, combine bacteria that are *Positive* with oncoviruses that are *Positive* and test again. *Testers, they must touch.*					
61. hemoglobin (HGB)	Neg				

---

* Salmonella

Test substance	should be	at saliva	at lymph	at organ with tumor	at tumor
	RESULTS				
62. complement C3	Pos				
63. stem cell factor (SCF)	Neg				
64. hypothalamus cells	Neg				
65. chlorogenic acid	Neg				
66. human growth hormone (HGH)	Neg				
67. pituitary cells	Neg				
68. phloridzin	Neg				
69. tumor nucleus	Neg				
70. pancreas cells	Neg				
71. gallic acid	Neg				
72. orthophosphotyrosine (OPT)	Neg				
73. tricalcium phosphate	Neg				
74. p53 gene	Neg				
75. isopropyl alcohol	Neg				
76. Clostridium (3 species)	Neg				
77. Fasciolopsis buski	Neg				
78. Fasciolopsis cercariae	Neg				
79. Carcinoembryonic antigen (CEA)	Neg				
80. Bacillus cereus	Neg				
81. Human Chorionic Gonadotropin (HCG)	Neg				
82. yeast, Baker's	Neg				
83. Fasciola	Neg				
84. Strongyloides	Neg				
85. Onchocerca	Neg				
86. Dirofilaria	Neg				
87. Paragonimus	Neg				
88. Clonorchis	Neg				
89. Eurytrema	Neg				
90. Ascaris lumbricoides	Neg				
91. Ascaris megalocephala	Neg				
92. Ribonucleotide reductase, (RRase)	Neg				
93. DNA	Neg				
94. DNA polymerase	Neg				

Test substance	should be	at saliva	at lymph	at organ with tumor	at tumor
	RESULTS				
95. fibronectin	*Neg*				
96. cadherin E	*Neg*				
97. laminin	*Neg*				
98. prostaglandin (PGE2)	*Neg*				
99. phosphatidyl serine (PS)	*Pos*				
100. cytochrome C	*Pos*				
101. ubiquitin	*Pos*				
102. caspase-1	*Pos*				
103. cathepsin B	*Pos*				
104. telomerase inhibitor II	*Pos*				
105. lipase-pancreatin	*Pos*				

Repeat the tests at the lymph after the saliva has cleared.

Repeat the tests at the organ with the tumor.

Repeat the tests at the tumor.

Test #99 tells you if apoptosis is being signaled to begin.

Test #100 tells you if apoptosis is underway.

Tests #101 to #104 tell you which essential link for apoptosis might be missing.

Test #105 tells you if external digestion by your own digestive enzymes has begun.

Next, test if the immune system's white blood cells are eating the tumor. To identify the tumor cells, put the regular tissue slide in series with (touching) the tricalcium phosphate sample. The tumor part of an organ invariably has tricalcium phosphate deposits, which mark it.

To test if the immune system (WBCs) is eating the tumor cells, choose only the CD14 and CD8 white blood cells. Place them near, not quite touching, the saliva sample, to indicate that more than those reachable by direct contact with saliva will be tested. Place tumor cells on opposite plate, for example, breast/tricalcium phosphate for breast tumor cells.

Test substance	should be	at saliva	at lymph	at organ with tumor	at tumor
	RESULTS				
106. tumor cells in CD8 cells	Pos				
107. tumor cells in CD14 cells	Pos				

Five days after PS, lipase-pancreatin, and "tumor cells in CD8s" (and CD14s) are all *Positive* together, you may **schedule a scan or new blood test**.

Search for WHAT and WHERE

*1. (**laundry bleach**) If *Positive*, search in water.

*2. (**water softener**) If *Positive*, search in water.

*3. (**motor oil**) If *Positive*, search in water.

*4. (**wheel bearing grease**) If *Positive* search in water and in CD4s, CD8s, CD14s.

*5. (**asbestos**) If *Positive*, search in water, house dust, food.

*6. (**mixed heavy metals**) If *Positive*, search in water, cookware, dentalware, supplements, foods.

*7. (**mixed azo dyes**) If *Positive*, search in water, supplements, food, drugs, enamel and plastic food containers, plastic teeth, toothbrush, etc. Search for Fast Red, Fast Green, Fast Garnet, Fast Blue, Fast Red Violet, DAB, Sudan Black B (find list of dyes on page 603).

*8. (**malonic acid set**) If *Positive*, search in water, cookware, dishes, utensils, food, dentalware.

*9. (**north pole**) If *Negative*, search in water for polarization, in saliva for SCF, nickel, and Fe_2O_3.

*10. (**south pole**) If *Positive*, search in water for polarization, in saliva for SCF, nickel, and Fe_3O_4.

*11. (**mercury, thallium**) If *Positive*, search for amalgam in dentalware, mercury and thallium in glass and Teflon food containers, tampons, medicine, supplements.

*12. (**gold**) If *Positive*, search in dentalware, jewelry, glassware, and in ovaries, pancreas, hypothalamus. Search for HIV (in P24), prions, Salmonella.

*13. (**uranium**) If *Positive*, search for water softener salts in water, medicines, supplements.

*14. (**copper**) If *Positive*, search in water, water pipes, dentalware, cookware, supplements, and in liver.

*15. (**cobalt**) If *Positive*, search in water, cookware, supplements, dish detergent, and in heart, liver, WBC and critical organ. Check blood test for low LDH, alk phos.

*16. (**chromium III & VI**) If *Positive*, search in water, cookware, food, supplements, and for yeast, Staphylococcus, Streptococcus in lymph, SV 40.

*17. (**germanium, strontium**) If *Positive* for germanium, search for hypochlorite (chlorination treatment) in water, saliva. If *Positive* for strontium, search distilled water, malfunctioning filter. Search for Mycobacterium TB, M. avium/cellulare, Mycoplasma, Pseudomonas, CMV, Strep pneumoniae, Pneumocytis, Chaetomium, HIV (in reverse transcriptase), SV 40. Search in bone marrow, RBCs, B-cells, platelets, lungs, megakaryocytes. Search for CORN.

*18. (**vanadium**) If *Positive*, search in cookware, plastic teeth, house dust. Search for E. coli, Mycobacterium avium/cellulare, Flu, in saliva, lymph. Search for CORN.

*19. (**selenium**) If *Positive*, search in supplements (vitamin C), cookware.

*20. (**nickel**) If *Positive*, search in water, dentalware, jewelry, cookware, and for yeast, E. coli, Staphylococcus, HIV, Clostridium. Search at CD4, CD8, CD14 WBCs. Test polarization.

*21. (**aluminum**) If *Positive*, search in water, body products, food, cookware; and at throat, cerebrum, skin.

*22. (**lead**) If *Positive*, search in water, drugs, supplements, and at liver, bone marrow, colon.

*23. (**bromine**) If *Positive*, search in breads, cereals, spices.

*24. (**cadmium**) If *Positive*, search in water, cookware, dentalware, supplements, drugs. Search at kidneys.

*25. (**thulium**) If *Positive*, search in water, vitamin C, supplements, drugs.

*26. (**formaldehyde**) If *Positive*, search in house dust, food. Also search for benzene in saliva.

*27. (**arsenic, ruthenium**) If *Positive* for arsenic, search in house dust. If *Positive* for ruthenium, search in distilled water, charcoal filters. Search for Salmonella ent., S. para; S. typhi. Search for S. ent. at pancreas. Search for prion.

*28. (**methanol**) If *Positive*, search in diet and at pancreas, eyes. Also search for benzene.

*29. (**benzene**) If *Positive*, search in water, foods, medicines, body products, supplements. Search for P24, reverse transcriptase.

*30. (**PCBs**) If *Positive*, search in water, foods, medicines, body products, supplements.

*31. (**hypochlorite**) If *Positive*, search in water and for germanium.

*32. (**ferritin**) If *Positive*, search for asbestos in water (see #5). Search for ferritin on/in WBCs.

*33. (**Flu**) If *Positive*, search for F. buski, Clostridium, salmonella, prion. Search for dyes, heavy metals in water, WBCs.

*34. (**prion** protein) If *Positive*, search for Salmonella. Search for PGE2, gold at lymph.

*35. (**mumps**) If *Positive*, search for casein and Ascaris larvae in parotid gland and lymph.

*36., *37., *38. (**Salmonella ent., para, typhi.**) If *Positive*, search for Salmonella ent. at pancreas, Salmonellas in WBC. If *Negative* here, search for dyes in

WBC. Search for gold, molybdenum, ruthenium in lymph. Search for oncoviruses inside bacteria.

*39., *40. (**Shigella**) If *Positive*, search in food. Search for oncoviruses inside bacteria. Search at bronchioles. Search for manganese at bronchioles.

*41. (**Staph aur**) If *Positive*, search at breast, skin, and teeth (bone). Search for yeast, SRC, chromium, Strongyloides, Adenovirus. Search for pink skin.

*42. (**Strep pneu**) If *Positive*, search at pain location, at teeth. Search for chromium, formic acid, hemoglobin (bleeding), benzene.

*43. (**Strep G**) If *Positive*, search for Ascaris, chromium. Search at respiratory organs (lungs, trachea, larynx, bronchi).

*44. (**Aspergillus**) If *Positive*, search for chromium, cobalt, nickel in water, cookware, foods. Search at liver for Aspergillus, aflatoxin, bilirubin oxidase. Search blood for bilirubin, bilirubin oxidase.

*45. (**Penicillium**) If *Positive*, search for copper, aflatoxin, bilirubin at liver.

*46. (**aflatoxin**) If *Positive*, EMERGENCY! Search for aflatoxin, copper, chromium, cobalt, nickel at each of 10 liver locations. Do blood test for total bilirubin and evidence of liver failure.

*47. (**E. coli**) If *Positive*, search for vanadium, molybdenum, manganese, chromium, nickel, all oncoviruses, and for E. coli bacteria with oncovirus inside.

*48. (**formic acid**) If *Positive*, search for HGB (bleeding) at pain, tumor, and effusate locations. Search for benzene (see #29). Search for Streptococcus pneumoniae.

*49. (**MYC**) If *Positive*, search for mumps, F. buski, Ascaris, casein.

*50. (**SRC**) If *Positive*, search for Strongyloides, linolenic acid (oil), potato.

*51. (**JUN**) If *Positive*, search for Onchocerca, myristic, oleic, palmitic acid (oil), cinnamic acid antigen, corn.

*52., *53. (**FOS, FOS / JUN**) If *Positive*, search for Dirofilaria, lactose, oleic acid (oil), coumarin (antigen).

*54. (**NEU**) If *Positive*, search for Ascaris lumbricoides, Ascaris megalocephala, linolenic acid (oil).

*55. (**RAS**) If *Positive*, search for yeast, chromium, cobalt, nickel.

*56. (**SV 40**) If *Positive*, EMERGENCY! Search for gallic acid, pancreatic fluke, limonene, chromium, gold, strontium. Search for combinations of SV 40 with other oncoviruses and bacteria.

*57., *58. (**CMV, EBV**) If *Positive*, search at lungs for chromium, strontium, aluminum, malonic acid, Streptococcus G and its combinations with oncoviruses. Search for Strongyloides, lauric acid, linolenic acid, potato.

*59. (**Hepatitis B**) If *Positive*, search for Clonorchis, Clostridium botulinum, combinations of Hepatitis B with other oncoviruses and bacteria. Search for oats, carrot (umbelliferone). Search at liver and pituitary.

*60. (**Adenovirus**) If *Positive*, search for Ascaris, combinations of Adenovirus with other oncoviruses, bacteria and hypothalamus cells. Find metal requirements of carrier bacteria and for oncoviruses using subtraction method with Syncrometer®. See text.

*61. (**HGB**) If *Positive*, signifies bleeding. Search for location of bleeding, Streptococcus pneu, formic acid, benzene, menadione, coumarin, ASA, dyes, and maleic anhydride.

*62. (**C3**) If *Negative*, search for PGE2 and food antigens. Search for combinations of C3 with food antigens. Search for F. buski.

*63. (**SCF**) If *Positive*, search for free hypothalamus cells, chlorogenic acid.

*64. (**hypothalamus**) If *Positive*, search for chlorogenic acid, Strongyloides, potato.

*65. (**chlorogenic**) If *Positive*, search for hypothalamus cells, Strongyloides, potato. Search food for chlorogenic acid.

*66. (**HGH**) If *Positive*, search for free pituitary cells, phloridzin, human liver fluke, oats

*67. (**pituitary**) If *Positive*, search for phloridzin, Clonorchis, oats. Search for combinations of pituitary cells with Flu, Adenovirus, CMV, EBV.

*68. (**phloridzin**) If *Positive*, search for free pituitary cells. Search in food.

*69. (**tumor nucleus**) If *Positive*, EMERGENCY! Search for chlorogenic, phloridzin, gallic acid, SV 40 virus, Strongyloides, Clonorchis, Eurytrema. Treat immediately. Retest in 3 days.

*70. (**pancreas cells**) If *Positive*, search for gallic acid, Eurytrema, limonene.

*71. (**gallic**) If *Positive*, search for SV 40, pancreatic fluke, free pancreas cells. Search in food.

*72. (**OPT**) If *Positive*, EMERGENCY! Search for OPT in suspected organs, also F. buski, isopropyl alcohol. Search for tumor nucleus.

*73. (**tricalcium phosphate**) If *Positive*, search for A. lumbricoides, A. megalocephala, vitamin D_2, vitamin D_3.

*74. (**p53**) If *Positive*, search for vanadium pentoxide (atomic absorption standard), azo dyes.

*75. (**isopropyl alcohol**) If *Positive*, search for Clostridium bacteria, OPT, Fasciolopsis cercariae, HCG.

*76. (**Clostridium**) If *Positive*, search for DNA, isopropyl alcohol. Search at colon, teeth, tumor.

*77. (**F. buski**) If *Positive*, search for OPT, Bacillus cereus, MYC, ONION, allyl methyl sulfide.

*78. (**F. cercaria**) If *Positive*, search for Bacillus cereus, ONION, allyl methyl sulfide, HCG.

*79. (**CEA**) If *Positive*, search for yeast, Onchocerca.

*80. (**Bacillus cereus**) If *Positive*, search for F. buski, d-tyramine, d-thyroxine, d- tyrosine, d-phenylalanine.

*81. (**HCG**) If *Positive*, search for Fasciolopis cercaria.

*82. (**Yeast**) If *Positive*, search for chromium, cobalt, nickel, CEA, asparagine, RAS. Search for red skin areas.

Search for Staphylococcus or Streptococci at breast, breast skin or teeth.

*83. (**Fasciola**) If *Positive*, search for lauric acid (lard), gluten, gliadin, beef, fibronectin.

*84. (**Strongyloides**) If *Positive*, search for linolenic acid (oil), potatoes, SRC, CMV, EBV.

*85. (**Onchocerca**) If *Positive*, search for JUN, JUN / FOS, liver growth factor. Search for cinnamic acid antigen, dilated veins and vein valves visible under skin, nodules under skin, myristic, oleic, palmitic acids (oil), corn. Search in non Hodgkin's tumors.

*86. (**Dirofilaria**) If *Positive*, search for FOS, FOS / JUN, liver growth factor, lactose, oleic acid (oil), coumarin antigen, purple patches (purpura). Search in Hodgkin's and abdominal tumors

*87. (**Paragonimus**) If *Positive*, search for lemon and limonene, zearalenone, benzene. Search for lung disease, Pneumocystis, EBV, CMV.

*88. (**Clonorchis**) If *Positive*, search for oats, Clostridium botulinum, free pituitary cells, phloridzin. Search at liver. Also search liver for Hepatitis B virus.

*89. (**Eurytrema**) If *Positive*, search for SV 40, gallic acid, lemon.

*90. (**A. lumb**) If *Positive*, search for quercitin, NEU, mumps, Adenovirus, cathepsin B, telomerase inhibitor II, linolenic acid.

*91. (**A. megalo**) If *Positive*, search for d-carnitine, NEU, laminin, telomerase inhibitor II, cadherin E.

*92. (**RRase**) If *Positive*, search for duration of RRase, thiourea, DNA, bcl-2 in minutes and seconds. Search for yeast.

*93., *94. (**DNA, DNA polymerase**) If *Positive*, search for Clostridium. Search for bcl-2, RRase, thiourea (check time of duration for each).

*95. (**fibronectin**) If *Positive*, search for Fasciola.

*96., *97. (cadherin E, laminin) If *Positive*, search for F. buski, Ascaris megalocephala.

*98. (**PGE2**) If *Positive*, search for food antigens, F. buski, Bacillus cereus, d-tyramine.

*99. (**PS**) If *Negative*, search for caspase-1, telomerase inhibitor II, cathepsin B, ubiquitin. All four must be *Positive* for apoptosis to proceed. Search for parasites, yeast, CEA, HCG, HGH, SCF.

*100. (**cytochrome C**) If *Negative*, search for PS, caspase-1, telomerase inhibitor II, cathepsin B, ubiquitin.

*101. (**ubiquitin**) If *Negative*, search for Onchocerca.

*102. (**caspase-1**) If *Negative*, search for yeast, CEA.

*103. (**cathepsin B**) If *Negative*, search for Ascaris lumbricoides, Fasciola, Onchocerca.

*104. (**telomerase inhibitor II**) If *Negative*, search for A. lumbricoides and A. megalo, yeast, Onchocerca.

*105. (**lipase-pancreatin**) If *Negative*, search for cathepsin B.

*106. (**tumor cells in CD8 cells**) If *Negative*, search at CD8 cells for nickel, wheel bearing grease.

*107. (**tumor cells in CD14 cells**) If *Negative*, search at CD14 cells for nickel, wheel bearing grease.

Changes to Make

1. (**laundry bleach**) Switch to NSF-bleach water, rainwater, well water.

2. (**water softener**) Disconnect; replace pipes and/or water heater.

3. (**motor oil**) Switch to NSF-bleach water, rainwater, well water.

4. (**wheel bearing grease**) Switch to NSF-bleach water, rainwater, well water. Remove from critical organs and their WBCs with homeography. Remove systemically with DMSO.

5. (**asbestos**) Switch to NSF-bleach water, rainwater, well water. Asbestos alone can be filtered out with homemade filter. If in dust, change dryer belt, remove gym equipment with treadmill belts, stop use of hair blow-dryers. If in food do 2 hot water washes.

<u>6</u>. (**mixed heavy metals**) Switch to NSF-bleach water, rainwater, well water. If using NSF water, also purchase metal-free (tested), distilled water and pitcher filter with tested activated charcoal. Test final drinking water for strontium, aluminum, hypochlorite. Do dental clean up, removing metal, followed by zappicating entire mouth. Replace all cookware, utensils, food containers with varieties that do not seep heavy metals using a conductivity indicator. Test all plastic, enamelware, paper ware, Styrofoam, glass, ceramics, Teflon, and metal food containers. Take only tested supplements and medicines. Test to find safe brands. Harden toothbrushes, dentures, filter pitcher, cutlery by placing in steaming hot water for 30 min. Retest or repeat twice.

<u>7</u>. (**mixed azo dyes**) Switch to NSF-bleach water, rainwater, well water. Double hot wash produce. Ozonate meats & dairy products 10 minutes. Purchase free-range, organic whole turkey, lamb, beef, tested for dyes. Avoid chicken, fish, seafood. Replace seeping cookware. Zappicate plastic teeth. Harden dentures, toothbrushes. Avoid colored foods, pills. Test body products for dyes.

<u>8</u>. (**malonic acid set**) Switch to NSF-bleach water, rainwater, well water. Replace cookware with safe varieties. Avoid foods that cannot be washed enough (sprayed potatoes, carrots, sweet potatoes, tomatoes) or tested.

<u>9</u>., <u>10</u>. (**wrong polarization**) Switch to NSF-bleach water, rainwater, well water. Remove all nickel in food, cookware and dentalware.

<u>11</u>. (**mercury, thallium**) Extract amalgam filled teeth. Replace cooking pots, supplements, drugs with safe varieties. Stop using paper goods inside the body.

<u>12</u>. (**gold**) Extract metal containing teeth, zappicate mouth later. Replace jewelry with non metal varieties.

<u>13</u>. (**uranium**) Remove water softener.

<u>14</u>. (**copper**) Replace water pipes with PVC; do metal clean up as in <u>6</u>.

15. (**cobalt**) Avoid dish detergent; remove metals as in 6.

16. (**chromium III & VI**) Avoid finely ground foods, supplements, herbs (choose cut and sifted variety); remove metals as in 6. Test for staph, streps, Yeast, SV 40.

17. (**germanium, strontium**) Avoid chlorinated drinking water or boil for 1 full minute in safe stainless steel pot. Test again. Avoid strontium by choosing different distilled water, repairing water filter pitcher, stop eating honey, corn, cornstarch-containing pills, dextrose in IV therapy.

18. (**vanadium**) Do metal clean up as in 6. Check for leaking or stored fossil fuel. Switch to all-electric utilities. Zappicate plastic teeth.

19. (**selenium**) Switch to safe varieties. Metallic form is toxic.

20. (**nickel**) Do metal clean up as in 6. Extract metal-repaired teeth, remove metal jewelry. Avoid finely ground powders as in herbs, nut butters, blender-prepared foods. Avoid untested food processors, graters and grinders. Avoid untested food, supplements.

21. (**aluminum**) Filter water through Syncrometer®-tested activated charcoal in pitcher filter. Avoid aluminum in food preparation, cookware, body products.

22. (**lead**) Replace copper pipes with PVC. Replace supplements, drugs with tested varieties.

23. (**bromine**)Avoid commercial breads. Find bromine-free varieties of flour, cereals, spices.

24. (**cadmium**) Do metal clean up as in 6. Change galvanized pipes to PVC. Avoid untested supplements, drugs, cookware.

25. (**thulium**) Avoid reverse osmosis water filters, supplements prepared with such water, unless tested by Syncrometer®.

26. (**formaldehyde**) If *Positive* in house dust, remove new furniture, foam bedding, excess paneling, unwashed suits from bedroom closet, newspapers.

27. (**arsenic, ruthenium**) Steam clean carpets, furniture, drapes without commercial treatments. Remove pesticides from house. Replace wallpaper. Avoid ruthenium by choosing different distilled water, boiling any new or used charcoal filter in a large volume of tap water for 5 minutes.

28. (**methanol**) Avoid commercial beverages, teas, bottled water, baby food, medicines unless tested.

29. (**benzene**) Switch to NSF-bleach water, rainwater or well water. Avoid processed foods, bottled water (unless tested), beverages. Double hot wash produce. Test all supplements, medicines, water filters.

30. (**PCBs**) Switch to NSF-bleach water, rainwater, well water. Use no filters or distillers unless tested. Avoid commercial body products. Double hot wash produce. Sonicate baby supplies, dental supplies.

31. (**hypochlorite**) Boil water (NSF-quality) 1 minute in tested stainless steel pan or ozonate 15 minutes. Test again.

32. (**ferritin**) Switch to asbestos-free water. Remove asbestos-containing treadmill belts, dryer belts, hair dryers. Double hot wash produce.

33. (**Flu**) Switch to NSF-bleach water or rainwater or well water to eliminate 5 immunity destroyers. Search for combinations of Flu with oncoviruses and with hypothalamus and pituitary cells. Stop organ erosions.

34. (**prion**) If feeling sick, dizzy, disoriented, search for dyes, heavy metals (gold) at WBCs, saliva, water (see 6., 7.). Search at saliva for food antigen causing PGE2 triggering of prion.

35. (**mumps**) Avoid dairy products in diet except butter and heavy whipping cream. Starve and kill Ascaris.

36., 37., 38. (**Salmonella ent., para, typhi.**) Sterilize food by cooking, ozonating. Rinse raw food in Lugol's iodine solution. Use HCl drops and citric acid with meals. Eliminate dyes; do metal cleanup as in 6. Remove gold, molybdenum, ruthenium from food and water. Boil carbon filter in tap water.

<u>39.</u>, <u>40</u>. (**Shigella**) Sterilize food by cooking, ozonating, and using hydrochloric acid drops. Rinse raw food in Lugol's water. Search food, supplements for manganese.

<u>41</u>. (**Staph aur**) Avoid soaps, lotions, body products; filter aluminum out of water with filter pitcher. Avoid oils in diet. Avoid chromium metal pollution from cookware, supplements, water, food.

<u>42.</u>, <u>43</u>. (**Strep pneu & Strep G**) Remove chromium and strontium from food, water, cookware and dishes. Avoid finely ground foods and supplements. Avoid benzene in food and water. Do metal clean up as in <u>6</u>. Starve and kill Ascaris.

<u>44.</u>, <u>45.</u>, <u>46</u>. (**Aspergillus fungus, Penicillium fungus, aflatoxin**) Do metal clean up as in <u>6</u>. If bilirubin oxidase is *Negative*, search for aflatoxin, Sudan Black dye.

<u>47</u>. (**E. coli**) Do metal clean up as in <u>6</u>. Filter distilled water, after boiling charcoal. Stop eating triggers for oncoviruses found. Remove fossil fuel from home. See #18. Search food, supplements for nickel, chromium, vanadium, molybdenum, manganese.

<u>48.</u> (**formic acid**) Avoid benzene in water, food, products, supplements, drugs, also formaldehyde, methanol which lead to formic acid. Switch to NSF-bleach water.

<u>49</u>. (**MYC**) Avoid chicken and eggs in diet in USA. Stop F. buski parasitism. Stop milk in diet (to stop mumps).

<u>50</u>. (**SRC**) Avoid all cooking oils. Test meats for linolenic acid. Switch to free-range, organic meats. Stop potatoes in diet.

<u>51</u>. (**JUN**) Avoid oils in diet. Stop cinnamon and corn in diet.

<u>52.</u>, <u>53</u>. (**FOS, FOS/JUN**) Avoid milk. Add lactase enzyme to whipping cream. Avoid oleic acid (olive oil). Avoid coumarin (clover honey, vanilla, fragrant rice).

<u>54</u>. (**NEU**) Give away household pets. Avoid quercitin (squash & pumpkin, unless very well cooked) and d-

carnitine (all meats, except free-range, organic). Test meat for bleach variety before purchasing. Avoid linolenic oil.

55. (RAS) Avoid live yeast in diet. Avoid commercial breadstuffs. Use bread maker. Ozonate all food to destroy asparagine. Clean up heavy metals as in 6.

56. (SV 40) Avoid gallic acid in food (commercial breadstuff, grains, and cooking oils). Use *Food Table* for help. Avoid limonene (lemons, pineapple, etc.). Stop triggering oncoviruses found. Stop providing heavy metals to bacteria found. Starve and kill Eurytrema.

57. (CMV) Avoid lauric acid (and lard) in food. Do metal clean up as in 6., particularly strontium.

58. (EBV) Avoid linolenic acid oils in diet. Do metal clean up as in 6., particularly aluminum.

59. (Hepatitis B) Avoid oats and umbelliferone (carrot) in diet; see *Food Table*. Stop Clonorchis parasitism and Clostridium invasion.

60. (Adenovirus) Avoid myristic acid (oil) in diet. Starve and kill Ascaris.

61. (hemoglobin) Test all food and water for benzene, menadione, coumarin, ASA. Test cookware, dentalware, supplements and food for malonic acid set. Also test for heavy metals, particularly chromium.

62. (complement C3) Avoid food antigens phloridzin, chlorogenic acid, gallic acid, ONION, and others found; use *Food Table*. Starve and kill parasites

63., 64., 65. (SCF, hypothalamus cells, chlorogenic) Stop chlorogenic acid in food. See *Food Table*. Starve and kill Strongyloides. Stop potatoes in diet.

66., 67., 68. (HGH, pituitary cells, phloridzin) Stop phloridzin in food, kill Clonorchis parasites, avoid oats in diet.

69. (tumor nucleus) Remove chlorogenic acid, phloridzin, gallic acid from diet. Starve and kill parasites.

70., 71. (pancreas cells, gallic) Avoid gallic acid in food, kill pancreatic flukes. Avoid limonene in diet.

<u>72</u>. (**OPT**) Stop tumor nucleus formation. Kill parasites. Kill oncoviruses.

<u>73</u>. (**tricalcium phosphate**) Kill Ascaris; stop d-carnitine and quercitin in foods to starve Ascaris.

<u>74</u>. (**p53**) Remove vanadium and dyes from food, water, cookware, dentalware. Avoid fossil fuels in home. See #18.

<u>75</u>. (**isopropyl alcohol**) Avoid body products, drugs, processed food. Kill Clostridium in colon, teeth, tumors. Kill F. cercaria with extra large doses of wormwood.

<u>76</u>. (**Clostridium**) Do dental clean up. Kill Clostridium in colon with betaine hydrochloride, in tumors with oregano oil and Eucalyptus tea.

<u>77</u>., <u>78</u>. (**F. buski and cercaria**) Stop ONION family in diet, and cooked foods with allyl methyl sulfide. Kill F. buski with BWT[*] program. Kill Bacillus cereus with nutmeg (but it has myristic oil, stop after 3 days).

<u>79</u>. (**CEA**) Stop asparagine in diet by ozonating all proteins. Avoid chromium, cobalt, nickel in food, cookware, dentalware to kill yeast. Avoid CORN and linolenic acid to starve Onchocerca.

<u>80</u>. (**Bacillus cereus**) Kill F. buski. Kill Bacillus cereus. Normalize magnetic polarization by removing nickel from water, food, supplements, dentalware, cookware.

<u>81</u>. (**HCG**) Avoid ONION and allyl methylsulfide in diet. Starve and Kill F. buski.

<u>82</u>. (**Yeast**) Ozonate all foods to destroy asparagine. Do metal clean up as for <u>6</u>. Avoid ground supplements and foods, blended foods.

<u>83</u>. (**Fasciola**) Avoid wheat, beef, lauric acid (lard) in diet. Kill Fasciola.

<u>84</u>. (**Strongyloides**) Avoid linolenic acid in cooking oil and foods. Avoid potatoes and lauric acid (fat).

---

[*] BWT means the green Black Walnut hull tincture plus wormwood and cloves as in text, without substitutions or alterations.

85. (**Onchocerca**) Avoid corn, myristic, oleic, palmitic acid (oils). Kill Onchocerca with levamisole and BWT program.

86. (**Dirofilaria**) Avoid milk, dairy products, lactose, oleic acid (olive oil). Ozonate butter and whipping cream, also add lactase enzyme to both to destroy lactose. Kill heartworm with BWT program and levamisole.

87. (**Paragonimus**) Avoid lemons and limonene in food. Kill Paragonimus. Avoid benzene in water and food. Avoid potatoes with ring-rot fungus.

88. (**Clonorchis**) Avoid oats in diet. Avoid umbelliferone (carrots, parsnips) to prevent liver disease. Kill liver flukes.

89. (**Eurytrema**) Avoid lemon and limonene in diet. Avoid gallic acid (in commercial breads, grains, and cooking oils).

90. (**A. lumb**) Avoid quercitin (squash & pumpkin) and linolenic acid (oil) in diet. Sterilize all food. Starve and kill Ascaris regularly.

91. (**A. megalo**) Avoid d-carnitine (all meats) in diet, except free-range, organic turkey, lamb, beef. Avoid linolenic acid (oil). Sterilize all food. Starve and kill Ascaris regularly.

92., 93., 94. (**RRase, DNA, DNA polymerase**) If duration is greater than 1 minute, search for SCF, HGH, wrong polarization. Search for nickel.

95. (**fibronectin**) Kill Fasciola. Avoid lauric acid (lard) in diet.

96., 97. (**cadherin E, laminin**) Kill Ascaris and F. buski. Sterilize all foods. Avoid d-carnitine and quercitin. Avoid linolenic acid (oil).

98. (**PGE2**) Kill F. buski, Bacillus cereus to prevent food allergies. Find and avoid allergenic food.

99., 100. (**PS, cytochrome C**) Kill the responsible parasites, bacteria, viruses for each missing item.

101. (**ubiquitin**) Kill Onchocerca; avoid linolenic acid.

102. (**caspase-1**) Kill yeast.

<u>103</u>. (**cathepsin B**) Kill Ascaris, Fasciola, Onchocerca.

<u>104</u>. (**telomerase inhibitor II**) Kill Ascaris, Onchocerca and yeast.

<u>105</u>. (**lipase-pancreatin**) If *Negative*, return to #103.

<u>106</u>.,<u>107</u>. (**tumor cells in CD8 & CD14 WBCs**) Remove sources of nickel in dentalware, jewelry, cookware, supplements, food. Do metal clean up as in <u>6</u>. Remove wheel bearing grease.

Clearing your Body

All treatments are meant for a 3 week period.

{1.} (**laundry bleach**) Will be automatic.

{2.} (**water softener**) Will be automatic.

{3.} (**motor oil**) Sodium selenite, 200 mcg, take 5 four times daily.

{4.} (**wheel bearing grease**) Take wheel bearing grease out with homeography at R and L kidney, R and L kidney WBCs, CD8s, CD14s followed by critical organs. Take DMSO on an empty stomach, before breakfast, highest concentration available, ¼ tsp. (25 drops) in ½ cup cold water, once a day. Test urine for excretion periodically till done (about 6 months). Test DMSO for thallium.

{5.} (**asbestos**) Levamisole, 50 mg, take 2 three times daily; glucuronic acid 200 mg, four times daily.

{6.} (**mixed heavy metals**) Take metals out with homeography after clean up. Take drops of metals-out-of R and L kidney, R and L kidney WBCs, CD4s, CD8s, CD14s, and lymph, also R and L adrenals if very advanced, followed by critical organs.

{7.} (**mixed azo dyes**) Take dyes out with homeography after clean up. Take drops of dyes-out-of R and L kidney, R and L kidney WBCs, CD4s, CD8s, CD14s, and lymph, followed by critical organs.

{8.} (**malonic acid set**) Drink parsley water, boiled 5 minutes in safe stainless steel pan, 2 cups in divided doses daily. Test parsley for bleach first. Increase vitamin C (or rosehips) to double amounts.

{9.}, {10.} (**wrong polarization**) Will be automatic.

{11.}(**mercury, thallium**) L-G, L-A, 1 tsp. to 1 tbsp. of each 3 x daily. Zappicate mouth 3 times after tooth extractions. Use *take-out* drops for liver or a critical organ that has mercury or thallium.

{12.}(**gold**) Continue taking out heavy metals, including gold, as in {6.}.

{13.}(**uranium**) Will be automatic.

{14.} through {24.} (**copper to cadmium**) Use *take-out* drops for any of these metals if present at a critical organ or at CD4s, CD8s, CD14s after metal clean up.

{25.}(**thulium**) Wear two 10-gauss ceramic magnets over each kidney, north pole touching skin, by daytime only. Use masking tape. Soak off in shower. Wear one magnet at back of neck over center spine bone. Test magnet polarity weekly.

{26.}(**formaldehyde**) Take taurine, 1 capsule 3 times daily for 3 days, cysteine 1 capsule 3 times daily for 3 days.

{27.}, {28.} (**arsenic, ruthenium, methanol**) Will be automatic.

{29.}(**benzene**) Zap. Start sodium and potassium bicarbonate mixture (or baking soda), ¼ tsp. 2 x daily. Take vitamin B_2, 300 mg, 2 before meals; also magnesium 300 mg, 2 before meals.

{30.}(**PCBs**) Zap. Take ozonated olive oil, ¼ to ½ cup, in a single dose for 1-2 days. Later, double lipase-pancreatin supplement to digest olive oil for 4 days.

{31.)(**hypochlorite**) Take organic germanium as hydrangea root ½ tsp. 4 times daily; Ge-132 150 mg, 4 times daily, 4 Brazil nuts, Hazel nuts or other nuts, alternating these to avoid build up of oils (see *Sources*). Take vitamin C, 1000 mg, 2 capsules three times daily.

{32.}(**ferritin**) Levamisole, 50 mg, take 2 three times daily before meals for 3 weeks, also glucuronic acid, 200 mg, twice daily, papain (optional, as much as possible).

{33.}(**Flu**) If ill, take Boneset tea, (c/s), 1 cup 3 times daily. Take Elder leaf tea, (c/s), ½ cup 2 times daily. Take

Eucalyptus tea, 1 cup twice daily. Take Oscillococcinum (homeopathic remedy) at bedtime, all until well. Do regular zapping or with vascular set on plate for several hours daily. Take selenite, organic germanium and vitamin C 5 times daily, or as in program. Do Lugol's-turmeric enema to kill oncoviruses.

{34.}(**prion**) Stop food allergens. Start drops to *take-out* gold and ruthenium from lymph and CSF. Zap CSF. Drink birch bark tea, (c/s), 2 cups daily. Take Reishi mushroom (Ganoderma), ½ tsp. 5 times daily till well. Take dyes- and metals-out-of-CSF if present.

{35.}(**mumps**) Lugol's-turmeric enema, daily for 3 days; lactase enzyme with meals. Digest casein with lipase-pancreatin as in program.

{36.},{37.},{38.} (**Salmonellas**) Take Lugol's, 6 drops in ½ cup water after meals and other times, totaling 6 times daily if sick, 4 times daily if not sick. Take citric acid with meals. Do Lugol's-turmeric enema once daily. Start *take-out* drops of gold, molybdenum, ruthenium at lymph for 4 days if present. Take Molybdic acid (4x) 3 drops, 6 times daily till well.

{39.}{40.}(**Shigellas**) Turmeric-fennel enema, 2 x daily for 3 days, can be part of larger enema. Take 6 turmeric and 6 fennel capsules by mouth, 3 times daily, preferably during enema. Take barley water (raw) for organic manganese.

{41.}(**Staph aur**) Do dental clean up to heal bone. Use only butter to cook, no oil. Zap all locations affected. Use *take-out* chromium drops at location of Staph invasion after metal clean up. Take IP6, 10 to 20 drops in water 3 times daily, and inositol, 1 tsp. 3 times daily till gone.

{42.}{43.}(**Strep pneu, Strep G**) Zap location of pain or bleeding. Use *take-out* drops of chromium at critical location and lymph. (See also benzene, formic acid, malonic acid.) Take ¼ tsp. bicarbonates twice daily for formic acid removal.

{44.}(**Aspergillus**) Use *take-out* drops for chromium, cobalt, nickel at all liver locations or other organs if present. Take out aflatoxin at all liver locations if present.

{45.}(**Penicillium**) Use *take-out* drops for copper at all liver locations or other organs. Take out aflatoxin at all affected liver locations.

{46.}(**aflatoxin**) Use *take-out* drops for any metals and dyes found and for aflatoxin and bilirubin from all liver parts and blood.

{47.}(**E. coli**) Use *take-out* drops for vanadium in lymph and critical organ. Take Lugol's-fennel-turmeric enemas once daily, can be part of larger enema. Take 6 capsules fennel and 6 turmeric by mouth 2 times daily and once to coincide with enema.

{48.}(**formic acid**) Give Na/K bicarbonate to excrete formic acid (1/2 tsp. 2 x daily) till formic acid is gone. Then stop.

{49.}(**MYC**) Do Lugol's-turmeric enema daily for 4 days. Take lactase enzyme, one with each meal and one between meals till gone.

{50.},{51.}(**SRC, JUN**) Levamisole, 50 mg, 2 capsules 3 times daily to kill Strongyloides for 3 weeks. Do Lugol's-turmeric-fennel enema daily for 3 days. Take lipase-pancreatin, 15 capsules, 2 x daily to digest oil deposits. Avoid corn to starve Onchocerca.

{52.},{53.},{54.}(**FOS, FOS/JUN, NEU**) Take Lugol's-turmeric-fennel enema daily for 3 days. Take lactase, one per meal and one between meals till gone.

{55.}(**RAS**) Take Lugol's-turmeric enema daily for 3 days. *Take-out* chromium at affected organ after clean up.

{56.}(**SV 40**) Take Lugol's-turmeric enema 1 x daily for 3 days and take Lugol's-turmeric-fennel enema 1 x daily for the same 3 days. Take 6 fresh seed recipe for 5 days, then 5 days OFF, repeating till gone. Take BWT parasite program daily. Stop powdered, finely ground foods.

{57.},{58.}(**CMV, EBV**) Take heavy metals-out-of-lymph and location of CMV or EBV with drops 3 x daily after metal clean up. If ill, start Eucalyptus tea, 2 cups daily till better. Drink only distilled-filtered water temporarily, as described in text, to remove strontium and aluminum. Avoid corn.

{59.}(**Hepatitis B**) Start milk thistle tea (tested for thallium), 2 cups daily and Eucalyptus tea as in program till better. Kill parasites with BWT program daily. Kill Clostridium with oregano oil, Eucalyptus, Birch bark.

{60.}(**Adenovirus**) Take Oscillococcinum at bedtime. Take Eucalyptus tea, (c/s), 2 cups a day, Boneset tea, (c/s), 2 cups a day, Elder leaf tea, (c/s), ½ cup a day. Stop all these when well. Take vitamin C, selenite, and germanium as in program.

{61.}(**HGB**) Give Yunnan payao (Chinese herb) ¼ tsp. 3 to 4 times daily in water to stop bleeding. Give Na/K bicarbonate (or baking soda) ¼ tsp. twice daily to eliminate formic acid.

{62.}(**C3**) Kill F. buski and remove nickel to stop allergies. Destroy remaining ONION deposits with double amounts of digestive enzymes.

{63.}, {64.}, {65.} (**SCF, hypothalamus, chlorogenic**) Kill Strongyloides with levamisole, 50 mg, take 2 three times daily before meals. Take lipase-pancreatin in large doses to digest potato residues.

{66.},{67.},{68.}(**HGH, pituitary, phloridzin**) Kill liver flukes with BWT program. Take lipase-pancreatin in large doses to digest oat residues.

{69.},{70.},{71.},{72.}(**tumor nucleus, pancreas, gallic, OPT**) Zap. Take 6 fresh, raw apricot seeds, pounded or rolled in zippered plastic bag, fresh from pit, daily for 5 days (if not available use peach or nectarine). Then take 5 days off and repeat till well. Use *Food Table* to avoid specific food allergens. Start BWT parasite recipe. Take lipase-pancreatin in large doses to digest food residues in tissues. Remove all metals as in <u>6</u>., particularly gold and strontium.

{73.} (**tricalcium phosphate**) Take vitamin D_3, 50,000 units daily. Take IP6 (10 to 20 drops in water 3 times daily) and inositol (1 tsp. 3 times daily) to dissolve hard deposits.

{74.} (**p53**) Use *take-out* drops for vanadium at lymph, tumor and any critical organ. *Take-out* dyes from each kidney and its WBCs.

{75.},{76.}(**isopropyl alcohol, clostridium**) Take oregano oil, 10 drops, 3 times daily for 3 days; take betaine hydrochloride for intestinal clostridium according to program; do dental clean up. Drink Eucalyptus tea, (c/s), 1 cup twice daily. Kill Fasciolopsis cercaria with wormwood, 10 capsules 3 times daily for 3 days.

{77} (**F. buski**) Take BWT-wormwood-cloves recipe while zapping. Take 6 fresh seed recipe.

{78.}(**F. cercaria**) Take additional wormwood, totaling 10 capsules, 3 times daily while zapping. Take 1 nutmeg capsule on empty stomach 3 times daily for 3 days.

{79.}(**CEA**) *Take-out* chromium from yeast-invaded area after metal clean up.

{80.}(**Bacillus cereus**) Take nutmeg, 1 capsule on empty stomach 3 times daily for 3 days. It contains myristic acid (see *Food Table*).

{81.}(**HCG**) Take additional wormwood, totaling 10 capsules 3 times daily while zapping. Take digestive enzymes as in program to destroy onion chemicals.

{82.} (**Yeast**) Use *take-out* drops of chromium, cobalt, nickel from affected organ besides lymph. Take digestive enzymes to remove asparagine. Eat home baked or bread maker bread to destroy its live yeast. Do turmeric enema daily. Zap affected area daily. Take IP6, 10 to 20 drops in water 3 times daily, plus inositol, 1 tsp. 3 times daily, for 3 days.

{83.}(**Fasciola**) Take BWT parasite program while zapping. Take lipase-pancreatin enzymes to remove wheat and oil residues. Take Molybdic acid (4x) to reduce allergies.

{84.},{85.}(**Strongyloides,   Onchocerca**)   Take levamisole, 100 mg, before each meal. Also BWT program. Use only butter and meat drippings, not oil in cooking. Take digestive enzymes as in program.

{86.}(**Dirofilaria**) Take milk digestant lactase, one with each meal. Take levamisole 100 mg, before each meal, also BWT parasite program.

{87.}(**Paragonimus**) Take BWT program while zapping. Take digestive enzymes. Drink Pau d' Arco tea, c/s-grade, tested for thallium, 2 cups, strong brewed daily. Eat only tested potatoes (for malonate and Ring Rot fungus).

{88.},{89.}(**Clonorchis, Eurytrema**) Take BWT program while zapping. Take digestive enzymes. Do Lugol's-turmeric-fennel enemas. Test grains, cereals for gallic acid. Bake your own breads. Use only butter and meat drippings.

{90.},{91.}(**A. lumb, A. megalo**) Kill Ascaris with levamisole, cysteine, besides BWT program, all while zapping.

{92.},{93.},{94.} (**RRase, DNA, DNA polymerase**) If *Positive* go to their respective numbers in this flow sheet.

{95.}(**fibronectin**) Do BWT program while zapping. Take digestive enzymes to clear food residues.

{96.},{97.}(**cadherin E, laminin**) Take levamisole, BWT parasite program, cysteine. Take digestive enzymes, eat only free-range, organic turkey, lamb, beef to avoid linolenic acid and d-carnitine.

{98.}(**PGE2**) Improve liver function with liver cleanses when possible, heavy metal removal as in <u>6</u>., BWT and 6 fresh seed recipe. Take nutmeg till Bacillus cereus is gone.

{99.},{100.}(**PS, cytochrome C**) When *Positive* proceed.

{101.} (**ubiquitin**) Take BWT program and levamisole; avoid corn and strontium.

{102.} (**caspase-1**) Do heavy metal clean up as in 6. Destroy asparagine by ozonating food. *Take-out* chromium from yeast locations. Take IP6 (10 to 20 drops in water 3 times daily) and 1 tsp. inositol 3 times daily.

{103.} (**cathepsin B**) Kill parasites with BWT program and levamisole while zapping. Take lipase-pancreatin in large amounts to clear away undigested food residues that feed parasites.

{104.} (**telomerase inhib II**) Use the BWT program, cysteine and levamisole. Avoid parasite's essential foods in the diet. Deprive yeast of chromium.

{105} (**lipase-pancreatin**) Take large amounts of lipase-pancreatin enzymes to digest the tumor.

{106}, {107.}(**tumor cells in CD8 and CD14 WBCs**) Use *take-out* nickel drops from CD14 and from CD8 lymphocytes for 4 days, but only after doing metal clean up as in 6. If nickel persists after 4 days, search for organs with leftover wheel bearing grease, and take this out first.

Flow Sheet Help

You may test the saliva instead of the actual person and therefore do all this testing in absentia. You should receive a homeopathic or homeographic copy of it (see page 584). You may also use a copy of a test substance instead of the real thing.

#1. through #25. Local supermarket laundry bleaches are a suitable test substance, having enough in common to be useful for other geographic areas, even countrywide. A few varieties are much higher quality, although not NSF-stamped. For example, they may not contain asbestos or only contain azo dyes. For this reason, never omit the asbestos and azo dye tests. Find which NSF-bleach is present, although this test is not listed. There are only a few in use throughout the USA. They do not cross-match. The local NSF-bleaches will be available at local pool supply stores. The water softener salts can be taken from locally available varieties found at hardware stores. They will be useful in other areas too, having in common, uranium, strontium, PCBs and aluminum. These make a strong cross-matching "frequency fingerprint". Fill amber glass test bottles half full of water and add about $^1/_8$ tsp. amount of liquid or solid. Cap tightly, label doubly, keep out of strong sunlight, heat, and magnetic fields. A motor oil sample can be poured, straight, or a small amount added to water in a test bottle. A wheel bearing grease sample can be made by copying the whole can into an amber glass or PE bottle. Use the copy. Or you could transfer some real grease using stainless steel. The can itself works fine, too. Wash and dry bottles carefully. Different brands give similar results. An asbestos sample can be made with a snipping of an engine gasket obtained at an automotive supply store. It should not be labeled "asbestos-free". Drop it into the test bottle and add water or use a plastic zippered bag. Mixed azo dyes and heavy metals can be obtained as copies. Our heavy metal sample was a piece of amalgam containing about 50 metals with 8 elements added (cobalt, uranium, radon, gold, antimony, strontium, chromium III & VI, ruthenium). It should contain these; test yours. You could make your own test substance the same way. Single elements are atomic absorption standards or copies of these. Bottles of north and south pole water were made as described on page 150. Germanium and selenium are the toxic, inorganic, semi-metal form, while the same name is often given to the organic essential form. This is, unfortunately, quite confusing. The malonic acid set was called the "5 M's" in previous books. After finding malonic acid in all laundry bleach and food sprays, their presence on produce could be expected. We can remove it with 2 hot washes, except in foods where deep absorption has occurred, namely potatoes, tomatoes, carrots.

#26. Formaldehyde is not only inhaled; it is also part of the benzene detoxification series (see page 353).

#27. Arsenic is a component of most pesticide sprays and wallpaper. No home should be sprayed with pesticides indoors.

#28. Methanol is part of the benzene detoxification series and could imply that benzene was previously present.

#29. A chemically pure grade or its copy is desirable for benzene testing.

#30. PCBs are a mixture of chlorinated biphenyls. In their capacity as direct immunity destroyers, they are much more deadly than commonly realized. Use a copy for testing.

#31. This is chemically pure liquid bleach. If water or food tests *Positive* for this, you know that some brand of bleach was used in it.

#32. This substance coats the WBCs after they fill up on asbestos. Touch ferritin to WBCs. This often causes <u>no asbestos signal</u> at WBCs. Search for asbestos at the tissue, not its WBCs.

#33. Use a copy for testing. Mine is Flu A and B combined.

#34. Use a copy for testing. Persons who show symptoms of Flu or prions have metal-filled or grease-filled WBCs and vanadium or gold and ruthenium in lymph. The grease harbors nickel, making the WBCs southerly. The WBCs should be cleared of these before continuing to kill parasites.

#35. People with and without symptoms can carry mumps at high levels. Mumps is associated with Mycobacterium avium/cellulare and acts as a carrier and protector of MYC virus. Mycobacterium/avium causes night sweats; it is dependent on strontium.

#36., #37., #38. These 3 salmonellas are often seen in any chronic disease, without causing typical symptoms. This may be due to their own viral infection. They are <u>always</u> seen after a F. buski is killed, not before. They only make you sick if your WBCs are incompetent due to one of the 5 immunity destroyers. It is part of detoxification-illness. It can be avoided by restoring immunity before doing intensive parasite-killing. They are easily killed with Lugol's solution, but seem to hide in the stomach (in the Peyer's Patches lymph nodes when these are incompetent). Salmonella ent. prefers the pancreas, and may be associated with all allergies. At least 2 varieties require gold, molybdenum, or ruthenium. The 3 varieties can be put into a single bottle from their slides.

#39., #40 These 2 intestinal bacteria are often seen in other chronic diseases, and also carry oncoviruses.

#41. This is a skin and bone bacterium that can spread to other tissues only if its needs are met there, as in the breast. They normally live <u>on</u> our skin but can penetrate when WBCs are disabled. They require chromium.

#42. This is the pain bacterium that appears to be attracted to minor bleeding sites, induced by formic acid. It requires chromium.

#43. This is a fierce bacterium that brings fever, fatigue and considerable illness. Viruses like Hepatitis B, Adenovirus, EBV and CMV can invade it, giving mutual protection. It requires chromium.

#44., #45. These are our 2 most common fungi; they take over dead matter in hours, extracting the metals for themselves. Depriving them of their metals is the fastest way to deplete their numbers. The liver is especially sensitive to the mycotoxin, aflatoxin, that they produce. Aflatoxin poisons the liver's ability to detoxify bilirubin, leading to jaundice. By dividing the liver in 10 or 12 pieces, metal *take-out* drops can be made for each part, followed by aflatoxin *take-out* drops. It takes only 4 days to lower the total bilirubin in the blood.

#46. Aflatoxin accumulation becomes an emergency in days. Speed in metal removal from each liver part is the emergency treatment. After that it can be removed from blood.

#47. E. coli requires vanadium, molybdenum, manganese, chromium, nickel. E. coli seems to be the most common cancer bacterium besides Clostridium, becoming loaded with nearly every oncovirus that can be transported by SV 40. Sickness can be turned around by depriving E. coli.

#48. If we speed up detoxification of the benzene series too much, more formic acid accumulates. There is a limit on how much bicarbonate can be given. Slower is better.

#49. through #58. MYC can join to CMV, Adenovirus and Hepatitis B, by some attachment that pulls them into tumor cells or into bacteria. I consider them, along with EBV, the <u>MYC group</u>. SV 40 pulls the other oncoviruses into cells. I consider this the <u>SV 40 group</u>. The MYC group is prominent in respiratory locations where staph and streps are also involved and get invaded. The SV 40 group is more prominent in other locations where E. coli and other intestinal bacteria are involved.

#51., #52., #53. Onchocerca and Dog heartworm are both filarial worms, as thin as baby hair. They often occur together, each making visible loops in the fecal contents. Their oncoviruses, JUN and FOS can fuse into a FOS/JUN combination that stimulates liver cell growth factor. Its role is not clear.

#59. Hepatitis B emerges constantly from the liver fluke, Clonorchis (also called Opisthorcis), by triggering with umbelliferone. But if Clonorchis is killed, Clostridium botulinum takes over the carcass, causing depression. When depression strikes the patient, particularly weeping, C. botulinum is found in the hypothalamus. It can be avoided by quickly taking oregano oil, Eucalyptus tea, Birch bark tea, along with more digestive enzymes.

#60. Adenovirus escapes from Ascaris when it is killed bringing common cold symptoms.

Bacteria that are chronic and produce symptoms, notably E. coli, Salmonella typhimurium, S. paratyphi, S. enteriditis, Shigellas, have a long list of attached oncoviruses. To test, place the virus sample touching the bacterium sample. When a small space is left between them, up to ¼" (½ cm.), you are testing for nearby (not internal) viruses.

#61. Free hemoglobin implies bleeding. It is quick to repair itself after causes (mainly formic acid) are removed.

#62. C_3 can be attached to food antigens as well as many other categories of intruders.

#63. SCF is pulled into tumor cells by SV 40 and by bacteria that have viruses or pituitary cells or hypothalamus cells attached to them. The significance of these attachments is not clear. None of this would be happening if chlorogenic acid and phloridzin had not been eaten. SCF is ordinarily detectable at night but only briefly during the daytime when a trauma has occurred. It is always excreted in nighttime urine.

#64., #65. Place the hypothalamus slide on opposite plate from saliva sample or from lymph (touching saliva). It is never seen unless chlorogenic acid is present, too.

#66., #67., #68. Although HGH is produced by everyone during the night and always excreted in nighttime urine, it is not detectable during daytime except in cancer. In this case there are free pituitary cells and phloridzin present in saliva and lymph.

#69. A tumor nucleus test can be made by touching 3 slides together: hypothalamus, pituitary, and pancreas. The pituitary must be in the middle. To make a copy of this, the blank bottle should stand touching one end, with the metal shield over it. Remember to add SV 40 to the bottle later, or you could get Negative results for a cancer patient. (In cancer the tumor nucleus is invaded by SV 40.) This trio becomes an independent unit bringing its growing force to whatever unlucky organ gets its fateful fusion (while it is producing PGE2 due to an allergic reaction). If 3 bottles are used instead of slides, they cannot be lined up for copying the way slides can. Bottles that touch each other will share their frequencies, spoiling each one's purity. This does not happen to slides. To copy bottles that must touch each other copy each one first so you keep your pristine set. Later, throw away the cross contaminated bottles. (You can rinse and reuse bottles.)

#70. & #71. Free pancreas cells are found only in the presence of gallic acid and the pancreatic fluke.

#72. OPT is not always produced by Fasciolopsis buski. There must also be isopropyl alcohol which appears to come externally and from Clostridium bacteria.

#73. This is difficult to dissolve even under acid conditions in a beaker, so patience and persistence is required. It may be doing little harm by itself so speed is not important.

#74. P53 is a part of the gene protein. Although we have this gene it does not normally produce so much gene-product that it is detectable. Metallic vanadium (pentoxide) is needed to bring about mutations in this gene that cause excess gene activation.

#75 & #76. Isopropyl alcohol is part of the stimulatory action on the free hypothalamus cells to make HCG in this abnormal setting. Since Fasciolopsis cercaria initiate this, possibly for their own protection, they must be acting in concert with local Clostridium bacteria that produce isopropyl alcohol, but this point is not yet clear.

#77., #83., #84., #87., #88., #89., #90., #91. These are bottles made with a frequency-generator only, not copied from slides of real parasites. The range of each adult plus its larval stages was included; then a 5 kHz extension was made at each end. Starting at one end of this extended range, every two kHz were chosen and combined in one bottle. These bottles were combined again, repeating till a single bottle was obtained containing every kHz of the parasite spectrum in the single bottle. This kind of bottle making is called "composite frequency". It allows testing for any stage in a single test.

#80. These common soil bacteria flow in a steady stream from a Fasciolopsis stage, not yet identified. In the vicinity of these bacteria d-tyramine is plentiful, l-tyramine is absent. The nearby amino acids, l-tyrosine, l-phenylalanine, and l-thyroxine which are normally present throughout the body get switched to the d-forms. The l-forms are then absent. This removes them from any role in productivity to make protein or hormones. I believe they are relegated to allergen status to be removed by WBCs. This is hypothetical. The switching process from l- to d- appears to spread to other amino acids, with a similar molecular structure, namely phenolic. I can speculate that the antigenicity of food phenolic substances is due to their tyrosine-like structure that is switched to a d-like structure along with d-tyramine. Becoming allergic to these is then a useful event, removing them from the territory where proteins should be made. This switch involves plane polarized light which is also affected by the magnetic field. d-histidine is part of this transformation, an amino acid that would normally chelate nickel in its l- form.

#81. The involvement of HCG in all tumors was already known to the embryologist, John Beard[20], 100 years ago. There are isomers (different forms) of HCG, not truly our own variety, as also found in classical research. This could be expected when it is instigated by a parasite larval stage. The cercaria stage of Fasciolopsis initiates its production by the hypothalamus (not the placenta). Other flukes' cercariae have not been tested for this action.

#82. It is bread yeast, Saccharomyces cerevisciae, not Candida, that plays a central role in cancer. A piece of its DNA is used to identify it exclusively. Its oncogene RAS is not always produced, requiring the trigger, asparagine. RAS disappears from the yeast genome if it is treated with sunlight or Frankincense. Yeast is particularly attracted to staphylococcus bacteria (or v.v.), so RAS invades them, too. Yeast and staphylococcus grow best in the breast skin giving it a rose color but it is not tender and painful till the streptococci join them later. CMV and Adenovirus are the common oncoviruses of staphylococcus and streptococcus,

---

[20] Search Beard embryology theory on Internet www.navi.net/~rsc

all of them being respiratory tract pathogens, transplanted to the breast by dental infections. Infections of teeth are swept up by neck lymph nodes that connect to shoulder and armpit lymph nodes, and from there directly across to the breast. This can often be felt as a "twinge". Yeast activates the enzyme ribonucleotide reductase which makes DNA out of RNA. It also causes carcinoembryonic antigen (CEA) to be made. Absolute deprivation of chromium is the best solution.

#83. This is said to be the most prevalent of all animal parasites in the USA. This speaks for lowered resistance in all domestic animals as well as ourselves. Giving cattle chlorinated water, without a mandate against laundry varieties with their added metals and dyes, has probably been the cause for them as well. My test sample is a composite frequency, so does not distinguish between the stages with this test.

#84. Strongyloides are also seen in migraine headache and addiction to alcohol and tobacco. In these addictions acetylcholine is regularly missing at special brain locations where Strongyloides exist.

#85. Onchocerca can produce small hard skin nodules that are not painful unless bacteria arrive there. The nodules are deep seated and cannot be cleared up except at the surface by zappicating it 20 minutes, or applying oregano oil dabbed on, or applying straight DMSO. These should not be rubbed in. Onchocerca leads to cinnamic acid allergy afflicting the bladder.

#86. Dirofilaria prefers the upper chambers of the heart, but lives in bowel contents quite well like Onchocerca. When free in a body space like the chest or abdomen it produces a snarl around a lymph node like a Peyer's Patch that traps free cells and starts a mixed mass of yeast, bacteria, parasite stages and loose human cells. These can grow after the tumor nucleus fuses to the lymph node that is producing PGE2 from SHRIMP allergy. These 2 filaria are the origin of Hodgkin's and non Hodgkin's masses.

#87., #88., #89. Drawings of these major parasites as they appear in the toilet bowl should help to identify most of them, see page 100. Clonorchis is small by comparison, about $^1/_8$ inch long in toilet expulsions, appearing to have a knob at one end like a midget clove bud. Eurytrema's 3 red dots identify it easily. Filaria are never seen loose, but as loops sticking out of the bowel contents, as if a hair had been eaten and expelled. The shadow of this loop can be seen easily with a flashlight. Also, the bowel contents are especially ragged and wispy.

#90., #91. These 2 Ascaris varieties can only be distinguished electronically. They each carry NEU oncogene, but have very different food requirements: quercitin and d-carnitine. While l-carnitine is essential in metabolism the d-form is considered an antigen. Free d-carnitine is not present in free-range, organic meats, possibly because the animals have not been drinking wheel bearing grease and nickel.

#92., #93., #94. These occur together in healthy people, being formed and then stopped after 20 seconds beginning at precisely :00 on a radio clock in every minute. Instead, in cancer, all are produced continuously, sometimes as long as 5 minutes followed by a 1 minute rest. The chance of finding any one in production at the time of testing is much less than 50% in health and is quite faint in sound. If you find them all *Positive* it is not normal. Time them. Clostridium causes DNA to be present continuously; yeast causes RRase to be present continuously.

#95., #96., #97. Fibronectin is not detectable in healthy people, perhaps due to its low concentration, perhaps not found in free form. Its presence always signals a nearby Fasciola fluke. Cadherin E is another adhesive molecule, and is always south polarized. Laminin, also adhesive, is produced after cadherin E. Both are produced by Ascaris megalocephala and F. buski.

#98. PGE2 appears where a food phenolic allergen appears, reflecting on its universal role as anti antigen.

PGE2 only appears when antigens have been made in a south pole location, namely turned into a d-structure in the case of amino acids. It disappears as soon as the location is changed back to north.

#99., #100., #101., #102., #103. Phosphatidyl serine, a normal part of the internal side of the cell membrane is loosened and sticks outward into the matrix as a signal when apoptosis is called for. Ubiquitin tags cell proteins for internal digestion. These 2 are usually detectable in healthy tissues, but never in tumors. Cytochrome C is not normally seen except in tissues already started into apoptosis, meaning PS is present. Cytochrome C has been set free from its mitochondrial home during the cells' internal breakup. Caspase 1 and cathepsin B are in the line of events that are needed for internal digestion. Cathepsin B can be blocked by an Ascaris nearby. Cathepsin B is also necessary to allow ordinary external digestion by our lipase-pancreatin enzymes.

#104. Telomerase inhibitor II is blocked by both Ascaris varieties but is instantly returned when Ascaris is gone.

#105. Ascaris has been known to inhibit trypsin enzyme (as in pancreatin) action for over 60 years. It was a standard experiment in clinical physiology at that time (search Internet for textbook by Hawk, Oser, Summerson in early editions, *Practical Physiological Chemistry*). For lipase-pancreatin enzymes to appear in a tumor we must be able to detect cathepsin B.

#106., #107. Apoptosis, external digestion by lipase-pancreatin enzymes and being eaten by CD8s and CD14s was our goal. After 1 to 2 weeks, a new scan could show reduction of tumors besides new well-being.

CHAPTER 13

BLOOD TEST RESULTS

Knowing how to interpret your own blood test results gives you insights that no doctor of the past was ever taught. There will be optional interpretations that can be settled with a Syncrometer® and can help you choose the correct path.

In earlier books, many blood tests were discussed in detail. Please refer to them for greater understanding of their meaning. In this chapter I will show you how to use your blood test to find your health problem and correct it.

People in the best health have results near the middle of the lab range. Values very close to the ends show that there is a health problem developing. If you can catch it, find its cause and remove it, you can prevent disease. Our working range shows you the limits we used to decide if a problem should get immediate action. You can set narrower limits. To protect your own health, you should search for the same causes when a test even begins to show an unhealthy direction.

For example, if your RBC is below 4.3 you could consider yourself anemic, although a therapist or clinic would not pay attention. Start to search for the same causes as would drive it down to 3.1.

To be useful for the very sick person, needing quick answers, a flow sheet format is used.

First find the problem in your blood test result by seeing if it is too high or too low. Then find possible causes in the alphabetized list that follows. When a cause is found, go to the *Tester's Flow Sheet* to find its source and its correction.

Blood Test Results

		Our Working Range	Our Lab Range	Units
a	RBC	3.1 – 4.8	4.5 – 6.5	MIL/mm^3
b	WBC	5 – 15,000	4.0 – 10.0	thous/μL
c	Plts	150-400,000	150 – 450	thous/μL
d	BS (non-fasting)	80 – 140	65 – 115	mg/dL
e	BUN	8 – 22	5.0 – 26.0	mg/dL
f	creatinine	.9 – 1.4	0.60 – 1.4	mg/dL
g	uric acid	3 – 4	2.2 – 7.7	mg/dL
h	cholesterol	200 – 250	130 – 200*	mg/dL
i	triglycerides	100 – 200	30 – 180	mg/dL
j	T.p.	6.5 – 7.5	6.3 – 8.3	gm/dL
k	albumin	4 – 5	3.9 – 5.1	gm/dL
l	globulin	2 – 3	2.0 – 5.0	gm/dL
m	GGT	10 – 45	0 – 57	U/L
n	AST	5 – 40	0 – 55	U/L
o	ALT	5 – 40	0 – 55	U/L
p	T.b.	.1 – .9	0.1 – 1.8	mg/dL
q	i.b.	.1 – .6		
r	d.b.	.1 – .3		
s	alk phos	75 – 95	39 – 117	U/L
t	LDH	120 – 140	91 – 250	U/L
u	calcium	9.0 – 9.7	8.5 – 10.4	mg/dL
v	phosphorus	3 – 4	2.2 – 5.6	mg/dL
w	chloride	100 – 110	95 – 111	m Eq/L
x	sodium	135 – 144	133 – 145	m Eq/L
y	potassium	4 – 4.5	3.3 – 5.6	m Eq/L
z	serum iron	50 – 100	30 – 170	μg/dL

Fig. 88 Checking your blood test results

The lab range depends on which test is used by the individual lab. If your range is different, use the top figure to compare the two and make an adjustment in your interpretation. For example, if <u>your</u> range for LDH is about twice as high as ours, double the working range, too.

---

* Cholesterol range not statistically set.

Common abbreviations

alk phos	alkaline phosphatase	**HGB**	hemoglobin
ALT	alanine amino transferase	**i.b.**	indirect bilirubin
AST	aspartate amino transferase	**K**	potassium
BS	blood sugar/glucose	**LD or**	lactic dehydrogenase
BUN	blood urea nitrogen	**LDH**	
Ca	calcium	**P**	phosphorus
Chol	cholesterol	**plt**	platelet
CK	creatine kinase	**RBC**	red blood cells
Cl	chloride	**T.b.**	total bilirubin
		T.p.	total protein
CO2	carbon dioxide	**trig**	triglycerides
creat	creatinine		
d.b.	direct bilirubin	**WBC**	white blood cells
GGT	gamma glutamyl transpeptidase		

Blood Test Flow Sheet

Spotting Your Problem From Your Blood Test

a	if RBC< 3.1	Give transfusion of packed RBC with plasma as needed. Search for vanadium, cobalt, Sudan Black dye, fructose antigen, malonic acid set, wheel bearing grease, other heavy metals in RBC, liver, bone marrow.
	if RBC >4.8	Search for vanadium, cobalt in RBC, bone marrow, reticular tissue. Search for hypothalamus or pituitary free cells attached to RBC.
b	if WBC< 5	Search for lead, cobalt, other heavy metals, DAB in bone marrow, WBCs.
	if WBC >15	Search for copper in lymph, bone marrow, WBCs, liver.
c	if plts< 150	Search for dyes, antigen (limonene), wheel bearing grease in plts.
	if plts >400	Search for HGB in saliva, lymph (bleeding).
d	if BS< 80	Search for yeast, chromium in saliva, lymph.
	if BS >140	Search for Eurytrema, limonene, phloridzin in pancreas and islets of Langerhans[*].
e	if BUN< 8	Search for azo dyes in saliva, lymph, WBCs.
	if BUN >22	Search for Clostridium in saliva, kidneys.

[*] Testers, to locate islets, put insulin sample touching pancreas.

		Search for cobalt, heavy metals in kidneys.
f	if creat< .9	Search for dyes in saliva, lymph.
	if creat>1.4	CHALLENGE! avoid KIDNEY FAILURE; search for methyl malonate at kidneys.
g	if uric acid < 3	Search for Clostridium, Yeast at saliva, lymph.
	if uric acid > 4	Supplement folic acid, 1 mg 3 times daily.
h	if chol < 150	Eat butter, cream, do liver cleanses, parasite program.
	if chol > 250	Do liver cleanses every 2 weeks, drink milk thistle tea, tested for thallium; do parasite-killing program.
i	if trig < 100	Eat butter, cream.
	if trig > 200	Supplement lipase-pancreatin, do liver and kidney cleanses, do parasite killing program till normal.
j	if T.p. < 6.5	Do parasite program, search for cobalt, vanadium, malonate set in liver[**].
	if T.p. > 7.5	Search for cobalt, vanadium, other heavy metals in liver, B-cells.
k	if albumin < 4	Search for cobalt, other heavy metals in liver.
	if albumin > 5	Search for heavy metals and dyes in liver.
l	if globulin < 2	Search for dyes, cobalt, vanadium at B-cells.
	if globulin > 3	Search for dyes and heavy metals in B-cells.
m	if GGT > 45	Search for DAB at WBC, liver; do liver cleanses, search for strontium, CMV.
n	if AST > 40	Search for lead at liver, bone marrow.
o	if ALT > 40	Search for lead at liver, bone marrow.
p	if T.b. > 1.0	EMERGENCY! Avoid jaundice and liver failure; search for copper, chromium, cobalt, nickel, aflatoxin at liver; remove with homeographic drops at each liver location. Also clear lymph and kidneys.

If aflatoxin is *Positive*, search for Aspergillus, Penicillium at liver locations. Clear liver and blood.

If Aspergillus is *Positive,* search for chromium, cobalt, nickel in liver.

If Penicillium is *Positive,* search for copper in liver.

q	direct	Is the detoxified portion of bilirubin. It reflects on liver function.

[**] To search in liver, divide liver electrically into parts shown on page 388.

	bilirubin (d.b.)	
r	indirect bili-rubin (i.b.)	Is the undetoxified portion of bilirubin.
s	if alk phos < 75	Search for cobalt, Sudan Black, Fast Garnet dye in liver, WBCs.
	if alk phos > 95	Search for DAB dye in WBCs.
t	if LDH < 120	Search for cobalt at saliva, lymph, liver, kidneys.
	if LDH > 140	Search for Sudan Black B dye in RBCs, kidneys. Search for Fast Green in WBCs.
u	if calcium < 9.0	Search for toxins in parathyroids.
	if calcium > 9.7	Search for toxins in thyroid.
v	if P < 3	Supplement vitamin D_3 tested for lead; search for vitamin D_2 in bone, lymph.
If vitamin D_2 is *Positive*, search for Ascaris in bone marrow, lymph.		
	if P > 4	Search for toxins in bones.
w	if Cl < 96	Supplement hydrochloric acid with meals. Search for toxins in adrenal glands.
x	if Na < 135	Search for toxins in adrenal glands.
	if Na > 145	Increase fluid intake to urine output = 2 L.
y	if K < 4	Supplement potassium gluconate. Search for toxins in adrenal glands.
	if K > 4.5	Search for toxins in thyroid gland.
z	if iron < 50	Supplement with ferrous gluconate, 10 mg, 1 to 3 times daily.
	if iron > 100	Do not supplement iron. Search for heavy metals in liver.

Dog Blood Test Results

CHEM 25	Results	Range	Units
Alk phos	322 (H)	10 – 150	IU/L
ALT (SGPT)	137 (H)	5 – 60	IU/L
AST (SGOT)	62 (H)	5 – 55	IU/L
CK	100	10 – 200	IU/L
GGT	9	0 – 10	IU/L
Albumin	3.0	2.6 – 4.3	g/dL
Total Protein	6.0	5.1 – 7.8	g/dL
Globulin	3.0	2.3 – 4.5	g/dL
Total Bilirubin	0.1	0.0 – 0.4	mg/dL
Direct Bilirubin	0.1	0.0 – 0.1	mg/dL
BUN	14	7 – 27	mg/dL
Creatinine	0.7	0.4 – 1.8	mg/dL
Cholesterol	156	112 – 328	mg/dL
Glucose	81	60 – 125	mg/dL
Calcium	9.1	7.5 – 11.3	mg/dL
Phosphorus	3.9	2.1 – 6.3	mg/dL
TCO2 (bicarbonate)	16 (L)	17 – 24	mEq/L
Chloride	110	105 – 115	mEq/L
Potassium	4.4	4.0 – 5.6	mEq/L
Sodium	146	141 – 156	mEq/L
Indirect Bilirubin	0.0	0 – 0.3	mg/dL
WBC	15.4	6.0 – 17.0	thous./uL
RBC	6.17	5.5 – 8.5	million/uL
HGB	13.4	12 – 18	g/dL
HCT	40.9	37 – 55	%
MCV	66	60 – 77	fL
Neutrophil Seg	85 (H)	60 – 77	%
Lymphocytes	6 (L)	12 – 30	%
Monocytes	9	3 – 10	%
Platelets	427	164 – 510	thous./uL
Absolute Monocyte	1380 (H)	150 – 1360	/uL
Remarks: Slide reviewed by technologist. WBC and RBC morphology appears normal. No parasites seen.			

Fig. 89 Checking your pet's blood test.

CHAPTER 14

PREVENT IMMUNE DEPRESSION-CLEAN UP

Our immune system keeps us alive from day to day. We are no match for a bacterium, a virus, or even a tiny bit of protein on the loose, like a prion in spite of our size.

Ships can be painted and gardens can be fenced to keep invaders out, but our bodies can't keep them out; there are too many holes to guard. So our bodies have brigades of special soldier cells to protect us from the inside instead, a kind of after-the-fact protection. They sniff out unwanted things, home in on them from far away, trap them, eat them and kill them, or kill them first and eat later. In light of this, many scientists have been doing research projects to find ways to fool your white blood cells so they do not attack our enemies (nor the metal tooth or implant or transplant). Such research is done in the dental and transplant industries and a lot is now known about immunosuppression, but it has not been applied wisely. It has not been applied to our pressing health concerns. Now, in the 21st century, we must quickly apply our knowledge to <u>rescue</u> our immune system, not suppress it, before the body dies of toxicity and new diseases. Three common diseases that can take our lives from immune depression are cancer, HIV/AIDS, and multiple chemical sensitivities (MCS). The Syncrometer® shows that many other diseases, even those called **genetic diseases** are actually due to immune depression. The immediate result of immune suppression, besides protecting the metal implant, is increased parasitism. In each case of so-called genetic disease, the Syncrometer® finds it is one or more of the five immunity depressors that is accumulated and has allowed a specific parasite to flourish. For example, cystic fibrosis is a so-called genetic disease where the CFTR gene has mutated. This stands for **cystic fibrosis transport regulator**. The Syncrometer® finds the parasite Gastrothylax in large numbers. This is based on only 5 cases but there were no exceptions. When it is killed this "mutant gene" disappears. The illness, of course, does not stop merely from this. A complex of bacteria and viruses already has a strong foothold. Immune depression must stop, namely, laundry bleach in the water and metals in the mouth to recover. Even autism and trisomy showed perfect correlation with laundry bleach water use. We can speculate that the different parasites bring different viruses that affect different genes, like in cancer. Having clean food and water is again most important in preventing genetic disease.

In earlier books I divided the chores of cleaning up your lifestyle into 4 parts: your dentalware, your body, your diet, your home.

Throughout this book, your cookware, dishes, glasses and food containers of all sorts have been singled out of your home clean up for special attention.

For help with the other parts, please go to the earlier books. There are many recipes for substitutes.

Food containers bring shocking toxicities, in such huge amounts, they must be removed at the very beginning of your curing program. It is quite easy to do, of course, but must be done to perfection for a very sick person. When the toxins seeping from your china cups and Teflon coated pans are thallium and malonic acid, you will always stay sick, even with tiny amounts. Getting a mouthful of dyes just from your toothbrush is way too much for a sick person.

Clean Up Your Diet

In this book you will be shown how to make food safe from toxicity, not just sanitary. The details depend on each food, so are given with the *Recipes*, page 507.

Clean Up your Body

We thought we were keeping cleaner than ever before with all the disinfectants put in our soaps and lotions. But we are not. We traded old-fashioned "dirt" for new fashioned chemical "dirt" that gave us immunodepression instead.

If you have very advanced cancer, use NOTHING that a mother would not put on her newborn baby.

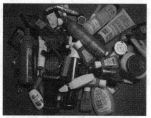

Check all labels for isopropyl alcohol. Throw those products away

Fig. 90 Some isopropyl alcohol-containing products

My recommendation is that you use NOTHING unless you can test it for laundry bleach, PCBs, isopropyl alcohol and benzene. A tiny bit <u>will</u> hurt you.

Switch to homemade recipes for soap*, toothpowder, shampoo, and use NOTHING more.

Don't use toothpaste, not even health-food varieties. Use tooth powder. To clean teeth, floss first, then brush. The homemade recipe on page 573 is quite enjoyable. Just a bit of powder picked up on a dry toothbrush is enough. Make your own floss.

Don't use mouthwash. Your mouth won't have an odor if there are no bacteria, not even in the morning. Keep your teeth clean with oregano toothpowder, once a day and Dental Bleach during dental work.

Don't use massage oils of any kind nor food oils as substitutes. Ninety percent (or more) of all the food oils in the USA market place I tested is contaminated with

---

* 20 Mule Team Borax™ works well for soap and is free of metals and other pollutants. It is antibacterial, inhibiting the enzyme urease.

benzene, PCBs, malonic acid, or antimony! Make your own starch lubricant.

Don't use hair spray or make your own.

Don't use perfumes or colognes. Don't use air fresheners. They pollute your lungs besides being themselves polluted. They contain coumarin, the antigen that invites cancer to the lungs. Test yours.

Don't use commercial lotions or personal lubricants no matter how many vitamins or herbs have been added. They are likely to have isopropyl alcohol and laundry bleach. Use NOTHING or a real avocado or butter.

Don't use cosmetics, mousse, shaving chemicals, nor rubbing alcohol. Use NOTHING.

Don't shave special places. Reconsider the real need for it. Any shaved place is severely scratched. This lets in bacteria and chemicals, where they were never meant to be, for instance, armpits and groin. This is where your precious lymph nodes are. Don't clog them with ANYTHING, nor damage the skin above them. You need to sweat.

Don't dye your hair with brand name varieties; their azo dyes are absorbed into your scalp and build up a large reservoir of dye here. Use henna varieties in bulk packages.

Don't polish your fingernails or toenails. The solvents penetrate the nails.

Don't attach fake nails. The acrylic acid becomes acrylamine, both carcinogens.

Don't get tattoos. The dyes seep constantly into your vital organs.

Don't put rings anywhere. Not even around your finger. There is a large amount of non-metal jewelry that can be hardened[*].

Don't wear a metal watch or watchband. Get plastic that you can harden in a sonicator or hot water.

Don't wear a metal necklace.

---

[*] Search the Internet for non-metal jewelry.

Don't wear glasses with metal stems or holders. Get all-plastic glasses and harden them in hot water like your toothbrush, or in a sonicator.

Don't wear metal earrings. You can harden plastic ones.

CANCER IS METAL-DISEASE. Even gold is deadly when your body no longer excretes it and Salmonellas can take advantage of this. Healthy people have not reached that point yet, but might not be far away.

Clean Up your Home

Your home was meant to be your "safe place". It is your little bit of universe, even heaven at times. But it has become your most dangerous place. Get it cleaned up while you are on your motel-vacation. This is an easy task because it mostly involves throwing things out. Hopefully your family and friends will jump to your assistance.

- The refrigerator gets checked or changed.
- The basement gets cleaned.
- The garage gets cleaned.
- Every room in the house gets cleaned.

Your refrigerator may still be one of the Freon-containing kinds. Happily our government has helped get rid of these. But if you were skipped in this upgrading process and still have a Freon refrigerator, wheel it outside the same day you read this. You may leave it on an extension cord and use it until you find a new non-Freon variety—totally, not partially, Freon-free.

You can remove freon from your body by drinking a glass of ozonated water every day. Be patient. The liver and kidneys should not be overwhelmed.

Clean Basement

To clean your basement, remove all paint, varnish, thinners, and related supplies. Remove all cleaners such as carpet cleaner, leather cleaner, brush cleaner, rust remover. Remove all chemicals that are in cans or bottles.

You may keep your laundry supplies: borax, white distilled vinegar, homemade soap, and chlorine bleach. This chlorine bleach will, of course, be polluted with azo dyes and all the remaining toxins. It can be used to clean the toilet and do the laundry, although the sewer system must surely become toxic at the end and detrimental to the environment. Find NSF 6% bleach at a pool store. Never use non-NSF bleach to wipe tables, counters or cutting boards. Its dyes and PCBs are left as a residue on everything. Having tungsten, nickel, chromium, motor oil and wheel bearing grease on your cutting board is not a good idea.

Also move any car tires and automotive supplies like waxes, oil, transmission fluid, and the spare gas can (even if it is empty) into your garage or discard them. Their volatile solvents permeate the house. Keep tools and items that are not chemicals.

Seal cracks in the basement and around pipes where they come through the wall with plastic cement. In a few days it will be hard enough to cover with a prettier color. Spread a sheet of plastic over the sewer or sump pump.

Clean Garage

Do you have a garage that is a separate building from your home? This is the best arrangement for an immunodepressed society. But if your garage is attached, as it often is, you have a problem. <u>Never, never use the door between the garage and house</u>. Tack a sheet of plastic over it to slow down the rate of fume entrance into the house. Your house is taller and warmer than the garage so garage-air is pulled in and up as the warm air in the house rises. You get so used to automotive fumes that you don't smell them.

322

Lung cancer is our most common variety. All lung cancer patients have two or three of <u>these air toxins in their homes</u> giving them lung disease besides the cancer:

- Freon (refrigerator, air conditioner)
- Fiberglass (drapes, open insulation)
- Formaldehyde (foam bedding, new clothing, newspapers)
- Vanadium (gasoline, leaking fuel, automotive exhaust)
- Asbestos (gym belts, dryer belts, hair blowers)
- Arsenic (pesticide used <u>indoors</u>, wallpaper)
- Beryllium (outside air pollutant)
- Strontium (outside air pollutant, water, corn, honey)
- Chlorine
- Tobacco smoke

After removing lung tumors with clinical or alternative treatments the lung destruction continues if you return to your home without cleaning up these toxins. Cancer must return, too.

Since these toxins cannot be guessed and there are no convenient tests, lung cancer patients are doomed. Learn to use a Syncrometer® so you can find your problem precisely. Or change it all; move. Chances are you would not land in the same air toxins as you have now.

Clean House

To clean the house, start with the bedroom. Remove everything that has any smell to it whatsoever: candles, potpourri, soaps, mending glue, cleaners, repair chemicals, felt markers, colognes, perfumes, and especially plug-in air "fresheners" (these usually have coumarin). Store them in the garage, not the basement.

Next clean the kitchen. Take all cans and bottles of chemicals out from under the sink or in a closet. Move them to the garage. Keep only the borax, white distilled vinegar for cleaning and bottles of concentrated borax you have made. You may also keep homemade nonfragrant soap. Keep fragrant soap in a double plastic zippered bag in the garage. Remove all roach and ant killer, mothballs, and chemicals that kill insects or mice. To wax the floor, get the wax from the garage and put it back there. A cancer patient should not be in the house while house cleaning or floor waxing is being done.

For cockroaches and other insects sprinkle handfuls of boric acid[*] (not borax) under your shelf paper, behind sink, stove, refrigerator, under carpets, etc. But some varieties of ants are repelled by borax, not boric acid (mix them). Pure clove oil or diluted with ethyl alcohol is best for ants but harms paint.

Chlorine from showers and faucet water can be reduced by filtering for the whole house, but only if the filter itself is tested for laundry bleach. Drink and cook with distilled-filtered water as described earlier.

The chlorine bleach is stored in the garage. Someone else can bring it in to clean the toilet (only). Toilet paper, tissues, and paper towels should be <u>unfragranced</u>. Family members should buy unfragranced products. They should smoke outdoors, burn their candles and incense in their own rooms with doors closed and windows open, blow-dry their hair outdoors or in the garage, use nail polish and polish remover outdoors or in the garage and not wear fragrance or fragrant shampoo or after-shave if you have lung disease. Air conditioners, but not fans, can be very helpful.

The cleanest heat is electric. Go "total electric" if possible. Have gas stove and furnace checked yearly.

Do not keep new foam furniture in the house. If it is less than one year old, move it into the garage until you are well. It gives off formaldehyde. Wash new clothing for the

---

[*] Boric acid is available by the pound from farm supply stores or see *Sources*. Because it looks like sugar, keep it in the garage, <u>labeled</u>, to prevent accidental poisoning.

same reason. Move unwashed clothing and suits to a distant closet. And do not sleep on foam pillows or a foam mattress, nor wool or feathers. Allergy to these play a large role in lung disease. Buy synthetic materials that you can wash in borax.

Take taurine and cysteine to help your lungs recover from formaldehyde damage (taurine 500 mg, two daily; cysteine 500 mg, two daily) after this clean up.

Avoid foods with air pollutants: water, corn, honey. For food use, avoid smelly plastic zippered bags. They are giving off phthalates, strong carcinogens! If your health food store uses them, let the managers know, and show them the plain kind you need to shop there.

Switch to plastic plumbing (PVC) before anybody in your home develops illnesses from copper, lead, or cadmium build up. Although PVC is a toxic substance, it gets hard enough not to seep.

Fiberglass in the air means that tiny microscopic bits of glass are going to your lungs and tumors. Merely covering holes to insulation does not work; they must be airtight—fill and paint them. Use duct tape to seal attic entranceways. Check the water heater. Check furnace, air conditioner fans, and dishwashers; pull out any fiberglass stuffed around them. Vacuum afterwards and throw away the bag right away. Best of all, find a contractor willing to remove all your fiberglass insulation and replace it with shredded paper or vermiculite insulation (see *Sources*). Don't keep gym equipment in the house, unless the belt is tested for asbestos. Baby powder contains talc, which is somewhat like asbestos. Have none in the house.

It is possible to get most of this house cleaning done in one day. Do all you possibly can. The more difficult jobs may take a week. This is a week of lost time if you are scheduled for a blood test or biopsy. If someone in the family can't part with all this "stuff", bag it all in double freezer bags of the largest size and store them in the garage.

When home is your hospital, you must be quite clear about your needs. One fragrant roll of toilet paper stowed in a drawer <u>will</u> hurt you if you have lung disease.

Suppose you have nobody who is willing to clean up the house, basement, and garage for you, or take on your pets for a month while you find them a new home. (Pets are too great a burden for your immune system at this time.) Don't delay for a minute if you should be invited to stay with a friend or relative who is willing to clean up their place for you and take you to the dentist. Test the tap water first—sending it to a Syncrometer® tester to find which kind of liquid bleach was used (be specific with tester). Or do it yourself by searching for grease collected at the top (see page 580). If the water is good, consider your life saved. You could even live nearby, later, to recover completely. If there are no invitations, go on your own vacation. Find a clean-water area by doing the water test. Put yourself into a smoke-free motel room (bring your own soap, sheets, and pillowcases, and ask that they not "clean" your room or spray it). Bring your own bug-deterrent so you don't create a problem for them. If you have a camper, remember to clean it up first. Send a dust sample to a Syncrometer® tester. Gas lines should be checked or closed off (use a hot plate), water pipes changed to PVC and a new hot water tank installed. Simply being outdoors is your safest place. A sunny beach, with shady places, where you can rest all day is ideal. Remember not to use any sunscreen or suntan lotions, only a broad-brimmed hat (see *Sources*). In fact, bring nothing with you that you don't need for the *3-Week Program*.

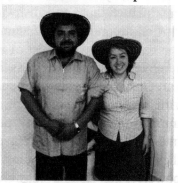

Fig. 91 Cancer curing or vacation?

But if friends and family mobilized to help you clean up, reward them with status reports on yourself. They have a stake in your success. You are most fortunate.

Clean Up your Dentalware

The Amalgam Era may soon be known as the darkest era in human history. Darker than cannibalism, headhunting, throwing Christians to the lions, burning non-Christians at the stake or having two world wars. The amalgam disaster was perpetrated on the very young and very old, on the sick and the healthy, and on women as well as men, much less selective than primitive atrocities.

The toll taken by persuading all these people to accept mercury mixtures to suck on day and night is unimaginable. It started the hundred-year slide downward of our immune power, our only defense against extinction.

The purpose of this dental clean up is:

- to get rid of the biggest source of heavy metals, plastic ingredients and dyes that are damaging your immune system, besides your laundry bleach drinking water.

- to get rid of Clostridium bacteria, that are part of the cancer cause, hidden under tooth fillings.

Our only defense against all the parasites, bacteria, viruses and even prions that try to grow in us is our immune system. We may think that cleanliness, intelligence, warm clothing and medicines protect us. But they do not. Our white blood cells have infinitely more power. Their job is eating our enemies and killing and removing them in a variety of ways: sometimes physically, sometimes through chemicals they make, sometimes through electrical (or perhaps magnetic) effects. When we accidentally damage our WBCs, it is a very serious matter.

Amalgam is producing a steady flow of mercury and thallium into our bodies, not to mention nickel, chromium, copper and dozens more. Even gold is extremely harmful, being an essential element for prions, Salmonella bacteria, SV 40 virus and even the HIV virus! None of the amalgam metals had to be disclosed even though nickel and chromium have had top rating as carcinogens for 30 years! Only mercury in California now has a warning.

Without disclosure, the entire amalgam-assault against humanity was a secret one. We did not know what we were putting in our mouths, although the manufacturers did. We thought "silver fillings" were mainly silver, and pure, when they were very impure and mainly mercury. The Dental Association knew all along what the results of scientific research was pointing to, and that the effects of eating such poisons, as one must when it is in the mouth, are cumulative so each passing year brings more toxicity.

It seems there was no concern for purity or health hazard by an organization that had the public trust. The Syncrometer® detected 50 metals in a single sample of new amalgam that was ready to be placed in someone's mouth.

Ag - Silver	La - Lanthanum	Se - Selenium
Al - Aluminum	Li - Lithium	Si - Silicon
Ba - Barium	Mn - Manganese	Sm - Samarium
Be - Beryllium	Mo - Molybdenum	Sn - Tin
Bi - Bismuth	Nb - Niobium	Sr - Strontium
Br - Bromine	Nd - Neodymium	Tl - Thallium
Cd - Cadmium	Ni - Nickel	Ta - Tantalum
Ce - Cerium	Pb - Lead	Tb - Terbium
Cs - Cesium	Pr - Praseodymium	Ti - Titanium
Cu - Copper	Pt - Platinum	Yb - Ytterbium
Dy - Dysprosium	Rb - Rubidium	U - Uranium
Eu - Europium	Re - Rhenium	V - Vanadium
Gd - Gadolinium	Rh - Rhodium	W - Tungsten
Ge - Germanium	Rn - Radon	Y - Yttrium
Hg - Mercury	Ru - Ruthenium	Zn - Zinc
Ho - Holmium	Sb - Antimony	Zr - Zirconium
In - Indium	Sc - Scandium	

Fig. 92 Elements found in "pure" amalgam by Syncrometer®

Notice the lanthanides in amalgam: Ce, Dy, Eu, Gd, Ho, La, No, Nb, Pr, Sm, Tb, Yb, Y. They are nearly all represented. As they diffuse out into our bodies, will their paramagnetic nature upset the delicate iron balance, will they be excretable? This should have been studied before putting them in our mouths.

The cancer victim must remove every bit of amalgam, however tiny, from the mouth. There is no way of getting immunity back without this fundamental act.

White blood cells that have eaten mercury and thallium can trap bacteria and viruses but never manage to kill them. They have lost killing power. They also do not make L-G or L-A (see page 570). A tumor full of seeped mercury/thallium has no chance to clear itself of SV 40 viruses and Clostridium bacteria or anything else.

In earlier editions of this book I recommended drilling out amalgam to replace with plastic for teeth that had fillings. I no longer do that.

Now that I see bits of mercury spattered all over the mouth, some large enough to see on x-rays, the safest solution is extraction. Tiny bits of amalgam created by drilling would add up to a much greater surface area for mercury seepage than before. The amalgam-diseases would not go away.

Plastic fillings shed azo dyes, heavy metals(!), bisphenol A (an estrogen-like substance, not good for boys or girls), and malonic acid, urethane, acrylic acid, DAP (a phthalate), all of which are carcinogens.

But a way has been found to stop plastic seepage, although the results are preliminary. If you have only plastic, not plastic-replacing-amalgam, you could choose this new and experimental path. It has been in use for 4 years but only used for 2 dozen patients. In each case, the new treatment stopped the seepage. It is done with a tooth zappicator, see page 344.

Extracting the teeth that once had amalgam and zappicating your plastic teeth is a compromise that should be monitored by each person choosing it. Have your saliva tested by Syncrometer®.

The Visit to the Dentist

Find an oral surgeon or dentist willing to clean up your mouth for you. Willing to search for leftover bits of old amalgam, called tattoos. It is more than "just pulling teeth." You may need to search hard for such a dentist. The alternative dentists have led the movement to ban amalgam from dental supplies. If you have cancer or other disease, find a **metal-free** dentist. This points to the progressive stance of this professional group. You may need to travel many miles and even visit other countries to find the right alternative dentist.

First, obtain a good quality panoramic x-ray of your mouth. A panoramic views the entire mouth including jaws and sinuses allowing you to see much more than single teeth (see page 335).

If your decision has been made, no delay is necessary. The dentist can see all the metal teeth at a glance. Then request in writing that she/he extract them, or sign the appropriate form (to legally protect the dentist).

Arrange for a friend to accompany you to the dental office. Ask for permission to have your friend nearby, just outside the cubicle with the dental chair. Your friend can hand you your antiseptic. Your friend should sit quietly, not wasting the dentist's time with talk or questions. Your friend can drive you home.

Treat yourself to a good meal before going for dental work. You will be on liquids for two days and should not lose weight. Do not take extra vitamin C on your dental-day. It detoxifies, that is, destroys anesthetic, so the dentist would have to give you much more of it.

If you have "dentist phobia", take a strong dose of painkiller (not aspirin), ½ hour before your appointment time (so you won't even feel the painkiller being given!).

Your Antiseptic is Best

Make your own antiseptic.

By far the best antiseptic to use during dental work is USP (NSF) chlorine bleach; <u>this is the kind that does not have the 5 immunity destroyers</u>. This excerpt describes it:

> Bunyan [in The Use of Hypochlorite For The Control of Bleeding, Oral Surgery, v. 13, 1960, pp. 1026-1032] reported that rinsing with 0.2% hypochlorite solution stops postoperative bleeding within 1 minute after a tooth extraction or other oral operation. The hypochlorite solution functions also to contract and harden the blood clots and make them more resistant to infection. In addition to the effective hemostasis and the change in the character of the clot, the author reported a reduction of swelling of traumatized gingival tissues and diminution of the postoperative pain.[62]

I have found this quote to be completely correct. There is essentially no bleeding, no pain, no swelling and no return of Clostridium.

<u>DON'T USE HOUSEHOLD BLEACH</u> because it is not safe for internal use! Obtain food-grade (USP) bleach from *Sources*. Purchase the same strength, (5 to 6%), as regular household bleach. Check the label. Then dilute it yourself. Use the recipe on page 572.

Bleach, whether USP or not is very caustic. You must not use it at full strength. You must dilute it <u>100-fold</u>. Follow the recipe exactly.

We will name your new <u>diluted bleach</u> that you have just made, Dental Bleach. It is only 1% as strong as regular bleach. Even this may be too strong for you. Try it at home first. You may dilute it further, in half. Then take it with you to the dentist, along with a safe cup. You will need ½ cup. <u>Rinse your mouth with it just before you sit down in the dental chair. Never swallow it!</u> Spit it into the receptacle. Hold your antiseptic in your lap. Later, when the dentist signals you to rinse your mouth, use your solution again. Also rinse one last time before leaving the office. The dentist will appreciate this extra care because she/he is less likely to see post-dental infection in you.

Second best would be Lugol's iodine solution (six drops of actual Lugol's iodine in ½ cup of water). This is not nearly as good. Use up the entire amount before leaving the dental office.

Third best is colloidal silver. Make your own colloidal silver solution since the commercially available ones I tested had the usual laundry bleach antiseptic.

As soon as the extractions are completed, the sockets left behind must be cleaned to remove leftover bits of tissue. This will prevent leaving a residue for bacteria to thrive on later. Then they are squirted with a dropper of diluted Lugol's iodine solution, or straight white iodine (see *Recipes* page 556). If you are allergic to iodine use Dental Bleach for this, too. You must supply these.

Commercial antiseptic made for the dental profession is not satisfactory. It invariably contains isopropyl alcohol besides dyes and other chemicals. These will enter your brain and tumors immediately through your new wounds. Strong salt water or straight ethyl alcohol (20%) would be better.

Save the Pieces

Tell the dentist before sitting down in the chair that you would like to keep the extracted teeth, root canals, and fillings, but they can all be tossed into a bag together. If the dentist tells you this is not allowed due to Public Health regulations, agree to fill out the proper application forms. (Were they safer in your mouth?) But they do belong to you. You may be curious in the future about what they contain, and could have been leaching.

If the odor from them is overwhelming you may understand how the internal infection of these teeth was poisoning your body! Finally, you may wish to look for the

Clostridium infection, which would be a darkened area or fine black lines under fillings.

Save loose pieces of metal and plastic because you may wish to have them analyzed at a later date, too. Or you may simply wish to gloat over the retrieved "treasure" as you identify corrosion and infection. Take a picture of them to remind you later how bad they really were.

When extractions are done, congratulate yourself for the achievement. **Start the *Dental Aftercare* program at once**. Do not eat or drink (besides water) for the rest of the day after an extraction.

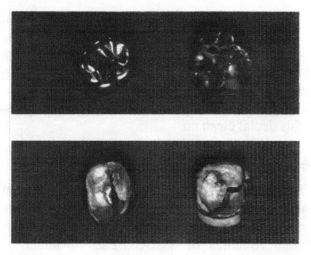

The top surfaces of fillings and crowns are kept glossy by brushing (you swallow the "brushings"). Underneath is tarnish and foulness. Ask to see your crowns when they are removed

Fig. 93 Tops and bottoms of some metal crowns

All root canals and dead teeth must be extracted, as well as teeth with metal fillings. Teeth with implants have not been studied enough to know which metals they shed or if Clostridium infections start in their vicinity. For this reason, you must use your own judgment on implants.

After extractions and cleaning the socket, the dentist or surgeon needs to do <u>two more things</u> before stitching up the wound: old cavitation cleaning and amalgam clean up.

Huggins Cavitation Cleaning

The tooth was held in the socket by soft tissues like tiny ligaments. Unless these are removed, too, they will decay and provide opportunity for bacteria to reside there, to create a future cavitation. This procedure was taught in the past by Dr. Hal Huggins and many dentists are familiar with it.

<u>While the new sockets are being cleaned, any old infected sockets, called old cavitations should be cleaned out as well</u>. Some cavitation sites are less obvious; they must be searched for by a knowledgeable dentist. Hidden cavitations, those that don't show up on the x-ray, nor develop at former tooth sites, often clear up without surgery after this dental clean up.

Arechiga Gum Cleaning

The second task after extracting your metal teeth and cleaning cavitations is to <u>remove imbedded amalgam</u> from the gums. This procedure has been developed by Dr. Benjamin Arechiga of Mexico. Each quadrant of your mouth needs an amalgam clean up. The top of the gum line will be gray from absorbed mercury. It is easiest for you to have this done while extractions are being done. The dentist begins by cutting a straight line on top of the bony ridge of the jaw where teeth once were.

Next, he/she snips away $^{1}/_{8}$ inch (3 mm) of the gum on each side of the incision. Two ribbons $^{1}/_{8}$ inch wide and extending from the wisdom teeth to the closest front teeth are discarded. The remaining gum tissue stretches over the top easily and is sutured over. Surprisingly, the new gum tissue is more elastic and heals <u>much faster</u> than the old, mercury-saturated gums. You can count on your gums being healed in two to three days. We call it the Arechiga technique, after the oral surgeon who invented it. While the dentist is cutting out mercury-drenched gum tissue, the exposed bone can be cleaned of old amalgam bits that are easier to spot now.

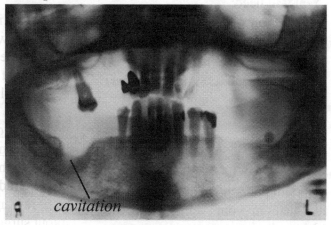

Fig. 94 Panoramic showing large cavitation at lower left

Dental Aftercare

One of the purposes of doing this dental clean up is to kill Clostridium bacteria that have invaded the crevices under tooth fillings. From here they colonize the rest of your body. Evidence for this may already be in your blood test results: **a low uric acid level**. This is associated with Clostridium invasions.

Extractions do not automatically clear up infections, though. And antibiotics cannot be relied on either. So a very vigorous program is needed to clear up infection even after the infected teeth are pulled. Deep wounds such as the base of the new socket is exactly where Clostridium bacteria prefer to be. This *Dental Aftercare* program is successful in killing Clostridium.

Copy the next few pages and carry them with you to the dental office. Your friend could review them while you wait.

You will need:
- a water pick
- hot water, towels
- pure salt (see *Sources*)
- Dental Bleach, USP (see *Sources*)
- one or two stainless steel strainers for food preparation

Purchase these <u>before</u> your dental appointment. Practice using the water pick beforehand, too.

The immune power of your <u>arterial</u> blood is much greater than in your <u>veins</u>. How can you bring arterial blood into the jaw area to heal it faster after dental work? Simply by hot-packing it from the start!

The first day of dental work is critical. If you miss this, a massive spread of infection can occur because the mouth is always a "den of bacteria", and your own tooth infection is itself the source.

Just <u>before</u> leaving the dentist's office, <u>as soon as you are out of the chair, rinse with Dental Bleach. Then, again, as soon as you get home</u>. Next, swish your mouth <u>gently</u> with a cup of warm water. Keep the cotton plug in place for you to bite down on and reduce bleeding, even while swishing. Don't <u>suction</u> the water forcefully around your mouth.

At the same time apply a hot towel to the outside of your face where the dental work was done. Wring a washcloth out of the hottest water you can endure, trying it out at a place that is not anesthetized first. Otherwise you might accidentally burn yourself. Or fill a plastic bag halfway with hot water, zipping it shut securely and enclosing it in a second plastic bag. Do this for 30 minutes, 4 times a day and every time you feel pain for a few days. Then 3 times a day for a week—even when there is no pain.

Don't suck liquids through a straw for 24 hours; the sucking force could dislodge the healing clot. Don't allow your tongue to suck the wound site, either; and <u>don't put fingers in your mouth</u>.

As the anesthetic wears off there will be very little pain. But you could introduce bacteria yourself, <u>by eating</u>, or by putting fingers into your mouth. Consider your mouth a surgery site, off limits to everything! But the mouth cannot be bandaged and you must eat! To be successful, <u>eat a big meal just before your dental appointment</u>. Then drink nothing but water later on, the day of extractions. You may need a painkiller on the first night; choose a non-aspirin variety to minimize bleeding.

Bleeding should have reduced considerably by bedtime. The cotton plug put in your mouth by the dentist may be thrown away. If you need another one, make it yourself out of a tightly rolled paper towel the shape and size of a finger. Rinse it several times with pure water by squeezing it. Rinse your mouth with Dental Bleach once more before bed.

Dental Day Two

The next day (the day after your surgery) you need to be well fed, yet eat <u>no solids</u>, <u>or liquids with particles in them</u>. The particles easily lodge in your wound. Your choices are:

1. Beef broth, strained, with HCl drops added (see *Recipes* page 545).

2. Herb teas, sweetened, strained, with HCl drops added.

3. Fruit or vegetable juice, strained, with HCl drops added.

337

4. Puddings made of starch or flour, thinned with fruit juice to be drinkable, with HCl drops added.

5. Cream shakes made with heavy whipping cream (and other beverages), with HCl drops added.

Run each through the finest strainer. All foods are ozonated, then zappicated, and given HCl drops last.

Drink through a large straw to get the food past the tooth zone. Immediately after eating, rinse your mouth with a cup of hot water to which you have added ½ tsp. pure salt. Do not be afraid to start some bleeding; this could be expected and is even <u>desirable</u> if an infection has already started. Bleeding washes bacteria <u>outward</u>. Water swishing <u>never</u> dislodges the healing clot. Only strong suction or infection dislodges it. If pain increases instead of decreases on the second day, you are already infected. Continue swishing and hot packing for one hour. Stop using sweetener. Devote the whole day to fighting this infection. If the pain subsides, the infection has been cleared. If not, you will need a more forceful stream of water. Begin using the water pick at its lowest speed setting. Water pick repeatedly until the pain clears. (It could take four hours!)

Hot pack the outside of your face just as on the first day. Even in the night, if pain strikes, hot pack it at once. If pain is subsiding on the second day, you are being successful. But the gums are <u>not</u> healed; you cannot take chances yet on eating solid food. Nearly all infections come from eating solid food on the second day.

Floss the remaining teeth with homemade floss, being extra gentle. For floss, cut strips of plastic shopping bags, ¼ inch by four inches. Clean and rinse them with very hot water. Fish line floss and toothbrush are too harsh after dental work. Clean remaining teeth by hand-rubbing, using paper towel wound around your finger and dampened, then dipped into oregano oil tooth powder (see *Recipes*).

Also rinse your mouth with Dental Bleach several times during the day and bedtime (at least four times).

Dental Day Three

On the third day, you may <u>drink</u> blended solid food; do not try to <u>chew</u> solids with remaining teeth.

Use your water pick now after each meal. It must be hardened first or you will get the seepage from it into your wounds and brain. Simply fill to the top with steaming hot water and let stand ½ hour. Repeat. Then fill the tank with hot tap water to which you have added a few drops of Lugol's iodine, or 1 tsp. colloidal silver, or pure salt. Set it at the gentlest level at first, squirting each site gently. Floss the front teeth and finger-rub them with oregano oil tooth powder.

No matter how carefully you eat, you will see food entering the gum spaces. Notice how difficult it is to squirt out any trapped food. Swishing is <u>not</u> sufficient! You need to water pick till all spaces are cleared; inspect each one. Continue hot packing. If pain returns and water picking has not succeeded in clearing it after 4 hours, you must <u>hurry</u> back to the dentist to search for the food particle. The wound will be opened and cleaned out for you.

Dental Bleeding

A moderate amount of bleeding is normal, even days later. Bleeding caused by water picking is not too serious. But if you sense an emergency, apply ice cubes wrapped in a paper towel or washcloth. Bite down on them till bleeding stops. Continue ice packing for 4 hours. Check your pills for aspirin. Stop taking these. After bleeding stops return to hot packing. If ice packing does not stop the bleeding, go back to the dentist or emergency room.

If you have a very low platelet count or are on a large amount of "blood thinners" which promote bleeding you need special attention. Yet, oral surgery is a very skilled profession. Dental work is safe in the surgeon's hands. Platelets can be given just beforehand; blood thinners can be temporarily stopped; and a transfusion can be given before or immediately afterward. These same patients often state that they feel better, immediately after the dental extraction, than they can remember in months! It was the dental problem that was poisoning their platelets and their blood! It may be the last transfusion that will be needed, in spite of some unavoidable blood loss with dental extractions.

Stitches should be removed earlier for immune depressed (cancer) patients than others because they will get infected by the third day! Do not use self-digesting sutures; you need the extra dental visit to be checked.

Be Vigilant the Next Week

Continue water picking, hot packing, and rinsing your mouth with Dental Bleach after each meal until the gums are healed over. This may take five to seven days, longer for some sites. Floss and brush your front teeth once a day. If pain stays away you can take credit for killing your mouth bacteria. You may reduce the treatments to 3 times a day, then twice.

Clostridium can return even after a week of steady recovery. If you detect an odor from your mouth, at any time, it is Clostridium making a comeback, even without pain. A crumb has lodged in a wound and is decaying. Try bleaching, swishing, and water picking for half a day, till odor is completely gone. Hurry back to the dentist if the odor persists. You cannot recover with a mouth infection.

If you got through the whole ordeal without needing more than one nights' painkiller and without needing to return to the dentist for extra clean up, give yourself excellent grades. And if you got through, in any way, still give yourself very good grades!

It is common for dentists to recommend cold packing to reduce swelling after dental work. I recommend hot packing because I consider swelling less important than infection or pain. It is also common for dentists to rely on antibiotics to clear up infection. I find this is not sufficient. The whole *Dental Aftercare* program is needed.

Plastic Fillings

> Plastic fillings may now be saved by the newly discovered technique for plastic hardening in the mouth. But risk is present since it is new and not yet widely used.

Fillings of plastic* can be spotted on a digital x-ray that could not be seen on the panoramic x-ray. If such a tooth has never had an amalgam filling, you could harden the plastic with the toothbrush zappicator (page 344) instead of extracting it. Several days later, a test of the saliva should show no plastic tooth materials. If it does, repeat the zappication. If it still does, extract the tooth. They can be kept clean by once daily brushings with oregano oil tooth powder.

> Only further research will reveal whether new plastic fillings can be so well hardened and kept so well fitting that no seeping occurs and no crevices develop.

New Cavities

Search your mouth yourself, every month, for a fresh cavity. It will be a small brown discoloration. Rub this spot twice daily, once with Dental Bleach and once with oregano oil toothpowder. Purchase a long-handled dental mirror (from automotive supply store) so your helper can see the backsides of your teeth.

---

* Testers, search for azo dyes, acrylic acid, urethane, bisphenol A, DAP. DAP is hardest to clear or harden.

There may be a time when dentistry can safely fill a small hole but it is not now. Research is progressing in other countries to bring healing methods instead of new kinds of fillings. Search the Internet to keep pace with it. Remember that teeth are bones! Your diet should have calcium and vitamin D_3 in it. Ascaris parasites soften teeth and bones. Kill them regularly.

Jerome Tattoo Removal

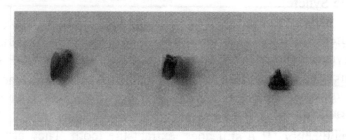

Bone fragments black with mercury should be removed.

Fig. 95 Tattoos

While the amalgam was being put into your teeth or taken out, tiny bits got away or flew away with great force into your cheek folds, into neighboring gums, into exposed bone nearby and down to the bottom of newly made sockets. Nobody will ever see these again, or so it was thought. (And guilt can never be laid.)

Larger bits of amalgam, called tattoos, can be seen on the panoramic or digital x-ray. Your dentist has already spotted them no doubt. But smaller particles do not show up. You must ask

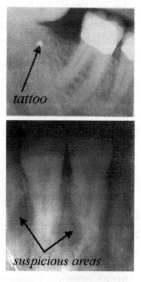

Fig. 96 Digital x-rays give superior view

the dentist whether he or she is equipped to search visually, with a **magnifier** and remove them all regardless how painstaking the job is. This and many more facts of dentistry are discussed by Frank Jerome, D.D.S. in his book, *Tooth Truth* (search Internet). Each quadrant of your mouth needs a careful examination for mercury.

It is quite easy to find tattoos using the newly developed "Dental Syncrometer® Probe" (see *Sources*) attached to the Syncrometer®. If your dentist is willing to remove these too, after you locate them with your Syncrometer®, you have a precious professional. If not, remove as much as possible yourself with the toothbrush zappicator.

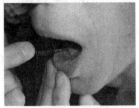

Find tattoos and cavitations in minutes.

Fig. 97 Dental Syncrometer® probe

Hidden Cavitations

These are not ordinary infected bone sites. They are primarily **bioaccumulation sites**. You can detect them easily by searching for mercury and other amalgam-related metals in the jawbone with the Dental Syncrometer® Probe. Here it finds dyes, acrylic acid and DAP from fillings, as well as silicones, tin, and strontium from toothpaste! Staphylococcus is there and if you feel pain Streptococcus is also there. The real reason for this bioaccumulation site is the presence of lanthanide elements that are abundant in amalgam and have drifted there. Wherever the lanthanides land, the white blood cells become "choked" with iron and calcium deposits. After this they stop "eating" any more toxins, ruining your immunity at this location. Healing is impossible here. They become pockets of mushy bone mixed with bacteria.

Even digital x-rays can scarcely picture these hidden bioaccumulation sites. Fortunately, many can be cleared without surgery, using a tooth zappicator.

Tooth Zappicator

A tooth zappicator is a small loudspeaker fastened to the end of a toothbrush. The speaker is attached to your food zappicator circuit, which produces a frequency of 1 kHz. The tooth zappicator is then placed over the hidden cavitation site for three minutes. All nearby areas are also treated for three minutes each. A surge of immune power is induced, which removes lanthanides, other metals, solvents, plastic remnants and bacteria all at once. The Syncrometer® sees these all in your white blood cells now. You should have taken germanium, selenite and vitamin C beforehand or you could give yourself detox symptoms.

Even when you are not able to search for them first, most hidden cavitations can be systematically cleared by zappicating along the whole ridge where teeth once were. Do it yourself to be sure it is thorough.

Repeat on inner and outer surfaces of the gums, making three treatments altogether. Don't miss the remaining teeth themselves.

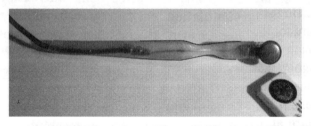

Fig. 98 Tooth zappicator and compass

The tooth zappicator can also be used to harden plastic. Press it against plastic teeth or teeth with plastic fillings to get this hardening action. For this purpose, treat for five minutes on top of each tooth location, then take a break for at least one-half hour. Drink water to help kidneys excrete. Repeat a second time on the inner surfaces of each tooth location. Take another break, and repeat a third (and last) time at the outer surfaces of the gums. The effect is permanent.

After these three five-minute zappicating treatments the plastic tooth no longer seeps dyes, and the stray amalgam that has saturated the tooth will be chemically changed so it can be more easily removed by the immune system. Build your own tooth zappicator, see picture.

Using your Tooth Zappicator

1. Insert a 9 volt battery into the 1 kHz zapper carefully, to be sure polarity is correct.
2. Connect the *Positive* output of the zapper to the *Positive* terminal of the loudspeaker. Do not use any *Negative* connections. They should not have hanging wires either.
3. Tape the zapper to the tabletop to guard against slippage while in use. A loudspeaker that falls to the floor could change its polarity.
4. Protect the tooth zappicator by placing it in a plastic zippered bag, with the loudspeaker in a bottom corner. Wrap the bag around it, handle and all, snugly. Tape in place. Be sure to keep saliva out of the plastic bag and off the bare tooth zappicator.
5. Wipe with ordinary ethanol or any alcoholic beverage or Lugol's water before first use. Do not get liquid inside.
6. Turn the zapper on. Place loudspeaker firmly on jawbone ridge for three (or five) minutes.
7. Start at the extreme end of one jawbone and work toward the other, skipping nothing. When you come to a tooth, place loudspeaker squarely on top of it. DO NOT TREAT METAL FILLINGS. Move to the neighboring location and repeat. When jawbones are both done on three surfaces, continue on all soft areas of mouth.

Divide the whole mouth, roof, sides, and back into imaginary little squares. Treat each square for 5 minutes. Leave no surface unzappicated. Don't miss the inside of the cheeks and the tonsils as far as you can reach. Drink water several times to help with excretion. Be sure to take a dose of hydrangea, selenite and vitamin C first. Be prepared for some detox-symptoms.

You are returning immune power to your mouth. Your white blood cells will deliver all these toxins to your kidneys and bladder. But your kidneys must be helped to excrete them; otherwise they quickly become south polarized and clogged. You will be instructed in the *3-Week Program* how to use magnets and to plate-zap the kidneys while taking kidney drops to protect them. Otherwise, use the *Kidney Cleanse* (see page 561).

For years, ever since you put amalgam in your mouth, the 50 metals you were sucking on have been dissolving and moving into the rest of your body in tiny deposits. I can estimate, by extrapolation from Syncrometer® tests, there are about 1000 such deposits in cancer patients, mostly in the brain and spinal cord. The majority of white blood cells already have mercury and thallium stuck in them, destroying their immune power. But the source of it all, your mouth, is finally clean. It is a huge accomplishment.

Home Dentistry

This beginning Home Dentistry is a creative innovation of huge significance. Being able to do simple check ups, using the Syncrometer® to guide you, may pave the way to <u>caries prevention</u> that has eluded us so long. You can find a tooth infection long before it becomes a cavity. And you may be able to clear it up with dental zappication, better hygiene and diet.

You are also able to clean up after amalgam removal yourself. You can stop seepage from plastic, and keep Clostridium away.

Your mouth is finally metal-free, plastic-free, dye-free, and Clostridium-free.

Solario Denture Making

For the quickest new teeth, impressions are made <u>before</u> extractions. The fitting is done as soon as your mouth is healed enough to tolerate it. For this, impression compounds are used.

Many new varieties have come into the marketplace with extremely toxic ingredients and so many dyes they even change color to let the dentist know when to take it out! The pituitary and hypothalamus glands in the brain, so nearby, are especially vulnerable. While the gums are healing, the tissue is open, so any dye or plasticizer can enter deeply and get stuck in your brain. If the impression compound used contains aluminum, dyes, and DAP[*] (although it may be called "alginate"), they will lodge there. If you just let it all happen, a strange new memory failure sets in about 6 months later. This induced dementia leads to gradual senility and cannot be reversed.

Dr. Solario of Mexico, uses dye-free beeswax as impression compound, and later hardens dentures with a sonicator. See *Sources*.

There are very many kinds of denture materials. Avoid porcelain. The choice of plastic and color is no longer an issue since it can be hardened enough not to seep (see page 573). Repeat it yourself at home, after every dental adjustment.

How can the dental surgeon who "cleaned up your mouth" ever know you became a cancer survivor? How can he/she be shown that their superior treatment is saving lives—such as yours and the dental profession played an important role? They might be very busy but never too busy to receive compliments and thanks. Send an email.

You will have made a friend.

---

[*] DAP is diallylphthalate, the same chemical as in DAP the window putty you purchase in the hardware store. It is carcinogenic.

> **Congratulations!**
>
> You have completed the hardest task required to get your immunity back besides changing your water. You have removed an assortment of about 50 heavy metals that were blocking your lymphocytes, neutrophils and macrophages, namely, all your immune cells. You have removed an assortment of dyes that were contributing to this. And you have evicted Clostridium from its fortress in your teeth.
>
> A glance in the mirror shows you a beautiful set of teeth, sweet-smelling breath at all times and chewing better than before. You have enabled your body to survive by stopping your immune depression.

On the Road to Recovery

Of course you have done a lot more than just clean up your teeth! You have cleaned up your whole mouth—your cavitations, your salivary glands, and your throat. You have learned to prevent tooth damage, the most important part of preventing breast cancer, bone cancer, and pain anywhere.

You might be wondering how much it will cost for this very special dental clean up. Although the dental work may seem straightforward, extractions being very common, the way you need them done is not at all common. Using homemade antiseptics, requesting cavitation cleaning and tattoo removal, using non-toxic impression techniques, but with digital x-ray equipment and a dental probe are all non-traditional. In Mexico, in 2004, the rate, including these clean ups, was about $85.00 per extracted tooth. Full dentures cost about $450.00-$500.00.

Thank You! Thank You, Dentists!

348

How to Make a Million Dollars in your Spare Time at Home: Sue!

Health problems should be solved by people themselves, not industry or government; the responsibility is too great. Now, even the planet's health is at stake. Only people's groups would not be influenced by other priorities. What I am suggesting is that people form their own groups, learn to use the Syncrometer®, find labs willing to do analysis of dental supplies, and form collaborations with dentists willing to work creatively. Then follow-up on the job done with analysis of saliva by lab testing. Peoples' groups could form similar collaborations with alternative physicians, including oncologists. Biopsy samples could be analyzed for heavy metals, plastic ingredients, and so on.

A rational approach to preventing illness and curing disease is within reach.

I was joking about making a million dollars, but maybe suing the American Dental Association and the AMA is the last resort solutions it will take to bring the problem of professional abuse to the attention of the agencies whose job it was. And to the American people, its suffering victims.

That is another reason for saving what was removed from your mouth (besides curiosity). Any extracted teeth with fillings could be analyzed. They could be set to soak in water overnight and the water analyzed for seeped ingredients. These ingredients were seeping into you. The real object is not to point out guilt but preventative—to find a developing problem before your entire family has been damaged, generation after generation. Before your family must spend half its generated income on health restoration.

Bad health underlies mental illness, addictions, and criminal behavior besides the customary diseases. Even reproductive disturbance is a state of bad health. It makes no sense to place a piece of estrogen-like chemical (as in bisphenol-A, used in dental plastic) in the mouths of children, to be sucked on day and night. Both girls and boys are likely to be affected, especially before puberty. Again, a people's group would not let this happen, if it were known, whereas a professional or governmental group is bound by laws and professional affiliations to have other priorities even when they know it is happening. <u>You</u> would not keep dark secrets as governmental groups do.

A list of labs doing analyses for metals, solvents, and other chemicals is given on page 604. Others can be found on the Internet. Be sure you understand the <u>sensitivity</u> of the testing each lab can do. Obviously, the ability to test to parts per <u>trillion</u> is better (more sensitive) than parts per <u>billion</u>. Avoid ppm tests.

Despite the lack of information amongst dental and medical professionals, the average dentist and doctor is devoted to human welfare. This is apparent in the movement, within each profession, to outlaw mercury, to outlaw all metal, to embrace new and better technology and to advocate better nutrition.

Not all agree. But that is my point. Progress is made from discussion and trying to achieve higher standards. If you find a dentist or a doctor willing to support your strange, new agenda, then you have truly found a treasure.

CHAPTER 15

SPECIAL PROBLEMS

Stopping Bleeding

Bleeding can be stopped even when it comes from an old ulcer that never heals or an old tumor, or internal location that could never be located. Often the only telltale evidence is a slowly falling iron (serum iron) level in your blood test along with anemia. The causes are the same for all locations.

There are 2 parts to bleeding: a small wound that lets blood escape, and a clotting problem that doesn't let it stop. You can cure both parts in weeks.

At first, you may only have one part. You may only have very tiny wounds I call "bleeds". All cancer patients have many tiny tissue bleeds; the only evidence might be chronic anemia. Your body can still manage its tasks quite well, in spite of this. Or you may only have a clotting problem. Your body is busy repairing and healing all its tiny bleeds all of the time. This is hampered when the blood refuses to clot quickly as it should. The blood test shows a slightly too long "clotting time" in the PT and PTT tests. You might have visual evidence from blue or purple spots under the skin, places where you tend to bump yourself, the thighs, legs, arms, and the backs of your hands.

You can stop making the wounds and stop upsetting the clotting times; then you have cured the bleeding problem. But if you only take "blood boosters", or iron pills, or herbs that supply wound healers and clotting corrections, you have not cured it. You can get profound, quick help from these treatments but they are only treatments. Unless the causes are stopped, the problem worsens with time, even when it appears to be under control.

The clinical solution is to quickly constrict (make narrower) the tiny blood vessels so they can't pass much blood. Adrenalin is one such treatment for emergencies.

Small bleeds that let blood escape consist of very tiny tears. They develop where **formic acid** has accumulated. Formic acid is extremely harsh—it is the same substance ants inject when they bite you.

Imagine having a hundred such tiny injections. They might be too tiny to give you pain yet, but they give you blood loss. They are really due to benzene that you have been drinking and eating. Drinking benzene-water or eating benzene-coated food gives you dozens of miniscule bleeds.

The Syncrometer® finds that benzene has a special route for detoxification by your body that leads to formic acid production. When this happens in the stomach or lungs, these will be the main bleeding organs.

The body is quick to detoxify it, using its own sodium and potassium bicarbonate. But if more formic acid is made than your body's potassium and sodium can keep up with, and always at the same place, a bleeding ulcer is formed. Blood in the sputum or bowel is obvious enough to be found. But when it happens in your tissues they are almost never found. The Syncrometer® finds them by testing for free hemoglobin at the saliva or in an organ.

Remember that the body can make benzene naturally from the mycotoxin, zearalenone, made by the fungus, potato ring rot (preceded by Chaetomium fungus). So it is no surprise that a detoxifying pathway has evolved for benzene.

First, benzene is oxidized to phenol, a very harsh, tissue-killing substance (used in fumigators). You must have enough oxidizing power in your body to do this.

Next the phenol is broken down to wood alcohol, which is particularly bad for your eyes and pancreas.

Wood alcohol gets changed to formaldehyde, another very harsh tissue killing substance (used by undertakers).

Formaldehyde is then oxidized to formic acid, the ant sting substance. This pathway was found by Syncrometer® in all cases of chronic bleeding.

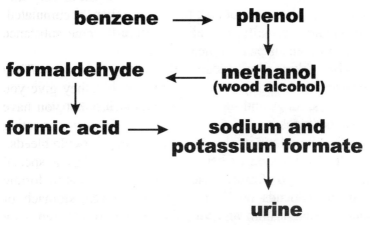

Learn this sequence the medical student way: Ben and Phineas met a farmer feeding a small fat yurt.

Fig. 99 Benzene detoxifying path

You already know where the benzene comes from: your water, your food, pills, supplements, IV bottles, in fact, everything made with benzene water. The benzene in air is negligible compared to these sources.

After you stop them all, it only takes 5-10 days to stop bleeding. It takes 5 days to move the last batch of benzene you ate along the path to formic acid.

But to remove the formic acid requires another 5 days because the body may be very short of its own bicarbonates. It has been using them up constantly on formic acid detoxification, by making sodium formate and potassium formate. Losing these strong alkalizers constantly could lead to an acid condition and a craving for salty food and soda beverages.

Fortunately, the tears heal quickly. After five days the formic acid can all be combined and sent through the kidneys to the bladder.

If there isn't enough sodium or potassium bicarbonate available, the body tries to push the formic acid through the kidneys anyway. Of course, bleeding then develops in the kidneys. All this formic acid makes them much too acid, besides, so they are not able to excrete other things as well. Toxins are normally neutralized before they are excreted. Not doing this is bad for the kidneys.

By taking low doses of sodium and potassium bicarbonate steadily, you can relieve bleeding kidneys, intestines, lungs and ulcers in the stomach or esophagus in days, not weeks.

Just how long it takes to stop bleeding depends on how much of a backlog of benzene is still waiting its turn for detoxifying to formic acid. The speed of detoxifying benzene depends on liver enzymes, as well as cysteine, taurine, magnesium and vitamin B_2. Speeding it up a lot only makes a bigger pool of formic acid at the end. Starting to take baking soda before speeding it up protects you from this. Patiently and steadily take the bicarbonates and a small amount of cysteine and taurine (one capsule a day).

In the same 5 to 10 days that you need to detoxify all the benzene in your body, you can cure your clotting problems.

The Clotting Problem

Vitamin K and coumarin play a role in bleeding.

The body has its own very complicated system of clotting quickly to stop bleeding. It uses calcium, thrombin, fibrin and many enzymes, all carefully regulated. There is also a complicated system of keeping your blood thin enough to flow well to prevent clotting! This is just as important. **Vitamin K** and **coumarin** play a role in these, as well as ordinary **aspirin**.

Vitamin K comes in different forms. The form that brings the clotting problem is called menadione. It slows down clotting. But it is not ordinary menadione. It is a "wrong form" of menadione. The Syncrometer® shows that its polarization is different. It is south polarized instead of north, implying that it is a different "isomer" (form). Of course, the body can change it back to north but this requires removing the nickel and the Bacillus cereus and even the Salmonellas which cause this magnetic and allergic transformation. Nickel is stuck in your wheel bearing grease and constantly seeps out from here. The Bacillus comes from F. buski parasites, whose eggs are trapped in the grease, too. A sick organ cannot remove these without help. Then the organ sets off its alarm and makes PGE2 instead. And vitamin K, a precious substance, will be treated like a common allergy, adding inflammation to the organ instead.

As if that were not bad enough, we could decide to <u>eat</u> some wrong form menadione!

Menadione is found in food, especially in <u>greens</u> and <u>grains</u> of all kinds (see *Food Table* page 36). When the greens are freshly picked they are north polarized and do not contain the allergenic form of menadione. Similarly for grains. But, in a day, for greens and in a few weeks for grains, the harmful south pole kind of menadione is already being made. This is the allergenic form. If you are bleeding you should stop eating menadione in greens and grains that aren't perfectly fresh. Temporarily stop eating <u>all</u> greens and most grains till bleeding has stopped. Grains <u>cannot</u> be fresh, so stick to barley only, as cereal, till bleeding stops. Your first green could be bok choy, and first <u>new</u> cereal, farina, packed under nitrogen. Store it in your freezer to slow down its aging. Cream and dairy products, too, are suspect, and must be tested.

As you remove wheel bearing grease, with its trapped nickel and parasite eggs from your body, and kill F. buski with its Bacillus cereus and Salmonellas, the allergy problem gets smaller.

But even after bleeding has stopped and any purple patches on the hands and arms have shrunk, you should stay off menadione-containing foods. Wait till they are completely gone and stay gone before eating the customary greens—this time only fresh from the garden. Experiment slowly with grains to see if bleeding returns.

Coumarin slows down the clotting process, too. Coumarin has a wonderful "cut hay" aroma and comes from vanilla, clover honey, fragrant rice and even air fresheners. Your wise body makes PGE2 to fight it off. Again, you get inflammation wherever the coumarin accumulates. Coumarin is the lung antigen. Inflamed cells let in viruses, and with SV 40 lurking nearby, this lung could be the next metastasis.

Our most common cancer location, the lungs, have a tropism for coumarin, so lungs bleed extra easily.

Aspirin, called **ASA**, is naturally present in very many plants, (wintergreen and willow trees, for example, but also in foods). Surprisingly, it is present in very many canned foods, and in candies. It is in green beans and many fruits after cooking. Painkillers are particularly treacherous; their small amounts of ASA may not be mentioned on the label. Test them or ask your pharmacist. Find one without aspirin.

Avoiding coumarin, menadione, and ASA, while stopping all benzene in your food, has stopped every bleeding problem we have encountered. Stopping bleeding can be helped further with the Chinese herb, Yunnan Paiyao (see *Sources*). Getting a vitamin K shot sometimes helps. Bleeding in the stomach is helped by drinking the alginate—moose elm recipe (see page 559). But these are all minor "helps" compared to removing the causes: formic acid and the three food antigens. There is one more contributor.

Where the bleeding is happening decides which extra food allergy to suspect and test for[*]. That will be where the formic acid accumulates. That organ will be inflamed, from its own allergy and invites benzene and bacteria to land there. For example, D-mannitol is allergenic for rectum. Stop mannitol in the diet when there is bleeding of the rectum.

The clotting problem has developed independently of the benzene and formic acid problem. Tiny wounds from formic acid may be healing but the blood may still be much too thin from the clotting problem. It will still trickle through the healed wound sites when normal blood would not. So you cannot expect a cure till both problems are gone.

Heartburn is an early sign of benzene arriving in the stomach. In this case the phenol has already started to build up. Phenol will eventually turn into formic acid and produce pain and bleeding, although while you were younger and healthier it did not. The bleeding attracts streptococcus bacteria and soon pain will accompany bleeding. Antacids and soothing potions do not stop the relentless march toward bleeding, pain and ulcer formation. As the ulcer site loses its immune power, the other pieces of the cancer puzzle gradually arrive and one day give the dreaded diagnosis…cancer of the stomach.

Hurry to eliminate all your sources of benzene and allergens. Your RBC can be 4.3 and HGB 13.0.

Summary To Stop Bleeding

First, check if it is a clinical emergency; find clinical help immediately if unsure.

Then:

---

[*] Testers, test the bleeding organ for its food antigen using the *Food Table,* or simply test it for all the foods being eaten.

1. Stop getting benzene from water, food, all pills.
2. Give ¼ tsp. sodium/potassium bicarbonate (or baking soda), tested for benzene or laundry bleach disinfection. Take it twice daily, upon rising and at bedtime, in water. This will remove formic acid.
3. Stop getting menadione and coumarin in food. Stop getting aspirin (ASA) in food and in pain killer.

Stopping Pain

If you are in chronic pain or even severe pain, start searching for the causes right away, even while you are on painkiller. Search first in your painkiller! Test it by Syncrometer® for benzene, dyes, laundry bleach, malonic acid, and aspirin. These will prolong your pain and prevent curing it. Search for a clean brand immediately.

The Humbler

Pain is the master of us all. It is the great humbler, rich and poor alike. In thousands of years of civilization, we have not developed a pain reliever that is safe, quick, and can stop the intense kinds of pain—not merely at the aspirin level. Yet, they had been discovered! Unfortunately, they became an item of commerce immediately, holding the sick person hostage instead. Even pain relieving herbs and spices became proprietary items and secret "professional" knowledge! So no simple research could be done by ordinary creative people to arrive at useful replacements. We still know almost nothing about pain, but we will make a beginning.

Special Pain Bacteria

Originally, we believed in ordained pain, a kind of punishment for "bad" behavior that "deserved" agony. And, recently, academic studies have encouraged belief in pain as a stimulation of pain receptors present in our tissues and activated by very special substances. But the chronic pain of cancer is not that. The Syncrometer® finds that cancer pain is due to a common kind of bacteria, **Streptococcus pneumoniae**, at a place where <u>formic acid</u> has accumulated. Bacteria, formic acid and blood are present here together, so that we can hardly tell which came first. Certainly, antibiotics for the "strep" bacteria do not work for pain, but when formic acid is gone, bleeding stops and bacteria leave, too, and the most excruciating pain disappears in the same day.

Streptococcus pneumoniae is always seen in places with agonizing pain or even the tiniest pain. That could explain why pain gets worse rather quickly and chronic later. But why do these bacteria come? What attracts them? Could it be blood since blood is always present with them? Bleeding is caused by formic acid which comes from benzene (see page 352). So benzene is really the cause of both bleeding and pain. Stopping bleeding should stop the pain. Amazingly, it <u>is</u> that simple. We already learned how to get rid of both benzene and formic acid. And we already know which allergens prolong bleeding. Knowing this, you won't need to wait an endless time to get off morphine, codeine, or other painkiller. We can look forward to a pain free time. But we will need about 10 days to accomplish it, five to detoxify all the benzene that is making formic acid, and five to detoxify all the formic acid. The bleeding stops within hours after formic acid is gone. Pain leaves a few hours after the bleeding stops. Hurry to get rid of your benzene sources and allergen sources so the clock can start ticking for pain relief.

Pain, Pain Go Away

Plain baking soda can neutralize formic acid. This is sodium bicarbonate. Of course, it cannot work if it was manufactured with laundry bleach because each dose brings you more benzene. If you cannot test, use NOTHING; it takes a week longer but you won't be contributing to your own failure. Any pill or food that still brings you benzene adds extra days of waiting for relief. A mixture of sodium and potassium bicarbonate is preferred, to balance these two elements, but if not available use the pure baking soda at hand. Don't expect fast permanent relief, though. There will be good days and bad days that tell you there are mistakes being made. Till then, use the least amount of drug painkiller necessary to let you eat, sleep, and get your cancer program started. <u>Do not choose a painkiller that includes an aspirin-like variety (ask the pharmacist) because it prolongs bleeding</u>. Read the section about bleeding.

Zapping Pain

Zapping pain is very helpful, too. You may even feel the zapper current for the first time if you have pain, since the current seeks out inflamed tissues. Zap continuously. If possible, zap the exact location of the pain, using a plate-zapper. The north pole field produced by the zapper's *Positive* offset current has pain-relieving effects all its own. This is besides activating the white blood cells and destroying the bacteria that cause pain.

Plain zapping, without a plate can clear up pain, too. The current can find the exact location by itself.

Spot zapping helps with healing at the same time as stopping pain. Place the *Positive* electrode (copper pipe from the plus side of the zapper) right over the painful spot. Press on it to make sure the current penetrates. Use a plastic glove on the hand that presses, not to steal away any current. Place the other electrode lower down, like under a foot. Or put the *Positive* electrode on the spine above the pain while putting the other electrode below the pain. Many kinds of electronic pain relief had already come into existence in the early 1920's, before the Dark Ages of medical suppression came over western civilization. A few of these methods are now in museums.

Starving Pain

Taking away the metals that are essential for the Streptococcus bacteria is more powerful than taking an antibiotic that blocks their metabolism. Sometimes more powerful than zapping...All living things need to be fed! Streptococci are dependent on chromium. Stop using all pots, pans, bowls, cutlery, and dishes until you have tested them for chromium seepage (see page 581). There may be little left—not even cups and saucers (see temporary place setting, page 241)! Test your food and water. Remove metal from your mouth. After this, making homeographic bottles that *take-out* chromium will be effective in 2 to 4 days. Make these, using your own zapper and a plain piece of aluminum sheet metal, about 3¼ inches square (see *Bottle-copying*, page 105).

Take-out chromium specifically from lymph and kidneys so it will be drained from the whole body slowly and steadily, and eventually deprive the bacteria. This could take 5 days. For a stronger effect *take-out* the heavy metal mixture, too.

It does no good to *"take-out"* the bacteria themselves because you are feeding them blood and metals. Feeding while fighting bacteria never works.

Pain Lurks Nearby

There are hazards to avoid that will certainly bring your pain back! If you drink or eat more benzene, even one polluted tablet (such as the painkiller itself), will make more formic acid. The pain will be delayed 5 days because it takes that long to reach the formic acid stage. All this obscures the cause, the one polluted tablet or an untreated toothbrush or "high quality" china cup. Do not take such risks. Do not risk a dab of lotion, an untested spice or a tea bag. Commercial products are being manufactured more and more with laundry bleach disinfectant, spreading benzene everywhere.

Prescription Painkillers

You can, of course, use prescription painkillers. The hazards are rather serious, though. Well over half of all pills I have tested were themselves bringing laundry bleach disinfectant, namely the 5 immunity destroyers. Their dyes are usually obvious, but even white pills contain numerous dyes that are invisible. When forced by emergency to take them, try to wash some dye off under the faucet. Let the washed pills dry on a paper towel. Alternate brands, if possible, so not so much of one pollutant accumulates. Take extra vitamin B_2 and coenzyme Q10 to help detoxify these dyes. Painkillers usually contain aspirin also, so bleeding and pain are worsened in the long run, but not suspected because it is delayed. A pharmacist can help you get aspirin-free painkiller. The morphine/codeine varieties slow down the intestine so much that constipation results. Then bacteria levels skyrocket, especially E. coli, greatly reducing your chance of recovery. Taking stool softeners and bowel activators helps but each brings its own laundry bleach toxins. Sodium alginate is a stool softener (see *Sources*) without this risk. The narcotic painkillers also disturb weight gain and general thriving. Try to switch to substitutes, even if you have to double or triple the amount.

But emergency need for pain relief has first consideration. Do not feel bad or guilty about needing it. Just be sure to zap your pain all day, take small amounts of baking soda for 2 or 3 weeks, and most of all avoid benzene-polluted food, water, cookware and dishes. Avoid commercial products of all kinds. If pain reduces, it shows you it will be possible. If it then gets bad again, assume you got benzene into your body, somehow, five to ten days earlier. Track it down. Suspect everything and eliminate it. Don't despair from repeated failures. You can have repeated successes, too.

Permanent Pain Relief

It may take several tries before pain stays away naturally because there are unsuspected benzene sources and mistakes must be made. Give yourself excellent grades for succeeding. Not only did you conquer pain, you rid your body of benzene, one of the 5 immunity destroyers; you stopped internal bleeding so your red cell count and iron levels can go up again. Now your energy will go up and life will look much better.

Every source of benzene or heavy metals that you find can lead to a permanent improvement for your health, not just for pain. You may have a dozen unsuspected sources. Finding them and eliminating them will help cure your other illnesses, too, besides the cancer.

Making your own Pain Killers

Taking drops of a copied pain medicine gives you about ¼ of its action, but gives it to you must faster (5 to 10 minutes).

There is no toxicity to worry about so you can take it over and over till you get relief.

Choose several varieties, up to 4 or 5, taking all of them one after the other in one session.

This is an example:

1. Copy several Advil tablets, writing the total dose on the label, with the name NOT-ADVIL.

2. Copy a few morphine-containing tablets the same way.

3. Copy indomethacin.

4. Copy Tylenol.

5. Find an aspirin variety, uncolored and tested for laundry bleach. Place several pills in a small, ½ oz. bottle, so they add up to about 4 times a real dose. Put this dose on the label. Add pure water to cover them. Place a similar bottle, almost full of water, beside the bottle with the pills. Place a metal pipe around each one on the copy plate and

zap 20 seconds. See copy making instructions on page 105. Label the new bottle NOT-ASPIRIN or FAKE-ASPIRIN, etc. Dump the real originals for safety from accidents by children. THIS IS NOT FOR PAIN WITH BLEEDING.

Take 6 drops of each, 1 minute apart. Repeat every 15 minutes till pain is tolerable*. No addiction or side-effects have been seen. Do not combine these into a single bottle. Include as many as you have available. Keep copying your copies to make more. Be sure to dump the originals for safety.

Beware of Anesthesia

Relieving pain without removing its cause is dangerous. It hides problems. The great relief also lulls us into thinking "things are better". Use your "window of relief" to hunt harder for your benzene or other sources. Use pain relief to get to sleep; you may follow it with Sleep Set. But next day, choose some suffering to keep your focus on pain causes.

Summary to Stop Pain

First, switch to non narcotic painkillers if possible.

Then:
1. Stop bleeding to remove Streptococcus pneumoniae.
2. Stop getting chromium; it feeds Streptococcus bacteria. Test all water, cookware, dishes, food and pills for chromium with a conductivity indicator, followed by a Syncrometer®.

---

* Testers, an organ in pain shows loud resonance with both acetyl choline and epinephrine at the same time. Many painkillers can "turn off" acetyl choline resonance. Morphine can "turn off" epinephrine, though more slowly, to give deeper relief.

Preventing Coma

Terminal illness is never too far away from coma to allow it to be "out of mind" for you. One day your patient, perhaps already scheduled by the clinical doctor for Hospice, sleeps very well. The caregiver mentions the improvement. The next day and the next sees no change. Is it leading to coma or is the sick body trying to make up for sleepless nights in the past and actually healing?

To answer this question, search for **acetyl choline** and **epinephrine** at the cerebrum or whole brain slide. Both should be *Positive* for the alert state. If one or both are missing for more than a minute search for tryptophane, melatonin, prions, and wheel bearing grease at CSF, cerebrum, pineal. You could expect to see wheel bearing grease everywhere, preventing both neurotransmitters from being made or used. You could expect to see prions everywhere, disallowing neurotransmitters to be present. You could expect melatonin everywhere as though the patient were asleep. But if tryptophane is *Positive* search for liver failure. There should be no free tryptophane in the brain.

The most serious possibility is liver failure. If the liver has turned into an Aspergillus and/or Penicillium fungus bed, nothing can wait. If one or both fungi are at the left liver (or any other liver location), the metals: copper, cobalt, chromium, nickel would be there. Use *take-out* drops for each one immediately for every liver part, even when only 1 or 2 locations were tested. Give copper-*take-out* drops first, because that dispatches Penicillium by itself. Be sure the kidneys and their WBCs are being treated with *take-out* drops for heavy metals, too. If not, take them out immediately. If the kidneys are clogged with wheel bearing grease take this out at the same time. You cannot wait for DMSO action.

From the fungus take over of the liver, the usual consequence is aflatoxin production at the liver, which spreads in a few days to aflatoxin at other organs and the blood. This inhibits **bilirubin oxidase** so that bilirubin now builds up at liver and blood. Take aflatoxin out immediately at each liver location and blood. Do a blood test to monitor bilirubin. If not caught very early, the whites of eyes will turn yellowish.

Bilirubin oxidase can also be inhibited by Sudan Black dye or cobalt in the liver. Remove both at all parts if present. Liver failure can be happening aside from jaundice, due to cobalt. Cobalt inhibits the early (glycolysis) part of food utilization so the liver is starved of energy.

Search for **fructose** buildup at saliva and liver, more evidence for a liver block; it should not be *Positive*.

Regardless of the cause of liver failure, the result may be lost ability to use tryptophane. Protein can still be digested to <u>make</u> tryptophane but <u>using</u> it is a different, more difficult process. It should be used to make neurotransmitters. A build up is seen in blood, at liver, and in cerebrospinal fluid. Tryptophane is a somnolent, inducing sleep, regardless of the time of day. If this is seen, search for all these causes immediately, and also make drops to *take-out* tryptophane from CSF, to avoid coma.

Somnolence can be caused by excess melatonin, seen at saliva, blood, and CSF. It is being overproduced by the pineal gland. Search for heavy metals at pineal, especially nickel. Wheel bearing grease at pineal and its WBCs brings nickel and other toxins. Take each item out immediately. Also take DMSO, the usual ¼ tsp. in ½ cup water, to remove the grease or motor oil. Check for the same toxins at kidneys and kidney WBCs, taking them out at the same time. Test for melatonin reduction after one day. If somnolence continues and melatonin is still present on the second day, take it out directly at blood and CSF for one day at a time. Test each day, otherwise you could bring about insomnia. If somnolence continues search for cobalt or nickel persisting at the pineal.

Stopping Effusions

"Water holding" is a common problem for cancer patients. Of course, it isn't really water. It is your precious lymph, full of body proteins and other important things your body made. Now you will throw it away as you drain it. But drain it you must until you can stop it from forming. If you don't, it will put pressure on neighboring organs till they can't do their work. We are very fortunate to have a clinical method available to drain, to put in a drainage tube, and sometimes to "patch" an effusion site. It buys you a little more time to find the causes.

This time the causes are malonic acid and dyes.

Dyes

We are inundated in dyes—not only the legal and accepted kind, but the illegal and unacceptable kind. How could DAB, formerly used to color margarine, but long ago banned, be everywhere in our environment now? How could Sudan Black, a tissue dye, never made legal, be so prevalent now that you can see its effect on nearly every cancer patient, even in their blood test? Fast Red and Fast Red Violet cause all the effusions in cancer patients. This makes them very dangerous. Why is there so much in our environment? We know, of course, that anything in the water supply becomes very prevalent. These dyes are in the laundry bleach water.

These 2 red dyes do not act alone. to cause the effusion. They seem to block an enzyme that we all have that can detoxify maleic anhydride. Maleic anhydride comes from malonic acid.

Malonic acid is an industrial chemical, used so much that you can find residues of it in almost anything made by industry (amalgam, food spray, plastic, laundry bleach, glassware, ceramic items, for instance). We eat and drink large amounts every day in laundry bleach water, sprayed food, and from seeping dishes. The body uses several steps to detoxify it, found by Syncrometer® in 1994. The steps are:

malonic acid ⟶ methyl malonate

maleic anhydride ⟵ maleic acid

D-malic acid ⟶ ?

Learn this sequence the medical student way: Mabel met a male malingerer doing a Main Street dance.

Fig. 100 Malonic acid detoxification pathway

Each step depends on having enough of the necessary detoxifiers. The first two require B_{12} and folic acid. The last three steps are the hardest, requiring a lot of vitamin C. Maleic anhydride will often stay backed up for long periods, till much more vitamin C is available. Where it is backed up it develops a porous spot in the tissues where fluids can pass through. Thin tissues like linings of the lung or abdomen will seep fluid if a thin spot develops in them. The fluid has no way to drain out again, so it fills up the lung or the abdomen. We call them effusions or "water holding" and need to drain them if we can't stop them.

The 2 red dyes are found wherever maleic anhydride builds up. Presumably, they are blocking an enzyme that could detoxify it further.

We can treat the problem with vitamin C in large doses; somehow this bypasses any enzyme that is needed. But treating a problem without removing the cause does not last. You will have to get IV treatments of 50 gms of vitamin C again and again unless you get rid of your malonic acid source and dyes.

Finding and eliminating the source of the dyes and the malonic acid is the permanent solution. Of course, that is made easier when they both come from the <u>same</u> source and they often do. Then the body drains <u>itself</u> with a little help from potassium, boiled parsley water, and vitamin C supplements.

The causes can be very hard to find. For example, your mashed potatoes! A cooked, peeled, organic tomato! Your beautiful, superior-rated toothbrush! A plastic strainer!

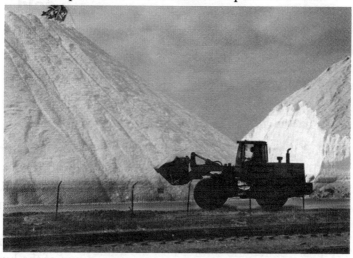

This salt pile goes to half the dairies and other markets in the USA, we were told. It is "sea salt" or "mineral salt". The ocean flats where this salt is harvested had a pink period during the summer for two years. The salt has pink stripes running down the length of it and pink patches here and there. Will your dairy herd get this dyed salt?

Fig. 101 Sea salt pile, a bearer of red dyes

The dyes and the malonic acid are deep inside the potato, too deep to come out with hot washes. The potatoes were sprayed with anti-sprouting chemicals. You can hardly find a potato that is not so sprayed! Tomatoes and carrots have the same problem. The colorful plastic toothbrush is made so soft, the colors and malonic acid diffuse into your mouth immediately, and every time you use it. These doses are much too great for the advanced patient.

If you have an effusion, switch to farmers' market produce, not store bought. Freeze it yourself for the winter so no glass or cookware is involved. Switch to a temporary place setting and stainless steel cookware till you have tested all other kitchenware.

This may be all that is needed for an early effusion—less than a year old. The dental clean up, water change, environmental clean up, and new diet might bring so powerful an immune recovery that the kidneys can drain it all without help. Then the thin spot heals and an x-ray shows a lung full of beautiful black (on the x-ray) air. Your body can still do miracles for you.

But if the effusion is older, and quite large, like half a lung full, you will need more help.

Help the kidneys and adrenal glands. Give them their missing frequencies by making drops of them to take, and zapping them. Give them parsley water, boiled 5 minutes (¼ cup, 4 times daily).

Assume the kidneys are partly blocked with methyl malonate. It is another part of the "malonate family", I previously called the 5 M's. It is the kidneys' special toxin. This would make the drainage much more difficult for your body. It would be like trying to pour water through a clogged strainer.

To unclog the kidneys of methyl malonate, take these supplements: **1.)** uva ursi capsules, 2, three times daily. **2.)** ginger capsules, 2, three times daily. **3.)** l-cysteine, (500 mg), 1, three times daily. This is besides the 5 supplements needed by all adrenal glands: vitamin C, folic acid, vitamins B_2 and B_6, and pantothenic acid. Adrenals and kidneys work together. After a day, increase the cysteine to 2 capsules three times daily. Then measure how much urine you are making in 24 hours, noting how often you got up in the night. It should be no less than 2¼ quarts/liters, with no need for nighttime relief. If your urine volume jumps up, it could be your new better kidney action at work. Check the effect on your effusion with a new x-ray in 10 days.

Prevent Hemorrhage

If your effusion also brings pain and bleeding, you will need still more help. It means there is formic acid and malonic acid arriving at the same place. You will need diuretic help. But set the stage carefully. Remove sources of malonate and dyes. Remove sources of benzene. Remove heavy metals; you are obviously getting chromium somehow. Remove kidney blockage by methyl malonate. Help the adrenals and kidneys with drops. Take the kidney herbs (Kidney Cleanse page 561). Remove the allergen for the organ that is seeping and bleeding. Then add a strong, but Syncrometer®-tested, diuretic, in correct amounts, together with potassium supplementation. The diuretic can be by IV or by mouth.

Because all this taken together is so powerful, you cannot stay on this treatment for long. After 10 days the action will be largely completed and the new toxicity from any drug or supplement will begin to pile up. Get a new x-ray or ultrasound that shows the new "water-line". If much remains, search for more sources, increase your compliance, switch to a different, tested diuretic, and different diuretic herbs and continue for 10 more days. If very little "water" remains, go off the diuretic, but stay on all the rest up to 3 more weeks. Add comfrey root and burdock root herbs (tested for thallium and laundry bleach), for their allantoin content to heal the thin spots.

Notice that bleeding, pain and effusates share their causes: benzene, dyes and malonic acid. They all came from your water. They interact in different ways, depending on where they accumulate. One problem can lead to the next, making it more severe, and seeming to be due to your advancing cancer. <u>Actually it is unrelated to the cancer</u>. These problems are <u>toxicity effects</u>. At first these 3 toxins only came from your water. But they wore out your detoxifying ability. Now you cannot detoxify nor tolerate <u>any</u> of these, not in <u>any</u> amount. Yet your body can heal you even at this late stage, by removing these 3 toxins completely. It is the miracle of life at work. Hurry, to clean it all up. Your effusions can go away.

Making your Own Diuretics

Find uncolored pills or capsules of popular diuretic medications. They must be tested for laundry bleach, dyes and malonic acid. Brands are not alike, nor are different batches. If you copy dyes or malonic acid accidentally, and take these drops, you will make your problem worse. Copy only clean varieties, preferably only the active ingredient from a manufacturer.

1. Copy Lasix (40 mg), use 4
2. Copy Miccel, a standard dose, use 4
3. Copy pure spironolactone (250 mg), use 4

The exact dosage is not important.

Make each separately in a ½ ounce bottle. Cover with pure water. Copy each and label: NOT MICCEL or FAKE LASIX. Dump the originals. Keep a spare copy as a "master" to make future copies.

Take 6 drops of each, 1 minute apart, every 2 hours at first, then only 3 times a day. If improvement gets stalled, or is barely noticeable, you are still eating dyes and/or malonic acid. Put NOTHING further in your mouth until it has been tested. You could find the culprits in 1 day. Remove these. Stop taking these homemade diuretics after 5 days. Switch to different varieties to avoid build up of unknown toxicities.

Summary To Stop Effusions

First, check if drainage would help your heart or other organs. Do this, or get a tube installed.

Then:

1. Stop getting malonic acid from water, food, pots, pans, dishes, cutlery. If you cannot test for malonic acid, test all for metal seepage. These toxins often occur together. Use nothing but HDPE♻ and stainless steel.

2. Stop getting dyes from plastic, food, dentalware, cosmetics, and water. Harden your plastic dentalware again. Even if you are getting drained every week, and can hardly breath or keep your heart stable, you can stop it all. Perfect compliance never fails.

Stopping Insomnia

A cancer patient needs his or her sleep more than others. Sleep is the time of healing.

Insomnia originates with the pineal gland. Bacteria and the immunity destroyers are arriving there to prevent it from making its melatonin. Melatonin normally puts us to sleep. And the WBCs work hard to clear the toxins or bacteria. When they catch up, your insomnia improves by itself. Unfortunately, the worst bacteria are the ones coming from your own bowel, so they are never far away, and you are never secure against insomnia. You must reduce their numbers and kill their oncoviruses to give your WBCs a chance to catch up with them. Start with Lugol's-turmeric-fennel enemas, plus the whole *Bowel Program* (see page 557). If you knew which oncoviruses are present, you could kill the parasite that brings these, but killing all common parasites is even a better approach.

Don't eat after 8 p.m. Don't take B vitamins at bedtime. Do take a hot shower. Do take digestive enzymes at bedtime.

If your cancer is advanced you have much more wheel bearing grease everywhere, and even on the pineal gland if you have insomnia. You must slowly dissolve it away with ¼ tsp. DMSO daily after removing it from the kidneys with *take-out* drops. If you don't remove it from the kidneys first you might only move the grease to a different location, like throat or lungs. Be patient. After 4 days of kidney improvement and taking the three WBC-foods (organic germanium, selenite, and rose hips), your body might focus on the pineal gland without your intervention. If sleep comes back, do nothing more except the program you had already started.

If it does not come back after 3 nights of no sleep at all, help the pineal gland by taking out wheel bearing grease homeographically. Make 3 bottles: one that takes it out a bit to the Right side, and one that takes it out a bit to the Left, besides at the slide you purchased. These will be *take-out* bottles, and are taken like other *take-out* drops, 6 times the first and second day, 3 times on the 3rd and 4th days. After this, continue once a day for a week and whenever sleep seems extra bad. Meanwhile, help your body to sleep with the homemade sleep set you can make yourself.

It is not uncommon for a cancer patient with advanced brain cancer to have no sleep at all for 20 straight nights, only brief dozes by day that aren't even felt!

Make your own Sleep Set

Herbs that promote sleep have been known for centuries, like chamomile tea. These could be copied into bottles and taken as a set of drops at bedtime. We will use items that are stronger. These are examples:

1. Drops of pineal gland. Copy the slide or another bottle-copy.

2. Drops of melatonin. Copy tablets that add up to at least 10 mg or some bulk pure powder, tested for laundry bleach and dyes. Copy the pure powder dry but cover tablets with pure water.

3. Drops of tryptophane. Copy the pure powder from a manufacturer or several capsules emptied into a bottle and water added.

4. Drops of ornithine. Copy the pure powder from a manufacturer or 10 capsules emptied into a container with pure water added.

For a more reliable "knockout" effect when thoughts are racing and emotions flaring, take 8 to 10 real ornithine capsules before the sleep set.

More powerful standard drugs could be copied for use in more extreme cases. Be sure all items are pure.

Use the standard dose of 6 drops of each, one minute apart, <u>after</u> you have gone to bed, not to miss the brief wave of action. The real ornithine can be taken 10 minutes earlier.

During times when you are taking the sleep set keep killing bowel bacteria, the real culprits.

Stopping Seizures

Seizures can begin at any time when a cancer patient has metastases to the brain. Growth of any sort inside the skull causes pressure. When "water-holding", or edema, occurs in the brain, this causes increased pressure. A scan of the brain might show that the midline is no longer straight, but pushed to one side, which is evidence of pressure against it.

Even without cancer, irritation of the seizure center by nearby Ascaris eggs or larvae, or by the natural food dye **malvin**, is always seen in seizures. This same dye is in plastic teeth, toothbrushes, processed food and any plastic utensil or object.

After cleaning up the kidneys, and stopping any dye from getting into your mouth, you can clear up the brain of dyes and Ascaris. This always stops seizures. But to stop them permanently requires several weeks of patience as mistakes are made in food selection and finding kitchenware that does not seep dyes. Toothbrushes and other small plastic items can be hardened by soaking ½ hour in steaming hot water. Repeat this. Of course, plastic teeth must be hardened immediately (by tooth zappication) to stop the flow of dyes from them (they even contain malvin!). Malvin is found in blue and red foods (see *Food*

Table). After these clean ups, *take-out* drops of malvin can be made for the cerebrospinal fluid[*]. Often the body removes it without this help.

Meanwhile, seizure control can be started by making a set of **Stop-Seizure Drops**, consisting of:

1. GABA drops. Copy gama amino butyric acid from pure powder emptied into a bottle or tablets with pure water added.

2. Phenytoin drops: Copy the pure powder. Do not copy a colored tablet or capsule; it may contain malvin.

3. Phenobarbital: Copy the pure powder. Do not copy a colored tablet or capsule; it may contain malvin.

Take 6 drops of each, leaving 1 minute between them.

If seizures do not stop after all this, you are still getting malvin (from your toothbrush?) or Ascarism is spreading. Kill Ascaris by starving both varieties, besides other methods discussed in earlier books. Seizures can return if the tumor is growing, or you are eating malonic acid, which causes effusates (edema) in the brain.

Stop taking the seizure drops before they put you to sleep instead. If seizures are not gone after 4 or 5 days you are actively causing them. Remove more causes.

Stopping Kidney Failure and Curing Cystic Kidneys

The hazard of kidney failure comes from the chronic drinking of malonic acid. The detoxification route leads through methyl malonate, and when the block is here there will be a buildup. The cause of the block is not known yet. But after the kidneys have used up their supply of vitamin B_{12} and folic acid they become swamped in methyl malonate. This causes obstruction of kidneys or a "cystic" condition. Supplying these vitamins does not relieve the condition fast enough if the creatinine and BUN are already

---

[*] Testers can use the set of brain "slices" to find where the last bits of malvin remain. That also identifies the seizure center.

rising past the top of their range. But homeographic *take-out* drops can bring relief in several days if all 5 supplements, known to be needed by adrenals, are given too. These are vitamins B_2, B_6, C, pantothenic acid, and folic acid. Take the amounts used in the *3-Week Program* plus B_6, 250 mg, 2 daily, and pantothenate, 450 mg, 3 daily.

Make *take-out* drops for methyl malonate out of R kidney, R kidney WBCs, L kidney, L kidney WBCs. Drink the Kidney Cleanse teas of marshmallow, gravel root, hydrangea, and parsley (boiled 5 minutes), while taking ginger and uva ursi in doses of 2 capsules, 3 times daily. A urine volume of 2¼ quarts is needed. If you get a sudden increase in urine you can be more certain of saving your kidneys.

If you have a raised BUN on your blood test it is partly due to Clostridium bacteria. Take oregano oil, 10 drops, 3 times daily and strong eucalyptus tea, 3 cups daily. Birch bark tea, 2 cups a day, also works. The crisis should be over in 3 to 5 days bringing down both BUN and creatinine. If it is not, more malonic acid is being consumed. Test cookware and dishes one by one while using only stainless steel and HDPE♳ containers. Stop microwaving; warm up food in hot water (see page 446). It conserves organic germanium, selenite and vitamin C.

Start taking l-cysteine (500 mg), one, 3 times daily the first day. Then take two, 3 times daily, watching for minor side effects. This supplement specifically affects kidneys to make new healthy tissue, which is, after all, what counts.

Be sure to avoid cheese in the diet; this is the kidney antigen. Also avoid chlorogenic acid and phloridzin so no new cysts can be made. After 3 weeks you may see kidney cysts shrinking. Keep taking wheel bearing grease and heavy metals out of the kidney set till they are back to normal.

Stopping Liver Failure

When an organ "fails" it cannot do the work it was expected to do.

Every organ has its genes busily making the correct enzymes for its jobs. Jobs are different for different organs. But the fuel that runs it all is the same, ATP. And the steps needed to make ATP are the same. They are called metabolism. By studying metabolism in any organ, a Syncrometer® tester could find where the block in metabolism is. Finding any buildup identifies it. Finding a toxin at the buildup site identifies one cause. For the liver, RBC, kidneys, heart, thyroid, and bone marrow, I have found cobalt to be the chief toxin. Cobalt is already known to block **glycolysis**, the first part of metabolism. Search for cobalt and quickly remove it with *take-out* drops at the failing organ. For extra assurance, double your efforts by also taking out mixed heavy metals.

Cobalt steadily seeps out from wheel bearing grease blobs in your body. The metals in the grease are *Positively* charged. Any organ with an inflammation is more negatively charged. The grease with its *Positive* charges sticks there instead of leaving through the kidney.

Stop eating carrots, which has the antigen for the liver, umbelliferone. This would inflame the liver.

Use *take-out* drops for wheel bearing grease from all the parts of the liver (at least 10).

Use *take-out* drops for heavy metals (including gold, ruthenium, molybdenum, vanadium, manganese, chromium, nickel, and cobalt) from all parts of the liver.

Keep kidneys cleared by *take-out* drops, too, so it can all enter the urine.

Automotive greases regularly block the neurotransmitters' arrival at any organ. Removing them brings back innervation to the liver as well as full metabolism in 4 days. The same routine can be used for other failing organs.

But failure of the liver has special importance. It leads to jaundice and coma (see pages 384 and 365).

Improving Appetite

To get well you need your appetite most of all. You need energy for healing.

A cancer patient gradually begins to lose weight. You believe your appetite is normal. Your weight loss seems unexplained. But the Syncrometer® shows the hypothalamus, which controls your appetite, is full of heavy metals.

Cobalt, nickel, gold and thulium have special effects on the appetite center in the hypothalamus. Now the appetite center cannot make **hydrazine sulfate**, your natural appetite stimulant. The Syncrometer® detects hydrazine sulfate made here in all healthy people. Without this you cannot feel hungry. You can remedy this, even after real **cachexia** (weight loss) has set in and you are down to "barely bones", by taking pills of hydrazine sulfate. Almost as good is an electronic copy of it called **placebo** hydrazine sulfate.

Hurry to clean up your kidneys so all the toxic metals can be excreted again. Start taking homeographic drops of "cobalt-out-of-hypothalamus" and "heavy metals-out-of-hypothalamus". Treating the kidneys and hypothalamus together can have you feeling new appetite in 2 days. But you don't even need to wait for this. Make your own **Placebo Appetite Drops** consisting of hydrazine sulfate. Copy the pure powder from a manufacturer to avoid pollutants, using about ¼ tsp. Or dump 4 doses of pills into a ½ oz. bottle, cover with pure water and copy. Take 6 drops, 6 times daily for 2 days, then 3 times daily.

Your helper and family will be thrilled to hear you say you are hungry for breakfast. It marks a turning point for the better.

CHAPTER 16

SPECIAL CANCERS-Liver, Brain, Breast

These examples are given to show more clearly how to find the problems and correct them in very advanced cancer patients. Although cancers are all alike in their causation, details are different for different organs.

Liver Cancer—Prevention and Cure

Metastases in the liver are some of the most common kind. This is because it is a collecting organ. It collects all the blood, collects food from the intestines, and anything toxic from some organ. It also collects more than its share of parasites. Parasites love to be in the liver. It is, after all, the body's kitchen and pantry. Sugar is made there; amino acids and fats are all available there. When bits of primary tumors from some other organ (which I called quads) have loosened and are circulating in the blood and lymph, they pass through all our organs. They can get caught in the liver if it has been building webs of cadherin E, fibronectin, and laminin. Now the tumor nucleus with its attached bit of primary organ can get very close to the actual liver cells. If the liver cells should get inflamed by a food antigen they will be standing with their doorway channels open, letting SV 40 viruses in, as well as bacteria with their gangs of oncoviruses. The liver has warned us many times about its inflammations long before the tumor nucleus or metastasis arrived but we didn't take notice. We thought it was indigestion and would pass.

Bits of liver tissue that are set free by these inflammations land in the skin. They turn into brown spots we call "liver spots" or "age spots". It should be our clue to strengthen our liver. Try not to get another one.

Not all our brown spots are liver bits, though. Round ones and those with a "halo" around them are not. When a real liver spot is formed it is reddish, not brown at first. It turns brown after a few days to weeks. It will go away if no more liver bits arrive. That means the body has digested it. If it does not come back, it means that the liver inflammation has stopped, too. The liver has gotten rid of the objectionable antigen. For the liver, the antigen is umbelliferone (carrots).

But not everybody's liver is allergic to umbelliferone permanently. It is Fasciolopsis buski's presence in the liver, bringing its *Bacillus cereus* that starts the allergy process (see pages 65 and 185). It coincides with wrong polarization due to nickel and the presence of Salmonellas.

When inflammations never stop the allergy develops and you will make PGE2. Soon a fusion with the roaming quads produces a quint (see page 188).

Liver cleanses, stopping eating carrots, killing parasites and stopping drinking laundry bleach water helps prevent liver inflammations. Getting vitamin A in every meal is important in protecting the liver. This means eating yellow fruit (apricots) and vegetables (carrots)! Liver attacks plague us from childhood, leaving their telltale marks, a new little brown spot after each one. Preventing them is what protects the liver from making a primary cancer or allowing a metastasis to develop. Does this mean we should never eat carrots? The umbelliferone is in the thin peel. Our parents always scraped this off. We should, too. Besides this, the top of a carrot often has green rings. This part has a different antigen that goes to lymph nodes, causing lymph node metastases. This allergen was found first in shrimp and is still called SHRIMP because its chemical name is not discovered yet. Besides all this, carrots in the market contain malonic acid from sprays. It does not come out with 2 hot water washes. We have lost carrots in our diet.

When you already have a liver tumor there is no time to lose. The liver stores food, so invaders here grow faster than in other places. Every day counts. Start right away to kill flukes

382

and roundworms, fungus and yeast. Kill clostridium and any other bad bowel bacteria. Kill viruses and oncoviruses. Use lots of digestive enzymes, between and with meals, to help the liver get rid of its undigested food deposits. Eat small meals throughout the day to avoid more food deposits. Remove copper, cobalt, nickel, lead and all other heavy metals with EDTA chelation therapy if it is available to you and with homeography, if not.

Often the liver has encased its tumor locations in round balls, called **hepatomas**. For you to digest the casing and clean it all up requires strong digestive enzyme action. But trypsin, a major part of our digestive enzymes, is blocked by the presence of Ascaris parasites! The classic experiment proving this is in the early medical-physiology textbooks (see page 310). Getting rid of Ascaris is necessary. Killing Ascaris larvae with cysteine and other methods was discussed in earlier books. But starving them is the fastest way. Stopping meat consumption (d-carnitine) and quercitin consumption (squash and pumpkin) reduces them to half their population in about one week. After that your own digestive enzymes can get to work. Surprisingly, free-range, organic meats did not have d-carnitine, not even after cooking.

It is easier to open and digest the hepatomas if the dyes inside have already been detoxified by vitamin B_2. It can be done with a few extra large doses of 40 capsules (300 mg each) in a single dose. Opening tumors should wait though, until Ascaris and other parasites, including yeast, have been starved for several weeks. It should wait till your body's immune power is up, at least 2 weeks. Then you can open them one at a time.

There will be surprisingly good liver tissue just outside the hepatomas. You can see this on any kind of scan. This good liver tissue is keeping your whole body going. Wait till the *3-Week Program* is nearly done and the blood test shows the liver enzymes getting better (coming down) before taking these 40 capsule doses of vitamin B_2. A fundamental principle in treating liver cancer is to build up the good liver before opening the bad liver (tumors). Cysteine builds more good liver.

After opening a tumor expect the LDH and alkaline phosphatase to go up on your blood test as dyes come flooding out. Sudan Black dye enters the red blood cells and DAB dye enters the white blood cells. After the 40 capsule doses, keep up a steady low dose of vitamin B_2 such as ten B_2 three times a day to detoxify the flood of dyes set free. Also take coenzyme Q10 to help detoxify dyes so the liver enzymes can come back down quickly. Keep the kidneys from clogging again with these dyes by zapping them and using *take-out* drops for dyes again.

Make special *take-out* drops to remove Sudan Black from red blood cells and DAB from white blood cells. After 5 days the LDH and alkaline phosphatase will be coming down again. Make 2 to 3 quarts of urine every day. After 10 days blood tests should begin to recover and could be repeated. The liver usually lets only one hepatoma open at a time. Wait till you see improvement before opening another hepatoma. Remember, life depends on the good liver, and is not so much threatened by the hepatomas.

Liver cancer often affects the bile ducts so they fill up with tumor cells and get blocked, which leads to jaundice. But just as often the liver is not able to detoxify your hemoglobin, which leads to jaundice, too. Why does that happen? Detoxifying your hemoglobin is required because a large number of red blood cells die each day leaving their hemoglobin behind. The body tries to salvage the iron in it. After this, it is the liver's job to detoxify the leftovers and push them out into the intestine. This detoxified form is called direct bilirubin on your blood test. Undetoxified hemoglobin is called indirect bilirubin (i.b.). An early stage of this detoxification makes a green substance, the color of bile. The green color is what makes our normal bowel contents dark colored. Otherwise, it would be yellow.

If the liver isn't healthy enough to keep up with this detoxification job, a large amount of i.b. is seen on the blood test, and the bilirubin gets backed up waiting its turn. The blood level rises. When it is high enough to shine through the skin you appear yellowish. The eyes tell this story first. Maximum effort is now needed to help your liver detoxify hemoglobin.

The Syncrometer® found that in <u>every</u> case (100%) of high bilirubin, seen on the blood test, **aflatoxin** was spreading through the liver. This is what is poisoning the liver's ability to detoxify hemoglobin even if blockage is physical, too, from tumor growth.

In earlier books I recommended stopping eating bread and grains. I could not guess that the aflatoxin was being made <u>right inside the liver</u> by 2 mold families. Aflatoxin is being produced <u>locally</u> in the liver because aspergillus and penicillium molds are growing in it. It does not come principally from foods, even though moldy grains contribute. These 2 molds are there because they have found dead parasites where you may have recently killed them. They are devouring them. Hurry to digest the dead matter with large amounts of digestive enzymes. Then there will be nothing for them to devour. Hurry to remove the copper, chromium, cobalt, and nickel, without which these molds can't grow. This means a total and complete metal clean up…food, water, teeth and cookware…in days! There is no time to lose.

Hurry to kill the oncoviruses and yeast in the liver with the special enemas (see page 269). Everything grows furiously in the liver and you have just opened a hepatoma cage-full of all these ferocious beasts.

Intravenous therapy, used by alternative cancer therapists, can clear up a jaundice swiftly with EDTA, B complex, laetrile and huge amounts of vitamin C…all with help from DMSO so they can penetrate better. Urea by mouth is often used, as well as milk thistle extract and digestive enzymes directly infused. Their success rates would be astounding if the IVs themselves were without PCB and laundry bleach pollution. Each IV should be tested for these, and then zappicated and delivered through a syringe filter from a glass bottle (This glass did not seep thallium). Other details are given in the earlier advanced cancer book. They would be astounding if the degreasing could be continued at home. And it would be permanent if the water at home was correctly disinfected.

Follow Lillian's case study of liver cancer. This was her second visit. At her first visit she came with ulcerated rectal cancer for which a colostomy was recommended. Three malignant lesions in the liver were metastases from the colon. It took 3 weeks to clear it all up the first time, both at the rectum and the liver, stop the pain and bleeding from the rectum, and find clean water. The plan was to live with one child who had clean water until her own well was fitted for delivery to the house. She was fortunate to have a well. But plans go astray when all seems well again so she didn't go home to clean water. Problems and pain reappeared in a few weeks. They were "bringing water in" from a good source which seemed safe enough in spite of many warnings against this. Soon it was too late to correct any mistakes. The cancer-fire had been lit again. They had to come back. Now she couldn't eat without pain and diarrhea. She couldn't sleep. But she could feed herself, and go to the bathroom, the most basic functions. And she did want to live. Her spouse and child both came with her to share responsibility for her, and showered her with the love of angels, tangible and determined.

#1 Follow Up Visit for Lillian	Liver Metastases

At her second visit her liver had been attacked more severely. Now 8 hepatomas were seen. The rectal tumor had revived, too, but more slowly. Her doctor at home had done a CT scan with "contrast" filling her up with dyes again in spite of our warnings. Now the dye-filled WBC could not kill even the simplest of bacteria, E. coli and salmonella. Her body was swarming with them. She could hardly eat, sleep or manage her

386

daily routines. No evidence of rectal cancer was found on the scan so it was barely mentioned in her summary by the doctor. The focus of her doctor was on the 8 liver tumors, which were to be biopsied and chemoed if possible, but in reality, totally hopeless.

Yet Lillian had escaped a colostomy, with a "bag" to carry her feces in at her first visit. Could she have another miracle?

After a 24-hour plane trip she came straight to the clinic before even going to her motel room. Her two caregivers were eager to get started. A blood test was done. A saliva sample was made by chewing a piece of paper towel till dampened, then

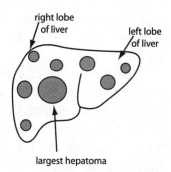

Fig. 102 Drawing of hepatomas

changed into homeographic form to copy its unique frequency pattern (see recipe on page 586). Now the real saliva could be discarded and a tiny brown bottle of pure water used instead. Transportation across the international border would be safe and legal if needed. The information about Lillian's state of health would be found by Syncrometer® inside this bottle.

She had brought 2 samples of drinking water, one from her own kitchen faucet and one from a son's. They were labeled MOM's and BILLY's. These were the tests run on the water samples:

Water Test		
Substance	Mom's	Billy's
PCBs	Pos	Neg
benzene	Pos	Neg
synthetic dyes	Pos	Neg
heavy metals	Pos	Neg
laundry bleach	Pos	Neg
NSF-bleach	Neg	Pos
motor oil	Pos	Neg

Water Test		
malonic acid	Pos	Neg
wheel bearing grease	Pos	Neg

Lillian had been living at home (at MOM's) instead of at her child's because she didn't want to live away from home while they were getting the well water in place; it might all take too long. Little did she know that she had chosen a suicidal course.

The lab test results arrived the same day. A low alkaline phosphatase and LDH were spotted (both due to cobalt toxicity), but one item, the total bilirubin, stood out like a sore thumb. It was over the top of its range, at 1.6. All attention had to be focused on the T.b. if we wanted to prevent jaundice and soon after, her demise. We had to get it down immediately.

Follow each Syncrometer® test now, and the treatment for each problem.

Syncrometer® Liver Analysis:

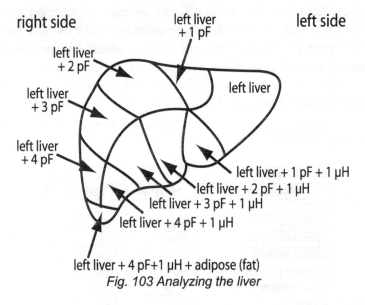

Fig. 103 Analyzing the liver

The liver was divided into 10 parts* and each part tested for OPT, which marks where Fasciolopsis buski parasite stages reside, together with Clostridium bacteria that make isopropyl alcohol and DNA.

Only two parts showed malignancy, though the scan showed 8 tumors and the report mentioned 6. This is not uncommon. Tumors are not necessarily malignant (yet).

Malignancy test at liver locations		
at left liver	OPT	Neg
at left liver + 1 pF	OPT	Neg
at left liver + 2 pF	OPT	Pos
at left liver + 3 pF	OPT	Pos
at left liver + 4 pF	OPT	Neg
at left liver + 1 pF + 1 µH	OPT	Neg
at left liver + 2 pF + 1 µH	OPT	Neg
at left liver + 3 pF + 1 µH	OPT	Neg
at left liver + 4 pF + 1 µH	OPT	Neg
at left liver + 4 pF + 1 µH plus adipose tissue (fat)	OPT	Neg

These two locations could be copied into a bottle of water for plate-zapping convenience. Another copy could be used for taking drops. When drops are taken at the same time as zapping at a particular location, a specially powerful return of immunity is seen there. What could we expect to see inside her hepatomas? These are the Syncrometer® results for one:

Left liver + 2 pF (has malignancy)	
OPT	Pos
PCB	Pos
benzene	Pos
asbestos	Pos
heavy metals	Pos
azo dyes	Pos
laundry bleach	Pos

---

* Plate-zappers put the liver slide from your anatomy kit on the zapping plate plus the correct number of capacitors or inductors. In this way you can construct each location for zapping or drop-taking.

Left liver + 2 pF (has malignancy)	
NSF-bleach	Neg
hypochlorite (water disinfectant)	Pos
malonic acid	Pos
wheel bearing grease	Pos

These results are a replica of her drinking water, showing how its toxins had accumulated at these hepatomas but not at the normal liver, nearby, given next.

Left liver (normal)	
OPT	Neg
PCB	Neg
benzene	Neg
asbestos	Neg
heavy metals	Neg
azo dyes	Neg
laundry bleach	Neg
NSF-bleach	Pos
hypochlorite	Pos
motor oil	Neg
wheel bearing grease	Neg

Notice how the normal left liver has already changed its bleach variety to ours (NSF-bleach) after only two days away from home. A healthy tissue can detoxify the chlorine (hypochlorite) too. The sick parts of the liver can no longer do this. It lingers, to oxidize nearby minerals, especially the organic germanium that is needed by the white blood cells. Her left liver was not malignant, but not well either. Lillian's normal liver could no longer detoxify the hypochlorite from water. Health will suffer even with the good NSF-bleach. She should ozonate, not chlorinate her water at home. Here at the clinic she could boil away the chlorine and filter out the aluminum and other metals. *Later, we used distilled water without chlorination and filtered out the remaining metals.*

Next, we tested for parasites at this hepatoma and compared it to good liver nearby.

Parasite[**] test at left liver + 2 pF (one of the hepatomas)	
Ascaris lumbricoides (pet roundworm)	*Pos*
quercitin (its required food)	*Pos*
Ascaris megalocephala (pet roundworm, another variety)	*Pos*
d-carnitine (its required food)	*Pos*
Fasciolopsis buski (human intestinal fluke or stages)	*Pos*
onion (its required food)	*Pos*
Clonorchis (human liver fluke)	*Pos*
oats (its required food)	*Pos*
Eurytrema (pancreatic fluke)	*Pos*
lauric (required fat for Eurytrema)	*Pos*
limonene (its required food)	*Pos*
Fasciola	*Neg*
Strongyloides	*Pos*
Onchocerca	*Neg*
Paragonimus	*Neg*
Dirofilaria (dog heartworm)	*Pos*
lactose (its required food)	*Pos*
Echinococcus granulosis (tapeworm)	*Neg*
Echinoporyphium recurvatum	*Neg*

Parasite test at left liver (outside of hepatoma)	
all above parasites	*Neg*
d-carnitine	*Neg*
lactose	*Neg*
asparagine (required food for yeast)	*Neg*
quercitin	*Neg*
oats	*Neg*

We can see that the bad things are housed inside the hepatoma, none are outside.

Notice that each parasite has its own food tucked in beside it!

Having parasites and other living invaders inside ourselves will give us their enzymes. The minerals from these enzymes

---

[**]All parasite tests were made with composite frequencies (see page 300).

will get oxidized into metals as they die or get killed. So little deposits of their metals will appear where they live. These will supply the next generation of parasites. If fungus is killed, it leaves behind its copper, cobalt, chromium and nickel.

Besides this, the laundry bleached water and any other source of heavy metals will bring a whole host of unnatural metals that will accumulate right there where the immunity has been destroyed. Notice the difference in metal deposits between the hepatomas and normal liver regions.

Metals * at left liver + 2 pF (the hepatoma)	
copper	Pos
cobalt	Pos
chromium III and VI	Pos
vanadium	Pos
germanium (metallic)	Pos
selenium (metallic)	Pos
nickel	Pos
manganese	Neg
ruthenium	Neg
molybdenum	Neg
tellurium	Neg
rubidium	Neg
thulium	Neg
indium	Neg
mercury	Neg
aluminum	Pos
iridium	Neg
iridium dodecacarbonyl	Neg
Fe_3+ (ferric iron)	Neg
Fe_2+ (ferrous iron)	Neg
Fe_3 dodecacarbonyl	Neg
Co_4 dodecacarbonyl	Neg
Fe_2O_3 (This is south pole iron)	*Pos
Fe_3O_4 (This is north pole iron)	Neg
south polarization	Pos
north polarization	Neg
motor oil	Pos

* Test substances for metals were atomic absorption standards.

Metals [*] at left liver + 2 pF (the hepatoma)	
cortisone (This should have been present.)	Neg

Not many unnatural metals were tested but aluminum is present from her drinking water as well as Fe_2O_3.

Metals at left liver (outside of hepatoma)	
copper	Neg
cobalt	Neg
chromium III & VI	Neg
vanadium	Neg
germanium	Neg
selenium	Neg
nickel	Neg

The normal liver tissue has not accumulated metals. The deposits of metals in the hepatoma make a very oxidizing environment. Things that enter this zone will get oxidized. As iron gets oxidized from Fe_3O_4 to Fe_2O_3 (ferrite) it switches its polarity (the part that the Syncrometer® detects) to south pole. Now this area will change to southerly. Some Fe_2O_3 comes directly from asbestos, which her water was bringing.

All invaders will be accelerated in their growth and reproduction at a south polarized location, discoveries made decades ago by independent scientists [*] when the study of magnetism as part of biology was still taboo.

At the same time DNA production is turned on and up. Compare the bacteria at the two locations.

Bacteria test at left liver + 2pF (the hepatoma)	
mumps	Neg
Salmonella enteriditis	Neg
Salmonella paratyphi	Neg
Salmonella typhimurium	Pos

---

[*] Read books by Albert Roy Davis and Walter C. Rawls, Jr. such as *Magnetism and its Effects on the Living System*, *The Magnetic Effect*, *The Magnetic Blueprint of Life*. Acres USA, PO Box 8800, Metairie, Louisiana 70011-8800

Bacteria test at left liver + 2pF (the hepatoma)	
Salmonella typhimurium / SV 40	Pos
The slash means SV 40 virus is touching the bacteria.	
Salmonella typhimurium / SV 40 / CMV	Neg
CMV does not attach itself to SV 40 to arrive inside S. typhi but it can infect S. typhimurium by itself.	
Salmonella typhi / CMV	Pos
Shigella dysenteriae	Neg
Shigella sonnei	Neg
Yeast	Neg
asparagine, its essential food	Neg
Staphylococcus aureus	Neg
Streptococcus pneumoniae	Neg
E. coli	Pos
E. coli / SV 40	Pos
Notice that SV 40 virus is inside E. coli bacteria.	
E. coli / CMV	Pos
E. coli / SV 40 / CMV	Neg
Again, CMV does not latch onto SV 40 although it can infect E. coli by itself. This suggests that CMV does not truly belong to cancer, but is part of chronic disease associated with cancer.	
E. coli / Hepatitis B	Pos
Hepatitis B virus is alive inside E. coli.	
E. coli / SV 40 / Hepatitis B	Neg
Hepatitis B does not latch onto SV 40 but it can invade E. coli by itself. It may only be part of chronic disease.	
Bacteria at left liver (outside the hepatoma)	
All above bacteria and Yeast	Neg

The hepatoma is heavily infected with bacteria, while the rest of the liver is not.

Bacteria bring their viruses; suggesting that the bacteria themselves are ill! Being infected with certain viruses makes a huge difference to the bacterial behavior. Bacteria, with their viruses, are seldom seen inside WBCs. The viruses seem to shield the bacteria from our white blood cells.

Viruses at left liver + 2pF (hepatoma)	
MYC	Neg
RAS	Neg

Viruses* at left liver + 2pF (hepatoma)	
SV 40	Pos
gallic acid, its trigger	Pos
JUN	Neg
NEU	Neg
FOS	Neg
oleic oil, its trigger	Neg
SRC	Neg
HIV as Reverse Transcriptase	Pos
P24	Neg
benzene, its trigger	Pos
Hepatitis B	Pos
umbelliferone, its trigger	Pos
CMV	Pos
lauric acid, its trigger	Pos
Adenovirus	Neg

Viruses* at left liver (healthy portion)	
MYC	Neg
SV 40	Neg
gallic acid, its trigger	Neg
FOS	Neg
Hepatitis B	Neg
umbelliferone, its trigger	Neg
RAS	Neg
HIV as Reverse Transcriptase	Neg
benzene, its trigger	Neg
NEU	Neg
CMV	Neg
lauric acid (food oil)	Neg
SRC	Neg
Adenovirus	Neg

This gives us a glimpse of the inferno raging inside the hepatoma although all seems quiet. It is understandable now, why no normal metabolism can be carried on here. No symptoms are felt, though. The hepatomas are forced to enlarge and grow by many forces at work: the incoming 5

---

* Three letter names are for oncogenes representing the oncoviruses, meaning tumor-causing viruses.

laundry bleach toxins, the arrival of south pole forces at close range, the increased parasitism and viral invasion from being fed so many of their essential foods and triggers.

Digestion gets worse and worse. As hepatoma cells get unable to do the fine chemistry expected of liver cells, life depends on how much good liver is still left outside the hepatoma. Giving a lot of l-cysteine is specifically helpful in growing new normal liver (2 capsules 3 times daily for 2 or 3 weeks), just as it is for growing new kidney tissue.

If the hepatomas are killed outright with x-rays or chemotherapy, the cancer cells, parasite stages and bacteria with their viruses will be killed altogether, leaving a ball of dead tissue to clear away. Even nonmalignant ones would turn into dead balls. A strong remaining liver could still clean up after them. But if the tumor nuclei, parasite stages, bacteria and viruses continue to be spawned far away from the liver and are again collected by the liver, it will become cancerous, again. After all, it continues to be inflamed by umbelliferone. And, even if the liver could recover and heal itself by not eating carrots, the tumor nuclei would simply find a new organ to attack. The eyes, brain, bone, the whole body, are at risk for attack as soon as an organ develops its own chronic allergy.

Although a temporary solution might be the drastic clinical one now in use, "kill all, remove all", unfortunately, it cannot bring a cure because the causes are not confronted.

When the causes are removed a true cure is put in place. You should then be able to see the hepatomas digesting themselves until they are gone on a new scan.

Lillian reached a satisfactory end point again in her curing program about 5 months later. Five tumors could still be seen in the new liver scan, a good result. Bout after bout of E. coli/oncovirus invasion took its time in clearing, always following a siege of heavy metals and malonic acid from food and cookware. These immortalized bacteria, in turn, reinvaded the remainder of rectal tumor, preventing complete healing there. It continued to bleed intermittently. The ultimate source of metals and malonic acid was not found in time for her departure date. But her family had learned Syncrometer® testing. Will they find it? (Since then, I have found the trigger for Hepatitis B to be umbelliferone, the source of it to be human liver fluke, and the favorite food of the fluke to be oats). Hopefully, she is staying close to her good water.

Brain Cancer—The Family Connection

#2 Mother-Daughter	brain cancer

Whether or not cancer is contagious has stirred a considerable amount of argument in the past. Now that we see the complex nature of cancer, with its 2 dozen or so contributors, we can answer our own questions.

Neither the contagion theory, inheritance theory nor environmental theory fits all the facts. But adding parasitism to the picture adds the missing link that ties the other 3 causes together.

When fleas bring heartworm to dogs, it is not obvious, even though fleas are outside parasites and easily seen. The heart disease could appear to be contagious, inherited, or environmental.

When a disease afflicts more than one person in a family and even more than one generation, we think of genes. But couldn't an infectious agent like bacteria or viruses or parasite larvae have crossed the placenta or come through the mother's milk? It is all too possible. We should take another look at inheritance of parasites. Our "genetic diseases" may not be genetic. Orphan diseases, new diseases, and old chronic diseases like diabetes, high blood pressure, and arthritis could be studied in simple ways. A Syncrometer® and a course in parasitology would bring many returns without using PCR techniques and microbiology.

When smoking-related and industry-related cancers are seen they would appear to be environmentally caused. And yet there are enough exceptions to make one think it is not that simple. If the person targeted was more heavily parasitized, particularly in the lungs, the exception would be explained.

Different theories are each likely to have some truth but how are they linked? I have studied several cases of parent and child where one of them had cancer. The links are easy to spot. Try to find them between Anita and her mother.

In this case study the child developed cancer, the parent not yet! But the risk factors are at work.

Anita and her mother came from Europe, hiring a translator to help change French and German into English (not a word of Spanish, the local language!) and vice versa for us all. Anita had a brain tumor that had been operated on at age 6 but now at age 14 was growing again and could not be operated on without risk of permanent paralysis or even death. Chemotherapy and radiation were not suitable either so with this dismal outlook she had gone to an alternative practioner before coming to our clinic.

It all started with seizures at age 18 mos. She was put on medication, but no contributing factors or causes were ever discussed. They were probably unknown to her doctors. She had 12 years to cure her seizures and could have been given electromagnetic treatments, invented and reported extensively in Italy's neurological literature, already 20 years ago (search Internet http://www.earthpulse.net/Sandyk.htm). She could have been tested for brain allergies, finding the food phenolic **malvin** to be the seizure antigen. Malvin is present in blue and red natural foods, as well as chicken and eggs. Such phenolic allergies have been found and extensively reported by ecological allergists. She could have been tested for the parasite, Ascaris, considered causative by the present author, having published this in her own books from 1994 to 2004. Both Anita's mother and doctors were unaware of any of these. All she knew was that her daughter's symptoms were increasing, until at age 12 a tumor was found. The diagnosis was malignant. Since then, alternative therapies had helped somewhat, but the clock was ticking for her lifespan. She was taking Topamax, 3 times a day when she arrived. If she even missed 1 dose it was noticeable with a beginning seizure attack. She had been warned not to miss any. In spite of medication, she had salivation attacks, eye attacks, arm immobility attacks, and headaches to warn of a seizure coming. She now had about 1 major attack in 10 days in spite of medication. They were told it was the result of both tumor growth and worsening seizures.

We told them she should stay on her medicine until the cancer was gone and then clear up the seizures.

Wisely, they had arranged a stay of 4 weeks instead of the regular 2.

Her first instruction was not to stray from the food provided at the special restaurant for cancer patients. No chicken or eggs were served and red or blue fruit or vegetables (tomatoes, strawberries, grapes, blueberries) could be immediately exchanged. Processed food (in cans or packages) were to be avoided since malvin is present in many, regardless of color, possibly from use of natural dyes. More importantly, the restaurant diet served food free of phloridzin, chlorogenic acid, gallic acid, apiol and the onion family. Avoiding the first 3 would stop production of the tumor nucleus. Learning to avoid apiol would protect her in the future from breast cancer and ovarian problems. Avoiding onions & garlic would starve and deplete Fasciolopsis stages. Besides all this, the special food chemical leading to brain cancer, caffeic acid, must be avoided, mainly citrus fruit. She began to cry. Her mother beamed with hope but disbelief. For a pizza, orange juice, and chocolate lover, like her daughter, this would never be possible without such a special restaurant, but here it was, a menu as flavorful and appealing as could be desired. She was a hungry child; hungry for all the old bad things. But seeing the other cancer patients, gasping for breath, pot-bellied with effusions, bent over from fatigue may have been a subtle deterrent. Seeing them improve from day to day and simply proclaim their joy in living another day would be a lesson, too. She had been taking life for granted.

At her first visit they supplied 4 water samples brought from home. These are the Syncrometer® test results:

Water sample #1 taken from Düsseldorf, Germany	
PCB	*Neg*
USA laundry bleach disinfectant	*Neg*
benzene	*Neg*
European laundry bleach disinfectant	*Pos*
heavy metals	*Neg*
NSF-stamped bleach	*Neg*
azo dyes	*Pos*
Triazo solid compound chlorine	*Neg*

Water sample #2 taken from a business location in Düsseldorf, Germany	
PCB	*Neg*
USA laundry bleach disinfectant	*Neg*
benzene	*Neg*
European laundry bleach disinfectant	*Pos*
heavy metals	*Neg*
NSF-stamped bleach disinfectant	*Neg*
azo dyes	*Pos*

Water sample #3 taken from a friend's home	
PCB	*Neg*
USA laundry bleach disinfectant	*Neg*
benzene	*Neg*
European laundry bleach disinfectant	*Pos*
heavy metals	*Neg*
NSF-stamped bleach disinfectant	*Neg*
azo dyes	*Pos*

Water sample #4 taken from her own home, kitchen faucet	
PCB	*Pos*
USA laundry bleach disinfectant	*Pos*
benzene	*Pos*
European laundry bleach disinfectant	*Neg*

heavy metals	Pos
NSF-bleach disinfectant	Neg
azo dyes	Pos

Her own water was of the worst kind, although returning home to any of the others would lead to disaster, too. She could not have synthetic dyes in her water and expect to get well, they would certainly include malvin. She was sent the results by special courier to let her start searching for friends and family members who would make a water sample for them. It had to be shipped "fastest way". After finding a safe water, she would still have to locate an apartment in that district and send a water sample from it to be tested, for complete certainty. Her husband immediately ended his business vacation to travel to his earlier home in France to search for safe water. There were many friends and relatives eager to help.

On her first day, a blood test was scheduled. Her blood tests at home had been justifiably skimpy since nothing on a blood test would have thrown light on her cancer or seizures anyway.

06/19/03 - Blood Test Results – Anita, age 14 seizures and brain cancer			
CBC		RANGE	
WBC	6	4.8 - 10.8	thousand
RBC	4.48	4.2 - 6.4	million
Hemoglobin	12.3	12 - 18	g/dl
Platelets	435	130 - 400	thousand

At once we can see from the high platelet count and rather low hemoglobin that she has internal bleeding chronically.

06/19/03 - Blood test results, continued			
WBC Analysis			
Segmented	42%		
Bands	0		
Lymphocytes	55%		
Monocytes	2%		

06/19/03 - Blood test results, continued			
Eosinophils	1%		
Basophils	0		

Here we see that the segmented kind is too low and lymphocyte kind is too high. It means she is overburdened by viruses. Having no symptoms of virus disease is quite misleading. I suspect mumps, which characteristically inverts the ratio of segmented to lymphocyte varieties. They should have been in a ratio of 70 to 25% in favor of segmented. We will test for viruses by Syncrometer® later.

06/19/03 – Blood test results, continued		
Blood Chemistry	Value	Range
glucose (blood sugar)	80	73 – 118
BUN (urea, kidney test)	15.9	8 – 23
creatinine (kidney test)	0.8	.4 – 1.6
uric acid	3.8	2.5 – 7.7
cholesterol	149	133 – 240
bilirubin, direct	0.28	.1 – .35
bilirubin, indirect	0.6	.2 – 1
bilirubin, total	0.88	.3 – 1.3
calcium	10.3	8.5 – 11.0
phosphorus	3.6	2.5 – 4.5
alk phos (enzyme)	73 LO	23 – 147
LDH (liver enzyme)	112 LO	71 – 195
AST (liver enzyme)	35	8 – 40
ALT (liver enzyme)	38 HI	5 – 35
triglycerides (blood fat)	122 HI	30 – 170
total protein	7.1	5.7 – 8
albumin	4.1	3.7 – 5
globulin	3	2 – 3.6
GGTP (liver enzyme)	42 HI	4 – 50
chloride	100	98 – 108
sodium	145	135 – 152
potassium	4.5	4.1 – 5.6

Reading Her Blood Chemistry Test

The LDH is rather low, suggesting cobalt toxicity. This would cause fatigue, which was one of her complaints. A better value would be 160.

The 3 other liver enzymes (AST, ALT, GGTP) are all slightly high. At her age they should be in the low 20s. The AST and ALT go up as lead accumulates in the liver. The GGTP goes up as the bile ducts clog, producing soft stones not visible with x-rays. We will recommend a liver cleanse quite soon. The calcium level is slightly high, meaning that toxins are accumulating in the thyroid gland. This suggests tooth filling material that arrives easily at the thyroid gland due to its nearness. A calcium level of 9.5 would have been better.

Checking the Dental Situation

Only 1 tooth, a molar, has a filling, plastic, not metal, and never was metal. We will test for seepage of the plastic into saliva, thyroid and brain.

All tests will be done on saliva since a saliva sample can be copied into water using homeography or homeopathy (see *Recipes*). This makes it safe, legal, and allows storage for very long periods of time. In this way a collection ("library") can be made of different cancers and diseases for future comparison. These are the results of her first Syncrometer® test done on a saliva sample prepared homeopathically on the day of her arrival. The test will take about 2 hours.

Although these results are standard findings for a cancer patient, a few details vary from patient to patient. Syncrometer® testing helps to find these. It becomes a useful tool to monitor progress although not necessary. By monitoring each step of treatment, the next step can be started sooner.

6/18/03 (day of arrival) - Saliva test		
tumor nucleus	*Pos*	the beginning of all tumors
Orthophospho tyrosine(OPT)	*Pos*	our malignancy marker

6/18/03 (day of arrival) - Saliva test		
SV 40	*Pos*	the cancer virus
RAS	*Pos*	an oncovirus
MYC	*Pos*	an oncovirus
FOS	*Neg*	an oncovirus
JUN	*Neg*	an oncovirus

Additional tests could be done but the tasks are already clear; all items should be *Negative*.

She was given a program (protocol) almost identical with the one used in this book. Several herbs will kill flukes and roundworms at the same time. Killing the pancreatic fluke will reduce her source of SV 40 viruses. Not eating gallic acid will stop triggering SV 40 out of the remaining pancreatic flukes. It will also stop "inflaming" the pancreas, so no cells are free to contribute to tumor nuclei. For this reason she is to eat only self-baked breads or machine-baked with bromine-free and gallic acid free flour (see *Sources*). Not eating chlorogenic acid-containing foods or phloridzin-containing foods will stop inflaming the hypothalamus and pituitary. Soon the tumor nucleus will be absent in her saliva.

Saliva is a systemic solution—it mixes with the other fluids, lymph, and blood quite quickly. But it does not reach the cerebrospinal fluid (CSF) of the brain quickly. So besides saliva testing we may do CSF tests on the same saliva sample. Further, OPT can be missed in the saliva test if it is just beginning in one organ. A urine test is more sensitive than a saliva test but less pleasant to handle, even when an electronic copy can be made to use instead. When OPT has already cleared from the saliva, a urine test becomes more important, to check if a leftover location of cancer still exists. The best test, of course, is a search for OPT in every organ, but this is not realistically possible, so only organs suspected are tested. A definitive test for beginning cancers at <u>all</u> locations in the body has not been discovered yet.

RAS comes from yeast growing in the body. Yeast is killed with the herb, turmeric powder, but to prevent its return the excess metallic chromium needs to be removed. A homeographic *take-out* technique for chromium will be used and monitored. By not eating asparagine, RAS will not be triggered, so this oncovirus will disappear at the same time as the yeast growth. She was told to eat only machine-made or homemade bread which raises the baking temperature and thereby makes sure all yeast was killed in her bread.

MYC comes from eating chicken and eggs, and from Fasciolopsis buski itself. She should stop eating chicken and eggs for the extra reason of avoiding malvin, the seizure substance. And of course, she should kill Fasciolopsis buski. Without MYC, any mumps virus will lose its shield from the immune system. Then, as soon as Anita's white blood cells get back their immune power they will eat all mumps viruses and kill them. By not drinking milk, mumps viruses will not come back.

Without mumps viruses the ratio of segmented WBCs to lymphocytes will come back to normal.

Meanwhile, she was given turmeric capsules and Lugol's iodine solution to do an enema of these daily. She would also take these by mouth at the same time as the enema, to reach the top and bottom of her body at the same time, considering how far away the brain is from the lower body. With this method, only a few enemas are needed.

Although the tumor nucleus will stop being formed by her new diet and be gone in 5 days, we should also kill it as fast as possible. She was told to take the 6 fresh seed recipe without any additions except barley flakes to give it some body. The wheat germ is stale and contains menadione and will be omitted since she already has internal bleeding (menadione worsens bleeding). After 5 days she was to stop the 6 fresh seed recipe for 3 days, then go back on if testing showed it was necessary. A second enema recipe, of 3 fresh seeds with barley flakes was to be done each day, too. It could simply be added to the regular one, before or after the turmeric. She was cautioned not to take more than 3 seeds to prevent diarrhea.

She was asked to keep a chart or use a calendar to mark every treatment she took and how much. News of the enemas brought her to tears. We reassured her it would be painless; she could learn it easily and not even need her mother's help. If she did 3 or 4 enemas, complete ones, holding them for an hour without expelling, she would be done and could stop them. It did not console here. But her mother was pleased with hope for quick results.

6/18/03 - Saliva test, continued		
p53	*Pos*	gene
This gene is "over expressed" in cancer, caused by vanadium toxicity. We will search for it and take it out homeographically.		
SCF	*Pos*	a south polarized growing force
Stem cell factor is excessive and reaching everywhere to stimulate cell division. We will stop the hypothalamus erosion that is responsible for SCF.		
CEA	*Pos*	cancer marker
Carcinoembryonic antigen is produced when yeast (S. cerevisciae) or Onchocerca or EBV are present.		
HCG	*Pos*	cancer marker
Human Chorionic Gonadotropin, is produced by the hypothalamus when Fasciolopsis cercariae and isopropyl alcohol are present.		
C_3	*Neg*	Complement C_3

The first four can be used as cancer markers. They should all be gone (*Negative*).

C_3, one member of the complement family, should be present in all body fluids. It is being used up by attaching itself to the parasite stages, food antigens, free-floating cells and tumor nuclei besides bacteria. When these are destroyed, complement C_3 will again be present.

6/18/03 - Saliva test, continued		
vanadium	*Pos*	stop gas utilities, test and change cookware and dishes, zappicate teeth
copper	*Pos*	stop copper water pipes

6/18/03 - Saliva test, continued		
cobalt	*Pos*	stop using detergent
chromium VI & III	*Pos*	stop using untested cooking pots and eating finely ground (by steel) powders and foods
selenium (oxidized variety)	*Pos*	stop malonic acid and metals from laundry bleach in water
germanium	*Pos*	stop chlorination of water

Of course, these metals came mainly from her laundry bleach water. But other sources are now just as important, because her body can no longer detoxify and excrete <u>any</u>.

Germanium deposits, which are metal-like, are made when the body is so over oxidized for years, that it can no longer keep reducing these or excreting them. Chlorine added to drinking water oxidizes organic germanium in the body. Toxic selenium seeps from glass cookware, along with malonates. We will supply fresh organic minerals that are not oxidized while at the same time removing the oxidized deposits and sources of oxidizing metals.

6/18/03 - Saliva test continued		
nickel	*Pos*	remove metal jewelry, discard seeping food containers
lead	*Pos*	replace copper water pipes, test supplements
Supplements and medicines often have lead. Copper pipes have lead soldered joints. Lead raises the transaminases on the blood test (AST, ALT).		
aluminum	*Pos*	filter the city water but only through a tested filter
Aluminum is added to all municipal water, good or bad. Boil 1 minute then filter with pitcher filter (a tested variety). Use a stainless steel pan OR start with distilled water; no need to boil before filtering.		
iridium	*Pos*	
This should be present but in organic form.		

Anita is more oxidized than the average cancer patient; it may have started at 18 months or even at birth from exposure to laundry bleach water. We advised her to seek a chelation doctor at home and get at least one series of chelations to drain many more heavy metals from her body with EDTA. With so much metal deposited in her, it is especially important not to add to it with regular sources of these metals in the modern lifestyle.

We also gave her EDTA powder to take, $\frac{1}{8}$ tsp. by mouth and $\frac{1}{8}$ tsp. by enema daily for 4 days. She was warned not to take more since it is very powerful. Meanwhile we would start taking out the metal forms of copper, cobalt, chromium, vanadium, germanium, and selenium as well as nickel and aluminum from lymph in a steady dose of homeographic "*take-out*" drops taken once daily (see page 112).

6/18/03 - Saliva test, continued	
urethane	*Pos*
This is tooth filling material. It implies seepage from her one plastic tooth. It is a carcinogen.	
acrylic acid	*Pos*
This is seeping from her one plastic tooth filling; it becomes acrylamine, a carcinogen.	
DAP (common putty)	*Pos*
This is diallylphthalate, part of tooth filling plastic and impression compound, a strong carcinogen.	
azo dyes	*Neg*
mercury	*Neg*
thallium	*Neg*

The absence of the last 3 showed that her plastic tooth was not seeping dyes, although it was seeping plastics. There was no amalgam. This will speed her recovery tremendously. We can zappicate this one tooth and retest the saliva for the seeping plastic ingredients. They should disappear.

The next test will be an organ search for the exact location of her brain cancer[*]. The organs are on stained microscope slides.

6/18/03 - Saliva test, continued		
at pituitary gland	OPT-*Neg*	no cancer here
at hypothalamus	OPT-*Neg*	no cancer here
at pons	OPT-*Neg*	no cancer here
at pineal gland	OPT-*Neg*	no cancer here
at cerebellum	OPT-*Neg*	no cancer here
at cerebrum	OPT-*Pos*	cancer is here
There is obviously malignancy at some location found in the tissue on this microscope slide. But it is not necessary to identify the location more precisely, because we will copy the entire slide as the location to be used in zapping or drop taking.		
at "whole brain" slide	OP-*Pos*	cancer is here
There is malignancy somewhere represented on this slide, too. It may be the same location as found on the cerebrum slide, but it may not. It is wise to clear it up using both slides.		
at choroid plexus	OPT-*Pos*	cancer is extra strong here

Other brain locations or body locations were not tested, although they should be. We will search for leftover locations with a urine test for OPT later because they may clear up automatically from our early treatments.

She will zap her three malignancy locations on a plate-zapper, which will reach them precisely with a resonant frequency coming from a ¼ volt *Positive* offset zapper.

---

[*]Testers, place the brain tissues to be tested beside her saliva sample on the test plate. This identifies the organ as hers and not the tester's. Leave a short gap, $1/16$ inch, to indicate there is no direct contact between saliva and brain tissues.

She will also take *"organ drops"* of these locations made by homeography. They will be taken at the same time as zapping them for maximum benefit.

By the second day she had already stopped making the tumor nucleus and delivering tiny tumor nuclei to these 3 brain locations. She had stopped eating caffeic acid, the brain antigen, too, so no primary "quads" could be found in the saliva, either.

The next test is for Fasciola, since this parasite invites metastases.

6/18/03 - Saliva test for Fasciola		
Fasciola composite *	at pons	*Neg*
	at pituitary	*Neg*
	at hypothalamus	*Neg*
	at "whole brain" slide	*Neg*
	at cerebrum	*Neg*
	at choroid plexus (her risk of new tumor formation continues here)	*Pos*

The risk of new tumor formation from approaching tumor nuclei stayed on at the choroid plexus because of fibronectin increase due to Fasciola.

Fortunately, the brain was not teeming with Fasciola stages, which would account for the rather slow progression of her brain cancer. We will stop the risk of metastases forming by getting rid of Fasciola with the parasite program and by not eating lard, the source of lauric acid, their food.

Next I searched for any locations with excessive "sticky" fibers. Fibronectin, laminin and cadherin E should all be *Negative*.

---

* Remember that our parasite testing system uses frequencies of all stages put into a single bottle, so only one test is needed to find any stage of a parasite or the adult.

410

fibronectin	at pons	*Neg*
	at cerebrum	*Neg*
	at "whole brain" slide	*Neg*
	at choroid plexus	*Pos*

Although the malignancy marker, OPT, had spread to neighboring brain organs from the choroid plexus, fibronectin had not. Good fortune for her!

laminin	at pons	*Neg*
	at pituitary	*Neg*
	at cerebellum	*Neg*
	at pineal	*Neg*
	at hypothalamus	*Neg*
	at "whole brain" slide	*Pos*
	at choroid plexus	*Pos*
	at cerebrum	*Pos*

Laminin is exactly where the cancer is, being brought by Ascaris megalocephala.

Ascaris lumbricoides is not present, so cadherin E is not present. Good fortune for her, again.

cadherin E	at pons	*Neg*
	at cerebrum	*Neg*
	at "whole brain" slide	*Neg*
	at choroid plexus	*Neg*

To kill both Fasciola and Fasciolopsis in the brain, she was to take 4 wormwood by enema, added to the turmeric-plus 3 seed recipe. She should also take 4 wormwood capsules by mouth daily, preferably at the same time as the enema was taken, and to hold it all inside for at least 1 hour. If she could avoid expelling any of it, success would come sooner.

After discussing these results and treatments she began to cry again; her mother was distraught, fearing the child would rebel. We discussed the reality of death and departure from dear ones with her and pointed to a 3-year old patient who was doing the whole program easily. She had brain cancer, too, and was held limply in her mother's arms at first, 2 weeks ago. Now she could already have her own bowel movements and sit alone. The weekend had arrived and our clinic medical doctor had just found a Mexican brand replacement for her Topamax anti-seizure tablet. Hers had been manufactured with disinfectant of the European laundry bleach kind so it had azo dyes in its makeup, not suitable for her recovery.

She could take the new pills and go to visit the local sights and enjoy herself, carrying her lunch and drops to take. The one day she had been off medication while searching for a dye-free variety reminded her she was a sick girl and needed to pay attention and do something for her future.

Three days later she had not accomplished anything. She did not like the food so didn't eat it. We encouraged the mother to keep trying and have nothing in the refrigerator to tempt her. She complained of right groin pain, inability to sleep and headache (like her mother's problems). She had taken one dose of Black Walnut tincture and only a few assorted supplements. She had considerable vaginal discharge, which annoyed her. I pointed to the probability that the enemas would cure some of these symptoms, too. This day her fresh saliva sample would not show much improvement with so little accomplished, so instead of searching for progress at the brain I searched at the kidneys to find any excretion problems.

At kidneys		
Dirofilaria	*Pos*	dog heartworm

They had never had a dog. I pointed out that we all have stages of dog heartworm, which is a strong contributor to our universal heart disease and die of it eventually. It is inches long, thin as a single silk thread and transparent as glass. If she could kill this she would probably lose her groin pain because the lymph nodes in the groin collect the heartworm stages. If the white blood cells in these nodes couldn't kill them, the nodes would enlarge, causing pressure and pain. Dyes that she had been drinking in her water at home would keep the white blood cells from killing the parasites.

At kidneys, continued		
synthetic dyes	*Pos*	from her laundry bleach water
lactose (milk sugar)	*Pos*	undigested milk
Milk sugar is heartworm's favorite food (its essential food).		

Without lactose the heartworms will leave. We started her on lactase enzyme capsules. Her mother said she never liked and doesn't drink milk but was a pizza (cheese) lover. The lactase capsules (see *Sources*) could be put into the heavy whipping cream she could still have (½ capsule per quart, left to stand overnight). To digest the lactose deposits already in her kidneys she would take 1 capsule with meals (3 meals a day) and 1 capsule between meals, altogether 6 daily for 2 days. But she must also stop using all oils in cooking, even olive oil, because **oleic** acid-containing oil triggers an oncovirus out of the heartworm, named FOS. Oils also have <u>malonic acid</u>, probably from the pesticides that were used in growing the crops and could never be removed before pressing out the oil (no matter how cold the process or "virgin" or "organic" the label states). Instead of oils she could use butter in all cooking. This appealed to Anita.

At kidneys, continued		
methyl malonate	*Pos*	derived from malonic acid
This is a severe kidney toxin, blocking its passage of many things and also causing cystic kidneys.		
maleic anhydride	*Pos*	comes from methyl malonate by the body's detoxification.

Maleic anhydride causes effusions, body lymph that escapes through its wall into a cavity like the abdomen or chest (lung).

Both of these compounds represent partly detoxified malonic acid. It takes huge amounts of vitamin C to detoxify them.

She admitted having pain off and on over the kidney at one side. She admitted she was not taking the supplements in our program. We pointed out 2 patients with huge effusions that had to be drained each week. This would be her fate soon. Meanwhile we made her 2 homeographic "*take-out*" bottles, one to take methyl malonate-out-of-both-kidneys and one to take maleic anhydride-out-of-both-kidneys. This would work now that she would no longer be eating oils. The dyes in the kidney white blood cells were blocking the removal of the malonate toxins. In fact, the heartworms themselves were even holding the dyes! So it all depended on her taking the Decaris capsules to kill the heartworms in our program. Would she?

Next day she arrived to zappicate her one plastic-filled molar with the toothbrush zappicator. Her new saliva test already showed improvements.

6/22/03 - Saliva test		
tumor nucleus at saliva	*Neg*	now gone
tumor nucleus at lymph	*Neg*	now gone
tumor nucleus at blood	*Neg*	now gone

These were unexpected good results. She was staying off the most important restricted foods.

Saliva test, continued		
OPT	*Neg*	(cancer marker missing)
The malignancy must be greatly reduced since it no longer shows up at the systemic level of saliva. We will search at brain locations.		
at cerebrum	*Neg*	
at whole brain slide	*Neg*	
at choroid plexus	*Pos*	
The malignancy is gone from 2 out of 3 locations. Is there a special hindrance at choroid plexus?		

Test at choroid plexus		
RAS	*Neg*	
The yeast oncovirus is gone.		
MYC	*Pos*	
This oncovirus requires the special enemas with turmeric and Lugol's.		
Fasciola	*Pos*	
Fasciolopsis	*Pos*	
SV 40	*Neg*	

She must have taken some enemas to kill the SV 40 virus and must not be eating gallic acid. These are most important.

Her mother stated she had only done 1 enema and had taken 2 capsules of freeze-dried green Black Walnut hull instead of the stronger tincture and other things. She also had one dose of 6 seeds by mouth. I pointed out to Anita that her body is very eager to heal; it is doing its best to heal her; she had an advantage of youth and health and could succeed. She should sit down with a fresh unopened 2 oz. bottle of BWT (ES) and pour it all into a glass. Then she should pour an equal amount of heavy whipping cream, already ozonated and treated with hydrochloric acid and lactase enzyme into the tincture and 1 tbsp. of syrup or sugar. It would be delicious. Drink it all while sitting down and try not to enjoy it so much she could become an alcoholic! She was to do this 2 days in a row and no more! She left in tears again.

6/25/03 - Three days later they came in smiling. Anita showed me (remember, none of us is speaking their native language) where her groin pain was gone, her kidney pains had left, her headaches hadn't returned, she felt energy, her discharge was gone. The mother beamed over her daughter's progress. She asked if I had seen her CT scans of the brain cancer she had brought from her doctor. I said I had, it showed nothing extraordinary besides extensive tumor. She beamed even more, in disbelief. I told her the growth would stop while she was with us but the tumor would not be gone nor even shrunk in the time she was here. They both must learn how to do everything so they could prevent a recurrence at home, using their knowledge. Most important of all would be staying in properly bleached water, with the NSF-stamp on the bleach bottle. This would have to be determined by Syncrometer® testing since the water department could not be expected to be forthright nor legally compliant.

The saliva test for this day showed:

Test at choroid plexus		
OPT	*Neg*	
Fasciolopsis	*Neg*	

She had killed the biggest flukes in her tumor; those responsible for making the malignancy marker, OPT. That was cause for joy but she could expect an attack of depression now from the Clostridium bacteria that would eat up the remains. She should quickly try to digest them with the 15 capsules of digestive enzymes twice a day, written on her program. Her mother said she had been crying, over nothing, at home, in spite of new joy. She was told to put a slide of Clostridium botulinum on the zapper plate permanently. These bacteria cause the depression.

Test at choroid plexus, continued		
3 Clostridium varieties* (C. perf, C. tetani, C. botulinum)	*Pos*	cause of depression
Fasciola	*Pos*	
Her other big fluke is still alive there.		

To kill her Fasciola would require much more wormwood. She should take 10 capsules twice a day for 3 days. Her mother said she had taken only 1 capsule once a day.

She zappicated her tooth, gums, inner cheeks, all soft surfaces in her mouth in a second treatment, to clear plastic ingredients from her mouth.

To kill Clostridium she would take 5 drops oregano oil, in a capsule, 3 times a day for 3 days.

She should also do a liver cleanse this very day. She had already done the hardest part—fasting all afternoon—because she had forgotten to pick up her lunch before coming to the clinic. Now it was 3 o'clock and she could only have one little bit of water (½ cup) before 4 o'clock, the deadline for even water. By the time she was home from the clinic it would be time to take the first Epsom salts. She had never done one. Nor had her mother. But another European patient, speaking another language they knew offered to help. Anita did not agree to all this. This time her mother was in tears, feeling overwhelmed and helpless, even with abundant good will and help around her. They were to use homemade apple juice, not citrus fruit, to avoid the caffeic acid in citrus while doing the liver cleanse.

Three days later they both gushed their way into the office door, demonstrating how large the stones were, "like hail stones", how many there were—first 50, then 100, then again 50. How the stones had covered the whole toilet bowl 3 times over! Anita had appetite now and could eat the food provided. (Thank you, to her friends and helpers).

The mother could hardly stop exclaiming that she didn't believe it possible, to have *these big green things, and so many coming out of her, and what a difference it could make*.

Their helpers explained that actually they had made many mistakes. But she did not accidentally eat. They cooked 5 apples and put them through a strainer to supply the fruit. The olive oil was not a special good kind; it had been grabbed off a shelf. She would need to digest the oleic acid oil promptly now with lipase and pancreatin enzymes. What was the worst part, I asked? The Epsom salts, she said. She had no effect from them, though, till a whole day later! So she thought nothing had worked. But she had drunk it all in the helper's kitchen and lay down at once and was asleep on the couch. We tested for effectiveness of her tooth zappicating she had done 3 days earlier.

Test for tooth plastic in saliva		
urethane	*Neg*	
acrylic acid	*Neg*	
azo dyes	*Neg*	
DAP	*Neg*	
The plastic tooth is not seeping any longer. But these toxins will still be in the brain tumor, no doubt.		

Test at choroid plexus, her remaining cancer location		
Clostridium	*Neg*	
These had been plentiful earlier.		
urethane	*Pos*	
dyes	*Pos*	
These dyes are still from her earlier drinking water since her tooth had been *Negative* for them.		
acrylic acid	*Pos*	
DAP	*Pos*	
Fasciola	*Neg*	

Plastic remnants are still in the tumor, as well as dyes, but Fasciola is finally gone.

She did drink 2 bottles of BWT 2 days in a row.

Test at choroid plexus, continued		
SCF	*Neg*	
No longer making excessive stem cell factor.		
HGH	*Neg*	
No longer making excessive human growth hormone. The live pituitary cells in the growing part of the tumor are gone.		

She had taken 10 wormwood capsules twice a day for 2 days to kill Fasciola in the brain. Now she should take 10 wormwood once a day to kill leftover parasites in brain locations not searched for; also coenzyme Q10, one every 2 hours till dyes are out of the choroid plexus.

But today she had a headache, severe, at left side, which is not normal for her. Her left arm was misbehaving, too, which was usually associated with seizures. It lasted 5-10 minutes. Her mother had taken her off the seizure medicine ahead of time just to "see if it was still so bad". That was days ago. Now she had eaten commercial pizza, with tomato, which has malvin. She also ate cherries, which have malvin. She must remember that she has a second health problem, seizures. She should read the food tables in my 2003 HIV/AIDS book to see which foods have malvin.

She has 1 week left with us. She has gotten rid of her cancer and only needs to keep up her program till the tumor shrinks or stabilizes and is turned into a cyst. She could conquer her seizures in the remaining time.

7/02/03 - Saliva test		
malvin	*Pos*	
She is so full of this food phenolic allergen, it even shows itself systemically in the saliva. This is the natural food-dye that triggers a seizure. It is present in red and blue foods of many kinds and in chicken and eggs. There are also Ascaris larvae in the vicinity, contributing their molting chemicals or bacteria and viruses. Both must be eliminated.		

She was told not to look for loopholes and eat near red, or near blue foods. And to eat no processed foods, which contain a lot of it. She could be grateful to a certain Dr. Robert Gardner who discovered and announced this finding, even though it cost him his job, his career, and his health. She should think about such personal sacrifices made for her. She should read about food phenolics and allergy on the Internet. There is more information in the 2003 HIV/AIDS book.

Test at WBC (immune cells)		
malvin	*Pos*	

This shows her immune system is working now, eating this toxin, malvin, for her. Her white blood cells have recovered from the bad water at home. But malvin should have been detoxified by the liver so it never needed to be removed by the white blood cells.

Test at choroid plexus, tumor location (no longer malignant)		
malvin	*Pos	food phenolic
The food phenolic is exceptionally high here.		
phloridzin	Neg	
chlorogenic acid	Neg	
gallic acid	Neg	
The 3 tumor nucleus-causing antigens are gone.		
urethane	Neg	
acrylic acid	Neg	
DAP	Neg	
dyes	Neg	
The tooth plastic is out of the brain tumor as well as dyes, but 2 dyes may still remain in small quantities in special white blood cells, Fast garnet and Fast green. They are too small a part of the whole set of dyes to test *Positive*, systemically, and will be tested separately*.		

At CD4 cells of choroid plexus		
Fast garnet dye	*Pos	(very high)
At CD8 cells, CD14 cells and RBCs		
Fast garnet dye	Neg	(each cell type tested)
At CD8 cells of choroid plexus		
Fast green dye	*Pos	(very high)
At CD4 cells, CD14 cells, and RBCs		
Fast green dye	Neg	

We will make *"take-out"* bottles for these dye remnants, by homeography, for her to take for 4 days.

Meanwhile her mother had made a decision. She would like to stay one week longer if I thought it possible to conquer her daughter's seizure disorder. I knew it all hinged on Anita's

---

* Testers, place the special lymphocytes, CD4 or CD8, in bottle-copy form, touching the choroid plexus slide. Do the same for other cell types. Test dyes one by one, not as a group.

self-discipline. I talked to her very plainly. I talked about her future, her desire to have a husband perhaps and a family. How embarrassing it would be to have a seizure in bed with him. And further, seizures don't stay nicely controlled by a medicine all your life. When they start as young as hers did, they worsen till the brain is destroyed or gets cancer or Alzheimer's at the young age of 50. Now was her chance to put the disease behind her so she could forget it all and live a normal life. The mother was showing tears but Anita showed no decisiveness. The thought of giving up pizza and her former life, as she knew it, was too much. I consoled her by saying that half a dozen liver cleanses might even cure the allergy permanently. She should do one every 2 weeks. And later, if she had a hint of a seizure to do a liver cleanse right away.

07/03/03 – Next day. The saliva was still full of malvin. The water samples from her father had not yet arrived. The mother was asked to call him to find out if they were sent.

07/04/03 – It is the big holiday in USA, July 4th. Everybody is partying. But Anita arrived on time with her mother. She had not had a seizure pill for 2 days (48 hours) and had had no seizures. Previously, missing even 1 pill brought on a state of seizures. She had been sternly warned by her doctor at home not to miss even one dose, because she was so intractable a case, as she well knew.

Now it was her mother's turn. She had become interested in her own opportunity for health. She requested to get some advice about her headaches, which were chronic and sometimes very severe. I asked Anita to help her mother now, since her mother needed help and nobody else could give it.

07/08/03 - Sylvia's (Anita's mother) headaches - Saliva test		
azo dyes	Neg	
heavy metals	Pos	
She should boil and filter her water to remove aluminum after she resides in a good water zone. And use only safe cookware and dishes.		
PCB	Neg	

07/08/03 - Sylvia's (Anita's mother) headaches - Saliva test		
benzene	*Neg*	
3 salmonella varieties	*Pos*	
These bacteria can contribute to headache.		
She had already detoxified the bad water she had been drinking at home, except for heavy metals.		
tyramine	**Pos*	headache toxin
This causes headache. It is plentiful in milk and bananas. Avoid milk unless ozonated 10 minutes. Add a pinch of nutmeg to all milk to destroy Bacillus cereus bacteria that make the tyramine. Bacillus cereus lives inside Fasciolopsis buski so these should be destroyed. Avoid bananas except the short kind without tyramine.		
Fasciolopsis buski	**Pos*	very high
This is a big risk factor for cancer. She should start to kill them at home after moving to safe water. Take BWT, cloves and wormwood. She could go slow like my first book describes, but she saw the quick results for her daughter when going faster. She could drink a whole bottle of the tincture with cream (but not while here, since she will be taking a long flight home in a few days and needs to avoid detoxification-illness).		
Clostridium	*Neg*	cancer bacteria
She has surprisingly few. Her body has not been killing the flukes.		
SV 40	*Neg*	cancer virus
She has the cancer parasite in large numbers (Fasciolopsis buski), but not the cancer bacteria nor virus.		
diallyl sulfide (onion)	**Pos*	
Her high level of Fasciolopsis is due to eating so much onion besides the immune destruction from her water. She should stop all onions and garlic, asparagus, cilantro, and beans.		

Next, tests were done at the cerebrum, her brain.

Tests at cerebrum (Anita's mother)		
OPT	*Neg*	no cancer
SV 40	*Neg*	no cancer virus
Fasciolopsis buski	*Neg*	no cancer parasite
diallyl sulfide (onion)	*Neg*	no food here for F. buski

Other locations in the brain were not studied, but an assortment of common cancer locations were tested.

Tests at colon		
OPT	*Pos*	
A cancer is just beginning here!		
diallyl sulfide	**Pos*	
The level of onion here is exceptionally high.		
Clostridium	*Neg*	
This is most unusual! Everybody in the USA has a colon full of Clostridium bacteria.		
isopropyl alcohol	*Neg*	
HCG	*Neg*	
tumor nucleus	*Neg*	

Although the colon is beginning a malignancy with so many Fasciolopsises there, a cancer also requires Clostridium, SV 40, and isopropyl alcohol, as well as a tumor nucleus. We have caught it at its earliest stage. A search in the immediate vicinity of Fasciolopsis would have found the isopropyl alcohol, but not in abundance like a typical cancer patient.

Is she not making a tumor nucleus at all, in spite of her daughter making so much? Surely they drink the same water and eat the same food.

Tests at hypothalamus gland		
Chlorogenic acid	*Pos*	starts tumor nucleus
Strongyloides parasites	**Pos*	causes migraine headaches
fibronectin	*Neg*	no glue is made
telomerase inhibitor II	*Neg*	should be *Positive*
Absence of telomerase inhibitor implicates Ascaris nearby.		

Tests at cerebrospinal fluid (CSF)		
tumor nucleus	*Neg*	
FOS, oncovirus	*Neg*	
JUN, oncovirus	*Neg*	
NGF (nerve growth factor)	*Neg*	
SCF (stem cell factor)	*Neg*	

SV 40 cancer virus	Neg	
MYC, oncovirus	Neg	
RAS, oncovirus	Neg	
CEA, cancer marker	Neg	
SRC, oncovirus	Neg	

She has none of these oncoviruses. Her immune system can keep up with devouring these free oncoviruses. But oncoviruses can be sheltered by attachment, or entrance into Flu virus and into many bacteria, making themselves and their sheltering hosts invulnerable. We will search for hidden oncoviruses.

Tests at CSF, continued		
Flu virus	Pos	free virus
These can contribute to headache. The presence of Flu shows that she recently killed a F. buski stage, spontaneously, without a special effort. Recall that she also had Salmonella. But her WBCs keep them low enough to prevent an ill episode.		
Flu/RAS	Neg	RAS-infected flu
Flu/MYC	Neg	MYC-infected flu
Flu/JUN	Neg	JUN-infected flu
Flu/FOS	Neg	FOS-infected flu
Flu/SRC	Pos	SRC-infected flu

SRC oncovirus comes from Strongyloid parasites, which she has so much of. They are triggered by lauric acid oil (lard). The oncovirus is extending the life of her Flu viruses so she has them chronically, contributing to her headaches. She should stop all oils and kill her Strongyloides regularly with levamisole.

Tests at CSF, continued		
copper	*Pos	excites brain
cobalt	Neg	
chromium	Neg	
nickel	*Pos	feeds pathogens
manganese	Neg	

Tests at CSF, continued		
aluminum	*Neg*	
thallium	*Neg*	
iridium	*Neg*	
iridium dodecacarbonyl	*Neg*	organic variety
vanadium	*Neg*	
mercury	**Pos*	destroys immunity
germanium	*Neg*	
selenium	*Neg*	

Her brain bathing fluid, the CSF, has heavy metals, copper, mercury and nickel. They are all very abundant. Nickel invites fungus, yeast and bacteria. She should stop cooking in ceramic, enamel and glass cookware and stop wearing metal jewelry. Of course, she should not have metal (dentalware) in her mouth. Copper, a brain excitant could magnify her headache pain. Nevertheless, she has fewer heavy metals than a cancer patient.

Tests at CSF, continued		
USA laundry bleach	*Neg*	
European laundry bleach	*Neg*	
After 2 weeks in laundry bleach-free water in our special motel for patients, she no longer has it in her brain or did she never have it?		
NSF-bleach antiseptic	*Pos*	our local variety
She is already carrying the safe local bleach in her brain or perhaps always had it, living at a different residence from the child.		
Fasciolopsis buski	*Neg*	
p53	*Neg*	
She had not accumulated vanadium to induce this mutation.		
Complement C$_3$	*Pos*	
She has normal complement without over consumption by allergies, etc.		
north polarization	**Pos*	
This should have been south because brain organs are normally southerly-polarized by daytime. Nickel is a direct cause of this inversion.		
mumps	*Pos*	

Tests at CSF, continued		
MYC	*Neg*	
This is a surprise. Without MYC to protect it, mumps should have been destroyed; maybe nickel and mercury are high enough to keep it chronic. But why is there no MYC? She has its carrier, F. buski, but maybe doesn't eat chicken and eggs. Anita did have MYC.		
Streptococcus G	*Pos*	pain cause
This bacterium causes pain and feeling of illness.		
E. coli	*Pos*	colon bacteria
E. coli/RAS	*Neg*	
E. coli/FOS	*Neg*	
E. coli/JUN	*Neg*	
E. coli/MYC	*Neg*	
E. coli/SRC	*Pos*	SRC-infected E. coli

Her E. coli bacteria are infected with SRC oncovirus, an advantage to both invaders. But altogether she is not overrun by oncoviruses, nor bacteria, nor parasites. SRC comes from her numerous Strongyloides. linolenic acid-containing oils, the unsaturated varieties trigger SRC. To eradicate it she should stop feeding her Strongyloides and also kill it at the same time with levamisole.

Tests at CSF, continued	
Salmonella enteriditis	*Neg*
Salmonella paratyphi	*Neg*
Salmonella typhimurium	*Neg*
Shigella dysenteriae	*Neg*
Shigella sonnei	*Neg*
Streptococcus pneumoniae	*Neg*
Staphylococcus aureus	*Neg*

A turmeric enema and a dose by mouth at the same time would kill a lot of the SRC oncoviruses. Adding Lugol's to the enema before or after (not mixed) would destroy both it and E. coli together. Taking levamisole 50 mg. 2 before each meal would help to kill Strongyloides. Liver cleanses at 2-week intervals would help clear Strongyloides from her liver as well

426

as leftover onion-chemicals. After 12 liver cleanses she should be losing her headaches, I am estimating.

How close is she to getting cancer like her daughter?

Tests at lymph		
hypothalamus (loose cells)	*Pos*	
This tells us she is shedding cells and must be eating chlorogenic acid. Strongyloides are present as we have seen.		
pituitary (loose cells)	*Pos*	
north polarization	*Pos*	wrong polarization for lymph
south polarization	*Neg*	
E. coli	*Pos*	
E. coli / SRC	*Pos*	
She has systemic E. coli invasion because the bacteria have advantages due to carrying SRC.		
phloridzin	*Pos*	
This is the food phenolic that brings about the loose pituitary cells.		
Clonorchis (human liver flukes)	*Pos*	very high
oats (food)	*Pos*	deposits
Oats is the favorite, perhaps necessary, food of human liver flukes. Stop eating oats. She is not digesting oats to completion which will lead to deposits in her organs.		
mumps	*Neg*	
Flu	*Pos*	
Flu / SRC	*Pos*	
She has systemic Flu invasion, due, no doubt, to their extra longevity from association with SRC.		

Let us check if she is releasing prions. Since prions come from Salmonella we will search for them too!

Test at pituitary gland		
prions	*Pos*	free prions
3 salmonella/prions	*Neg*	
salmonella-prion association is never seen.		

Testing the region right around her salmonellas, she showed prions. But she is not dizzy or disoriented. Her white

427

blood cells are probably keeping up with the prions, but the test for prions captured inside her WBCs was not done. I could still go back to her sample and search for this because it was a homeographic sample, not perishable.

Tests at pituitary, continued		
3 salmonella varieties	Pos	
3 salmonella/SRC	Neg	
The salmonella bacteria are not infected by SRC.		

We can draw some interesting conclusions from studying this mother-daughter pair. Anita may have been infected by Ascaris at birth, through the placenta, in the same way as puppies. She could, of course, have gotten them from her fingers, food, or parent's fingers. It could have taken 18 months to develop levels that could cause seizures. Maybe she was given dyed sugar water, too, so she got malvin at an early age. The water then, as now, could have played a critical immune-lowering role. But the child deteriorated rapidly while the mother did not. The mumps test was accidentally left out, but she had a lot of MYC. Her mother did not.

The eating habits of each, though rather similar for any family, clearly led to cancer in Anita, but only to the extent of duplex formation in the mother, not the tumor nucleus. If she had eaten gallic acid-type foods like her pizza-loving daughter (commercial breads, cheese), she might have had cancer, too. And, of course, a cancer has just begun. There are just enough missing links in the whole chain of events to obscure the infectious nature of the parasitism and the SV 40 virus. The genetic impact is clearly derived from parasites with their oncoviruses. These enter her tumor cells to affect her own genes. The environmental contribution from laundry bleach is obvious. So infection, genes, environment are all at work to decide the outcome, cancer, for Anita, but not yet clinical cancer for her mother.

Anita, continued

In spite of Anita's successes, it would be unfair to the reader not to reveal the truth about Anita's recovery, both her cancer and her seizures. She was in the lowest percentage of compliance. What Anita actually did is this:

- left her home
- drank only unpolluted, yet chlorinated water
- stopped eating the foods she was used to
- took levamisole (50 mg), 1 a day for about 1 week
- sodium selenite (200 mcg), 1 a day
- rose hips powder, ¼ tsp. daily
- Lugol's iodine, 6 drops twice a day
- lipase-pancreatin, 1 with each meal
- thyroid tablet (1 grain), 1 a day
- betaine hydrochloride (350 mg), 2 a day
- magnesium, vitamin B_2 and iron, once a day
- turmeric, 1 with each meal
- HCl drops, 4 on each meal
- zapped 60 minutes without a plate daily for 1 week
- wore kidney and neck magnets for 1 week
- 6 peach seeds, chewed up, daily
- vitamin D_3 (50,000 units per drop), 1 drop daily
- 3 enemas of turmeric/Lugol's, total
- 1 liver cleanse with raw apple juice & citric acid

This rather extreme non-compliance was revealed as a surprise at the end of their stay by her mother, who knew it all accurately. It shows how much easier it is for a young person to throw off parasitism and even a disease as serious as cancer.

And it keeps us humble, both writer and reader. We do not know much yet.

In my opinion, leaving home, changing the diet and drinking clean water were the decisive factors for her. And so it will be again. If she returns to clean water, and stays there, she could shrink the tumor and live seizure free. We hope her parents can provide the clean environment for her. We wish them well.

Breast Cancer...Prevention And Cure

We only need to pull one link out of the chain that leads to breast cancer, to prevent it, and this could be **apiol**. But it is hard to be perfect and hard to <u>know</u> if we are perfect. There would be much more security in pulling out several links.

Apiol is the food phenolic substance that has a tropism for the breast.

There was no case of breast cancer that did not have apiol accumulation in the breast. The breast was always inflamed and produced PGE2 although none of this could be felt or seen.

The chief sources of apiol are oils. The *Food Table* shows that common cooking oils all have apiol although a number of truly pure oils do not. Since plain uncooked soybeans contain it, I believe soybeans are the true source of apiol, having become mixed with other foods and oils for marketing.

Read labels carefully to avoid apiol brought into your diet with soy products. Traces of soy oil in other oils would not be on the label. Guarantees of purity should never be heeded.

A wise policy would be to use only butter and meat drippings, not even lard or margarine. Not even olive oil because of the malonic acid that was unavoidable in its production. The butter should be chosen for its purity, uncontaminated with laundry bleach and dyes.

Breast Lumps

If you already have breast "lumps", avoiding apiol should be a very high priority. Removing the apiol that has already accumulated in the breast is the next highest. There are only two ways to remove it: by detoxifying it or by helping the immune cells to remove it.

To detoxify apiol requires better liver function. Help the liver with liver cleanses every two weeks till all lumps are gone. A huge help for the liver is killing its parasites and removing its heavy metals in ways we have learned in this book. All problems for the liver are current—not past! It is the ongoing assaults that are damaging it.

Move to a clean-water zone. Remove the metal from your mouth. Clean up your products, home, and diet.

The other way to remove apiol from a breast with lumps is by the white blood cells. But first they need their immunity destroyers removed. Finding clean water and clean food does this all by itself if it is early, that is the lumps are very new or small. After this, it is best to help the immune cells with:

1. regular zapping to return their north polarization
2. plate-zapping to be sure the lumps themselves get the electrical treatment
3. chelation treatments to remove the heavy metals, particularly nickel
4. an assortment of digestive enzymes to digest lumps
5. feeding the white blood cells organic germanium, rose hips and selenite while removing their azo dyes (vitamin B_2 and coenzyme Q10)

If apiol is now gone, no new tumors can form in the breast.

But old lumps don't necessarily go away, you can assume Clostridium has already colonized them and you must do a dental clean up, bowel clean up (with betaine hydrochloride) and body clean up. Lumps cannot heal if anything is still living in them. It is easy to kill Clostridium in the lumps with oregano oil and Eucalyptus tea.

If you do succeed in getting rid of benign breast lumps just with the parasite program and stopping all oils in the diet, it is a good sign. Your risk for breast cancer is certainly reduced. But if you did it without checking into your own water pollution and without dental amalgam removal, your security could be temporary. A different kind of cancer, not breast cancer, could surprise you instead. Removing apiol from your diet only protects from breast cancer.

Sometimes your only clue to breast disease developing is a **twinge** of pain or sensation in the breast that is very brief.

It means that something is <u>arriving</u> in the breast. It is always something coming from the top part of the body. It is probably arriving through the lymph nodes of the armpit or from those of the upper chest. It may be metal, dyes, plastic, hair spray or any cosmetic, along with a few staphylococcus and streptococcus bacteria. These have found a route to your breast because the kidneys' WBCs are slowed down with their own wheel bearing grease, with its nickel, that switches them to a south polarization. It also means that your WBCs are not keeping up with the multiplying streptococcus bacteria. This is the time to act.

Clean up your body, clean up your diet, clean up your home, clean up your teeth, move to clean water. The move is most important. Collect water from different parts of town to find the NSF-bleach. Apply hot, wet cloths to your armpits to help the white blood cells there. Improving the circulation improves the cleaning of the area. Do this 3 or 4 times a day. Certainly, avoid shaving or applying any chemical. You may clip with scissors. Then assist sweating with the hot, wet treatments. The armpit needs arterial blood with its oxygen and nutrients. The skin of the armpit and below should be reddened by each hot, wet treatment. The twinges should go away or you missed something very important. Continue your clean ups till <u>no</u> twinges <u>ever</u> are felt.

Being able to prevent breast cancer is now within reach for the first time. But how can you be sure you are preventing it? For greater certainty you should learn to use the Syncrometer® and test for apiol and the tumor nucleus antigens yourself.

Estrogen Status

Women who get breast cancer have much too high estrogen levels. The body accommodates to this by making more receptors for it. After this, more estrogen can get in to stimulate the breast into growth. Women should test their estrogen and progesterone levels once a year. It must be done with awareness of your cycle time. If yours is much too high,

432

you can conclude that the hypothalamus and pituitary glands are disturbed and their duplexes are at large, making extra hormones in your glands. Hurry to stop inflaming the hypothalamus and pituitary (stop eating chlorogenic acid and phloridzin). Retest your hormone levels after a few months.

Still Preventing

Breast cancer is beginning to attack men and for the same reasons as in women. But in men an initial injury is usually remembered. It may have started as simply over exercising. In women the bumps and bruises and other pains are so frequent she does not remember them.

At first the tumor is just a small mass hardly big enough to feel. But if you do feel it, make an appointment with your doctor; then race the appointment to get rid of it first. Enjoy the foolish feeling of having to cancel the appointment. Zap, clean up, change your water zone.

The "inflammation" in the breast that comes before the tumor, is not felt. It is chronic because of apiol accumulation. The Syncrometer® shows there is no cortisone in the breast but too much estrogen instead. The adrenal production of estrogen is a major source of this extra estrogen since it is mostly the carcinogenic form, namely **estrone**. This, in turn, seems to reduce thyroid levels because breast cancer victims are nearly always low in thyroid, have a low body temperature, and slightly high cholesterol. Often this leads to slight overweight, which increases breast size. This increases the fat in the breast, making it able to take on more apiol, to its disadvantage. The habit of wearing a brassiere which holds the breast up instead of allowing it to hang freely, could contribute to poor circulation in the chest where much lymph needs to pass. Wear the expandable "athletic" variety or nothing at all.

Breast Injury

A physical injury happens very often to women. A recurrent breast abscess in nursing women or chest exercise in men requires that the body often <u>heals</u> this location. This means that stem cell factor is sent there often. The body will at first make excellent attempts to heal these. But parasites and bacteria can home in on clotted blood (the bruise) in such places. Lowered immune power gives invaders the advantage. Fasciola is the most plentiful parasite of the breast. Their telltale sign is a small brown spot in the skin. The Syncrometer® finds a Fasciola stage within centimeters of these spots and often quite deep. The stages cannot be killed if mercury or nickel is inside the CD8 lymphocytes, or CD14s, our macrophages. Moreover the C_3 is used up by the apiol there, so these 2 WBC types are not being helped. Yet, the body keeps healing the wound again and again, laying down quite a mat of fibrous tissue to do this. The breast begins to feel hard instead of super-soft, as it should. Fasciola produces special fibers by causing a big increase in fibronectin. Ascaris arrives later to increase laminin and cadherin E. These hold cells firmly in place so a higher density tissue is made. But that is not all. Aluminum arrives to add hardness to the healing zone. Aluminum is well known for this property (it is added to pickles to make them hard and to injections to keep your tissues so hard that the inoculating fluid can't disperse)! Cosmetics are full of aluminum. The aluminum is now flowing into the breast. Make your own aluminum-free cosmetics.

Cyst, Mass, Or Tumor?

If the body now encases all this completely, so no tumor nucleus with its SV 40 can get in, the tumor will have a rounded appearance on the ultrasound or mammogram and be considered a "cyst". If not, the fibers keep on being formed and can extend farther and farther from the original wound till quite a large "fibrocystic" mass is made. This is ragged in shape, not round and dense. It is considered simply benign fibrocystic disease.

The hazard now is further accumulation of toxins at the fibrocystic lump. The Syncrometer® sees a wrong magnetic polarization developing there, becoming southerly as bacteria grow, SCF arrives and iron gets oxidized to Fe_2O_3.

A healthy young woman can easily kill these bacteria by a dental clean up and hot packing the armpit and breast, but the fibrous mass and toxin collection will not leave. Obviously, digestive power and immune power has been lost. These would normally clean up the location.

Dead parasites and decaying blood invite a special class of bacteria, Clostridium, and special classes of fungus, Aspergillus, Penicillium, and Sorghum mold. These leave their copper, chromium, cobalt, and nickel behind them each time a generation dies. They are now in oxidized metallic form. But new fungus can use them while they are toxic to our enzymes. The lump will grow new generations of bacteria and fungus.

Telltale Signs

Generation after generation of the same fungus uses the same copper, cobalt, chromium and nickel finally giving you a brown round spot on the breast. Clostridium bacteria find it an easy trip to make from under tooth fillings and in the colon to the new benign mass in the breast.

In the breast everything repeats itself again and again, from bruising to bleeding to new parasites, and then bacteria and fungus, eventually including yeast (bread yeast).

Yeast Arrives

If you are a heavy bread eater, a lot of live yeast spores arrive with each bleeding event and with our habit of eating slightly decayed (has asparagine) food. RAS oncogene is soon triggered from each yeast bud.

MYC Arrives

If you are a hefty chicken eater, especially ground chicken, which is left slightly raw, MYC oncovirus enters the body again and again. While you are young and making enough HCl in your stomach MYC is immediately killed, but when HCl levels go down, MYC survives and spreads. There is already MYC virus in the F. buski parasite but new ones arrive constantly, too, all still held in check by your immune cells. They seem to wait till mumps virus appears in the parotid (cheek) salivary glands. MYC viruses invade (or join) the mumps virus. But the MYC-infected mumps does not behave like ordinary mumps at all so we have no way of knowing this is happening. Meanwhile MYC has a safe place to live for the rest of our lives. Milk casein (protein) gets into the salivary glands easily and does not get digested there. Milk casein in the salivary glands is the trigger for mumps to come out of an Ascaris stage. If it is the first time, around age 5, the mumps makes you sick, but later on no symptoms develop, or, at least it seems so. The Syncrometer® sees mumps virus everywhere, in seemingly well and chronically ill people, in blood, saliva, lymph, and in every tissue. Always it has its tag-along, the MYC oncovirus. Together they are quite invincible, contributing somehow to each other's longevity. Since milk casein is always arriving and chicken is always being eaten, the viruses find each other, and turn into a "dynamic duo" of mumps and MYC. This can go on for years. Is the mumps not destroyed by the antibodies we have built up? Does the MYC oncovirus ruin the lock-and-key principle that guides the antibody to the virus? Is the "mumps-shot" so many of us got helpful or harmful? This inadvertent human experiment should be carefully assessed.

MYC and RAS, with their mumps and Yeast, live on and on, without doing obvious harm. Then a change takes place.

Middle Age

In middle age, digestion gets worse; we burp and hiccup, overeat, and eat non-food. Wheel bearing grease and motor oil has accumulated in our vital organs due to slow-down in the kidneys' excretion. They coat the nerve endings, so acetyl choline and epinephrine are not transmitted (not seen by Syncrometer®). Our digestive organs depend on neurotransmitters and are not being stimulated enough. Nor are other organs. We gain weight instead of making energy. The Syncrometer® sees that exercise, deep massage, chiropractic adjustments, and chelation programs mobilize better degreasing through the kidneys. Better spontaneous detoxification can happen. But it is not enough to keep up with the non biological oils and greases being drunk and eaten each day. Digestion deteriorates and bits of undigested food land everywhere. Parasitism booms. Tumor nuclei swarm. SV 40 virus is triggered by undetoxified gallic acid and soon the barrage of SV 40 and tumor nuclei manage to fuse to inflamed breast lumps. The race begins between them and you for ownership of your body—longevity.

Still Preventing

At an early stage you could still kill it all and stop it all. You know the links. You know what to kill and remove.

Otherwise, the breast is being set up for an inferno of growth without an iota of apoptosis, digestion, or immune system action.

What is unique about breast tumors is that Staphylococcus bacteria always join in. They arrive from infected teeth. Staphylococcus can be seen swimming everywhere, in blood, in lymph, in saliva. But Staphylococcus is not a pain bacterium. The whole mass is not yet painful so they are not yet discovered.

Beyond Prevention

Staphylococcus enlarges the breast lump rather quickly so you now become aware of it. It brings epidermal growth factor to help it colonize your skin and lump. There is pressure and a bulge. But a visit to the doctor results in yet another bleeding event—by biopsy, this time a substantial bleed. Spores and eggs and parasite stages spill out. Bacteria and oncovirus spill out along the trail left by the needle and spread throughout the body, riding the vascular system. A biopsy serves a technical

437

purpose, and has its value, but the disadvantages seem much greater.

If surgery, radiation, or chemo is used, massive destruction leaves new bleeding, new trauma, new immune cell damage and fresh stem cell factor everywhere. You get temporary relief from the pain and pressure in the breast, but the whole process must, and does, repeat itself. Thankfully it will give you enough time to do the clean ups, diet and water change, and bring your immune system back to work to ward off a recurrence. But only if you jump to the task. If you believe the "surgeon got it all" or the chemo and radiation killed every cancer cell, you are probably quite right. They do an excellent job. But that is not what was needed to prevent recurrence, even though it saved your life.

Cancer Comes Back

The advanced breast cancer shows the bulge, shows the redness, the heat, the swelling and sensitivity that tells you cancer is back. But this time it has a different appearance. There are new actors.

The infected teeth have advanced too. They now have Streptococcus besides Staphylococcus, and Streptococcus brings pain.

When the breast bulge is painful you have reached this stage.

Staphylococcus and Streptococcus are especially "friendly" toward Yeast. In breast cancer these 3 become prominent together. Staphylococcus brings swelling and redness; streptococcus brings pain, yeast brings a waxy looking, rough skin surface. Each brings its growth factors, like CA 125, Epidermal Growth Factor, CAA-B, and CEA.

The breast has become an inferno of activity. Fasciolopsis is flourishing because its favorite food, ONION, is everywhere. Orthophosphotyrosine is being produced massively, turning the breast into a wildfire of growth. Breast cells are inflamed with bacteria, viruses, apiol and PGE2, and totally helpless.

The internal lump bulges out to enormous sizes, though the skin may still be containing it all. The body is desperately trying to contain it in a tumor wall. The entire breast is south polarized reflecting the growth going on inside. Drinking southerly water and eating southerly food is like pouring more gasoline on the fire.

Pain Rises

As pain increases, you reach a point where life is not worth living. Only morphine, pumped in repeatedly, brings partial relief.

If you are in a hospital, all the food and water may bring more benzene, the very morphine patch or pill brings benzene, and the port or delivery tubing brings even more, together with its seeping dyes and plasticizer. All have laundry bleach disinfection perpetuating the disease and pain. The surgeon's knife and anesthesia bring blessed, blessed relief once more.

But only Hospice (at home) can still save your life.

Preventing Disaster

As you convalesce, find a caregiver who can give you the new lifestyle you need. Study pain, page 358. Notice there is just one requirement...staying away from benzene. Find a helper who is precise with compliance so you can be confident of success. If possible, get the help of a Syncrometer® tester, he or she does not need to be on site. Give yourself and caregiver 5 days to reduce painkiller in half. Then another 5 days to reduce painkiller in half again. Then you are ready to do the *3-Week Program*, because you can still succeed. This time it will be a cure.

CHAPTER 17

CURING CANCER IN PETS

Our pets suffer in silence when disease strikes. It is heartbreaking to keep your pet company in the last weary days and hours when nothing more can be done, but wait. Instinctively, we humans know it is our fault. We did not provide. But what? What did we not provide? If only we knew. We all agree our animal friends deserve wellness. They deserve as much of their wild heritage as possible—and health and long life in trade for their loyalty.

Animal cancer has been increasing along with human cancer. Are the same forces at work? If so, we could apply our new knowledge and begin to prevent their cancers, too.

Searching for similarities and differences from the human species was my first project. It seems promising. Animal saliva can be used the same way as human saliva to give us a window into their well being. It can be copied electronically, made into a homeopathic or homeographic form and studied with a Syncrometer®.

Cats, **dogs** and **horses** have remarkably similar blood to ours (see page 316). Notice how complete their testing is. Clues to their condition can be read in it as easily as in ours. They too, have been struck by the 5 immunity-destroying toxins in the recent past. They now get new diseases as a result of this, like we do. But there is a difference between them and us. They recover much faster! If you are gazing with long glances at your terminally ill pet, given up by your compassionate vet, and would like to give it one more try, here is how you would do it.

As soon as you have decided, JUMP into action. Rush to the grocery store for bottled water that has been distilled but nothing more! No extra filtration or treatment of any kind should be listed on the label. Purchase NSF quality if available. It should have no chlorination as if for aquarium fish. Use a chlorine test kit for this. Also purchase a conductivity indicator to test for heavy metals (see *Sources*). There should be none. Get several brands of distilled water so you can be sure to find one that is good. The bottle should be the 1-gallon size made of polyethylene which is opaque like milk bottles. Different size bottles of an identical brand can be produced by different bottlers and get different disinfection. Next, order several packages of activated charcoal and a pitcher filter. Almost all the activated charcoal in the market has laundry bleach contamination. If yours does not you only need to boil it for 5 minutes in a quart of the distilled water to get the ruthenium, rubidium, and rhodium out of the charcoal itself. Pour off the water. Do not rinse. Just replace it after heat treating the pitcher and plastic filter holder (see page 587). This can now remove leftover metals in the distilled water. Next, order the two ingredients for Lugol's solution (see *Sources*). Do not buy ready-made Lugol's solution. Do not believe the pharmacist who promises to make it from scratch. You must see the dry ingredients yourself from which it will be made. All ready-made solutions have significant amounts of methanol and isopropyl alcohol, now, as 10 years ago. Buy inexpensive diet scales, plastic cups and spoons to do it yourself. Use the recipe on page 554.

As you rush about, give your pet meaningful glances and a few words telling it to hang in there; something marvelous is going to happen. Communicate with a very light touch, not to be oppressive. Promise it that if he or she gets well you'll do something for its **cat cousins** or **dog family**. Its eyes may be closed, but this promise will keep you both strong. You will be the natural doctor and **cat** or **dog** will be a good patient. It is a subtle bargain they both understand after the vet has offered it eternal sleep.

We will treat a **cat** first, then a **dog**. Although numerous people have sent faxes about how they successfully treated their horses for cancers, I do not have enough cases to write a general recipe. But **cats** and **dogs** have provided more. They respond remarkably well to natural doctoring. Follow **cat-Tinkerbell's** case on page 453 to learn the details.

Cat Cancer

There will be 3 parts to curing cat cancer. How much you do depends on how advanced she is. Stop treating when she recovers.

Part I of curing **cat's** cancer is with diet and supplements.

Buy a steak platter of stainless steel to feed **cat** on; test the platter for seepage with the conductivity indicator. There must be none. Or you may cut a temporary dish from a water bottle (see page 241). Throw away old dishes or anything washed with your sink water. They have PCBs, benzene and motor oil smeared over them. Your kitchen faucet is bringing laundry bleach to your pet's water[*] and dishes. Purchased pet food already has this bleach 9 times out of 10.

> The principle is this: Feed NOTHING that is toxic—not in water nor in solid food. It is a huge challenge.

Buy polyethylene dropper bottles and pipettes without rubber bulbs, see *Sources*. To clean the pipette, cut an X in the round end, using scissors. Squeeze the end while pouring distilled water through it. To feed, put your thumb on it. Use stainless steel or HDPE♳ pans, bowls, water dish and cutlery.

Wipe her dishes with an uncolored, unfragranced paper towel after rinsing in distilled water (not your tap water) or discard.

---

[*] Yes, for every fax about a **dog** or **cat** with cancer I received, I requested a sample of the tap water. It always had laundry bleach in it.

First of all, provide clean water. This means chlorine-free, heavy metal-free, asbestos-free, solvent-free, dye-free, motor oil-free. Such water does not exist. Your own tap water <u>has</u> all of these and **cat** must have none. Immediately call some friends who live in a rainy area and ask for two quarts of rainwater collected in plastic zippered bags, or stainless steel, or HDPE♲ containers (see page 114). Have it shipped in the original plastic bags placed inside other

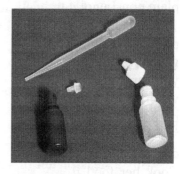

Fig. 104 Polyethylene (PE) dropper bottles and pipette

containers for leak proof shipping. But it should not be collected until it has been raining about ½ hour to be sure any chemicals have already rained down. When it arrives test for strontium, beryllium, vanadium and chromium.

While you are waiting for rainwater, pour her distilled, home-filtered water into a stainless steel or HDPE♲ bowl. Replace it every day. Such water absorbs the air quickly and tastes pungent with air pollutants and carbon dioxide from your kitchen. Pour hers fresh several times a day. As soon as the rainwater arrives, and if it is free of toxic metals, replace the bottled water or give both. Only now have you provided clean water. Rainwater provides the iridium healing factor. You should not filter this out; but if air pollutants exist, you must filter it through your filter pitcher.

If she does not lap any of it give her a dropper-full every hour using the PE pipette and slipping the pipette through the sides of her jaws. The water should be room temperature, not refrigerated, although your supply of rainwater should be refrigerated. Do not give her any rainwater shipped in glass, plastic, or other containers. If you are feeding by pipette, put one drop of Lugol's iodine into ½ cup of **cat's** water. Keep this in a separate plastic bag. Do not let **cat** smell the Lugol's water or she will suspect you of tampering. Give one dropper-full of the Lugol's water 4 times a day. Use a different dropper for the plain non-Lugol's water.

As soon as you have given her rainwater, you will have provided healing water, as she should have. In 2 days the new water will have exchanged with her own toxic body water. If you can't get any Lugol's water down her, give only the pure water. We will sneak the Lugol's into her food later. The purpose is to kill salmonella bacteria in her body.

Feed nothing canned, packaged or frozen. It was all disinfected with chlorine bleach, likely of the laundry variety. Cook her food from scratch. Buy a whole turkey, free-range, organic; lamb free-range, organic; or free-range, organic beef, or buffalo. Cook all the meat till it falls off the bones. Cook regularly in a stainless steel pan, using her pure water and no salt. After cooling, divide up the meat into single portions. Package each in double zippered bags for freezing, then in a larger sealed bag to keep out freezer odor. Throw nothing away, including the fat. Before serving cut the meat into very small pieces that she can lick and swallow without chewing.

All other meat will need to be detoxified of its laundry bleach. Purchase an ozonator and zappicator. You can build your own zappicator.

Arrange to ozonate on the counter top in a plastic shopping bag, see page 518. Open but do not unwrap any food. Hang the ozonator hose into the bag, not into any food. Close the bag with a twist tie, including the hose, to keep the ozone inside. When it is turned on you should see the bag puff out slightly, showing that a slight pressure has developed. All the better to penetrate butter, meat, and tall containers of cream. Turn off ozonator after 7 minutes. Close all containers and set on zappicator to give the food a north polarization for 10 minutes.

Meats and butter need a final soak in cold water right after ozonating. Use separate HDPE♲ bowls. Each will float. Heavy metals from the laundry bleach spray will dissolve in the water and soak out in 5 minutes after they have been oxidized by the ozonator. Flip the foods over and soak another 5 minutes. Shake dry and package in triple zipped bags for the freezer. They will keep a fresh taste much longer now! Leftover ozone can be blown away while reheating later.

Reheat frozen food in hot water, not the microwave. A higher temperature oxidizes the minerals she needs. Fill a larger size stainless steel pan, that can float an HDPE♴ bowl, up to 1" with distilled water. Do not contaminate her dishes with your tap water. If you do, discard them. Place frozen food in the bowl. Heat at moderate setting, covered.

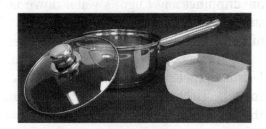

Place food in HDPE♴ bowl cut from bottom of 1-gallon water jug. Pour hot water in saucepan to 1 inch depth. Set bowl in saucepan. Cut bowl short enough so pan-lid can be used to cover.

Fig. 105 Hot water warmer

This is almost as fast as the microwave.

Cook where **cat** can smell your cooking.

Feed nothing else, not even a crumb of previous food. Keep it all out of sight. You, as the doctor, must stand your ground. Choose IV feedings if you think she is starving but otherwise feed by dropper and wait. Pour any broth and drippings into a plastic bag for storage and feed by dropper. If **cat** does not start to eat, switch to bone marrow. Serve a portion, the size of a marble, of lamb bone marrow that you dig out of one of the bones (see recipe page 545). Walk away to let her try to eat alone for 15 minutes. If nothing is eaten, prepare the mixtures below to feed by dropper. Prepare each one in a large stainless steel spoon that does not seep. Wipe clean later.

Feed only this special turkey and lamb for 2 days. Do not substitute other meats. (Remember these were selected to avoid linolenic and lauric acid which nurture Strongyloides and trigger CMV and other viruses. These are particularly common in cats.) If **cat** is willing to eat more of it, continue day after day. Other meat has all been sprayed with bleach and dipped in red dyes called "Beef Blood". Foods that have been ozonated will need to outgas before serving. Thaw and warm them briefly. Supplements will be fed by dropper, stirred into broth or drippings. Feed dropper after dropper-full as follows, stopping when she stops and trying again in an hour. Feed all of these once a day.

1. Minced bone marrow plus an equal amount of broth. Add 1 drop Lugol's, straight, and mix well with hardened plastic spoon[*]. To mince use a stainless steel knife on top of a HDPE⬦ cutting board. Do not use a blender—the blades give off chromium and nickel.

2. Plain broth plus ½ capsule lipase-pancreatin enzymes, unflavored, and ½ capsule vitamin B_2.

3. Finely minced meat plus broth plus 1 drop HCl (5%). HCl will ruin stainless steel.

4. Minced giblets plus lamb meat mixed with broth plus ½ capsule lipase-pancreatin digestive enzyme, ½ capsule turmeric and ½ capsule coenzyme Q10.

5. Minced turkey plus lamb meat plus ¼ capsule vitamin C and ½ capsule hydrangea powder (or a Ge-132, 100 mg capsule) and ½ capsule sodium selenite. Add broth to correct consistency for dropper. This is sour. Omit vitamin C if she gags. Switch to ground rosehips instead.

6. Minced giblets plus bone marrow plus ½ capsule mixed digestive enzymes plus ¼ tablet Decaris (about 10 mg levamisole) plus ½ capsule turmeric.

7. Minced turkey plus bone marrow plus ½ capsule coenzyme Q10 and 1 drop HCl. If she is coughing, give ½ capsule taurine.

---

[*] To harden small plastic items bring distilled water to near-boiling. Dump all plastic items into it, cover, turn off heat. Let stand ½ hour. Repeat for flexible and colored plastic ware.

Notice that amounts are not given precisely; you must use your judgment.

If nothing is eaten willingly, purchase a growing catnip plant or the dried herb. Add tiny amounts to each preparation.

8.   Pour a freshly opened 2 oz. bottle of green Black Walnut hull tincture into several polyethylene dropper bottles. Keep in freezer. Add 1 drop of tincture to ½ tsp. cold unozonated heavy whipping cream. Draw it up into the polyethylene dropper and stick the wet dropper into the catnip to coat it before feeding.

9.   Put a pinch ($^1/_{16}$ tsp.) of wormwood in another ½ tsp. cold whipping cream. Draw it up and coat with catnip to feed.

10. Put a pinch of freshly ground cloves (grind them yourself in a coffee grinder for 3 seconds only and store in freezer) in another ½ tsp. cold whipping cream. Add a pinch of mint leaves or catnip. Draw it up in a single dropper-full and feed.

Do not give larger amounts of #8, #9, #10, even if she is willing to eat more.

Get all these feedings into her in a single day. If she vomits she will feel much better and might eat more for you right afterwards. Feed right away again, to take advantage of this "settled" period. Choose #8, #9, and #10 preferentially. Do not force feed without a vets' help. She could easily choke. Let her swallow little bits.

Watch for detox-symptoms. If she develops a fever it is Salmonella: give ½ drop Lugol's, 6 times daily (put 1 drop in a spoonful of water or cream and draw up half of it). If she develops sneezing and aching, give ¼ tube Oscillococcinum. If she staggers and stares, it is prions; give her Reischi mushroom, a pinch in each dropper full of food.

Feed water with Lugol's between the food feedings if she will take it; plain water if not.

On the second or third day, if she has not moved her bowels, ask a vet to teach you how to give a **cat** or **dog** an enema. Use the correct equipment or ask your vet to help.

Empty the bowel first with 1 or 2 pre enemas of Lugol's water (2 drops Lugol's in ¼ cup of very warm water), adjusting the volume to whatever will stimulate a bowel movement. Insert the rubber hose (plastic is too stiff), lubricated with butter, filled with the Lugol's enema solution but closed off at the valve. Do not fill **cat** with air accidentally.

After she expels this, repeat right away, this time filled with the real enema solution.

First let in ½ capsule coenzyme Q10 dissolved in 2 tbsp. very warm water. Run it in slowly not to cause the bowel to move again. Next, run in 2 capsules turmeric stirred into 2 tbsp. very warm water. Run it in slowly not to cause the bowel to expel it. If it is expelled, repeat immediately with less water, warmer temperature and slower input. Use well buttered soft rubber tubing to be sure no pushing is felt. At the end of the turmeric dose, add 2 drops straight Lugol's solution to the tube to enter last. Be patient, to avoid any expulsion. Encourage pet to doze off if possible. Cover pet with blanket.

The total volume of enema liquid should be small enough to be totally absorbed. The back-to-back technique for the ingredients of this super enema provides the various substances needed in two forms: separate and mixed. Each form acts on a different virus, so that 2 forms become 3 different treatments. We must kill free bacteria, free viruses, viruses inside bacteria, viruses inside tumor cells (oncoviruses), free parasites, parasite stages in the white blood cells, viruses and bacteria alive inside white blood cells and more, each quite difficult to kill. And all this with a huge handicap: **cat's** white blood cells are full of motor oil, wheel bearing grease, heavy metals, and synthetic dyes, just like ours, which paralyze them. Her immunodepression has allowed parasites to increase; these bring their oncoviruses; the oncoviruses infect her intestinal bacteria, which extends their lives and gives them roaming rights. It then allows these super-bacteria to infect **cat's** body cells and white blood cells, handing on their oncoviruses to each. Cells with so many virus-induced alterations are useless for metabolism which requires numerous enzymes to be made in very specific ways. But cell division is made easier, which is

449

exactly the purpose of viruses (to trigger cell division so they will be reproduced). To kill free and sheltered viruses of different kinds inside a variety of bacteria and tumor cells simultaneously, a dozen clinical treatments would be needed. The herbal enema does it in several treatments and is mild, without side-effects.

If she does not seem much better the day after the enema, give another one, this time adding 2 capsules of fennel at the end, followed by Lugol's.

Do not try to kill parasites with drugs at the same time as herbs. The systemic effect of killing massive amounts of parasites in the tissues would leave too great a toxicity behind. The herbal enema way acts mostly on the intestinal tract, which has an exit. Tissues do not. The return of immune power and the starvation of parasites will be relied on to kill parasites in the tissues, because this causes much less toxicity.

Part II of curing **cat's** cancer is homeographic. This part may not be necessary if cat is already getting better. But if she is not getting better or has not begun to eat, it is very necessary. Use polyethylene dropper bottles (with built-in dropper cap, not rubber), your rainwater or distilled-filtered water and a *Positive* offset zapper. We will make *organ drops* and *take-out* drops. You can construct the device easily, or purchase it (see *Sources*).

If we can remove dyes, heavy metals and wheel bearing grease from **cat's** kidneys, kidney WBCs, lymph, and organ with the tumor, she can do the rest. We will not need to remove the asbestos, PCBs and benzene, as is necessary for humans.

Make all your "bottles" in the convenient form of ½ oz. polyethylene dropper bottles (see *Sources*) so no pouring needs to be done. Caps can not be switched, no water added; in fact, nothing can be done to a bottle of drops, once made, without ruining them. But the bottles can be rinsed and reused. They are colored brown to prevent light penetration. Light changes the polarization. Do not refrigerate them, nor set them within inches of a magnet or other electronic equipment. Make these first (see page 105):

1. Right kidney

You may use an actual kidney sample from the supermarket if a slide is not available. Purchase an inductor and capacitor set to make right and left sidedness.

2. Left kidney
3. Right kidney WBCs
4. Left kidney WBCs

Next, make *take-out* bottles:

5. *Take-out* dyes from Right kidney
6. *Take-out* dyes from Right kidney WBCs
7. *Take-out* dyes from Left kidney
8. *Take-out* dyes from Left kidney WBCs
9. *Take-out* wheel bearing grease from Right kidney
10. *Take-out* wheel bearing grease from Right kidney WBCs
11. *Take-out* wheel bearing grease from Left kidney
12. *Take-out* wheel bearing grease from Left kidney WBCs

Give **cat** 3 drops as soon as each bottle is made, not 6, as for humans. Leave 1 minute or more between different drops. They can cancel each other out if mixed in the mouth. They should not be given in the back of the mouth, but rather in front. Merely bare the teeth and let drops fall on top of them or on gums or inside lip. Do not touch her mouth with the dropper. If this happens, rinse the dropper and use a new dry one, otherwise it will destroy the whole bottle.

Give drops 6 times a day for 2 days, then once a day for 1 week or until she is too well to cooperate.

Often *taking-out* wheel bearing grease takes out dyes, heavy metals, and motor oil with it. You could tell by checking urine. If any of these is still present in the saliva after 4 days, she is still eating them! Search water, food, supplements and medicine.

Pets are surprisingly responsive to even a little bit of help for their health. Just a few days of removing oxidized elements (metals) and greasy insulators that block innervation may be all that is needed to bring back life and energy. The reduced elements that are essential as minerals for life will be arriving in food.

Part III of curing **cat's** cancer is electrical, called zapping.

Zapping is another way to empower your pet to shed its parasites, conquer bacteria, remove viruses and somehow, almost miraculously, to become well again. It only seems miraculous to us when the mechanism is not understood. But **cat** cannot wait. Her life is dear and should not be sacrificed in the name of science or what it is not.

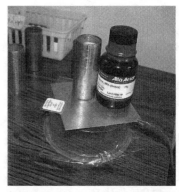

Taking a specific substance out of a specific organ (on the slide) can save a life. Blank is at center in metal shield.

Fig. 106 Making take-out drops

Animals should not become victims of a backward, albeit sophisticated, medical science or attitude. **Cat** is counting on your common sense.

A small pulse of *Positive* voltage applied to the skin repeatedly empowers the white blood cells to overcome their obstacles and devour whatever enemy is nearby. But to accomplish this the white blood cells must have been nourished with organic germanium, selenite and vitamin C (rose hips) to do their job. **These 3 WBC-foods are the highest priority treatments.**

Zapping a pet is easy when they enjoy it. **Cats** and **dogs** seem to feel playful right after zapping, or at least energized. Collars and holders for zappers have been designed, but holding your pet's paws on the damp electrodes is the simplest way. You can avoid draining any of the current into yourself by wearing plastic gloves or holding the copper tubes with a

452

plastic sheet cut from a grocery bag. A few minutes of zapping, done repeatedly, throughout the day has an additive effect. Soon your pet may be strong enough to vomit and move the bowels, showing her innervation is coming back. She may go for a little walk, search for a different bedding place, jump on the couch, or wish to see what is going on. You are gaining ground. Now **cat** will want different food. She will rebel against any medicines and resist all treatments. It is a mark of recovery. You will need to be more ingenious.

Cat cannot be set free yet; recovery is not yet certain. Taking parasite-killing herbs, doing virus-killing enemas, taking dyes and automotive grease out of kidneys and their WBCs, besides zapping…while drinking clean water and eating food that can be completely digested is a powerful approach. **Cats** and **dogs** rally easily. But going back to her former food and water would be disastrous. She is handicapped, probably for her lifetime. For slow, long-term improvement, ask your vet about giving DMSO, by mouth, 1 drop daily. I find it superb and without toxicity when given in a dropper full of cool water, on an empty stomach. It will dissolve and mobilize her automotive greases so she can excrete them, slowly and steadily. But it is not essential for getting well. And you must give kidney drops, once a day, too, with this long-term DMSO treatment. If you are her human-parent and her natural doctor, you must set the rules for her freedoms and health routine.

Let us see how **cat-Tinkerbell** got through his cancer adventure.

Cat-Tinkerbell

This is the water that **Tinkerbell** had been drinking. It was a 6-day sample taken from the kitchen faucet and tested by Syncrometer®.

Tinkerbell's water test			
PCB's	*Pos*	motor oil	*Pos*
benzene	*Pos*	laundry bleach	*Pos*

Tinkerbell's water test			
asbestos	*Pos*	NSF-bleach	*Neg*
heavy metals	*Pos*	azo dyes	*Pos*

Actually, only one test was necessary, taken from one sample. Identifying which bleach is used, automatically decides whether the other pollutants will be present. But in his case, no short cuts were taken.

Notice that drinking people's so called "safe" water has brought the 5 immunity-destroying toxins to him, just like for people.

Major toxins in Tinkerbell's saliva			
PCBs	*Pos*	heavy metals	*Pos*
benzene	*Pos*	motor oil	*Pos*
asbestos	*Pos*	laundry bleach	*Pos*
azo dyes	*Pos*	NSF-bleach	*Neg*
water softener salts	*Pos*		

Notice that **Tinkerbell's** saliva, representing his own body's water, is full of the same things as his drinking water. And somewhere a water softener had been installed, though not tested in the water sample.

Heavy metals in Tinkerbell's saliva			
copper	*Pos*	cobalt	*Pos*
chromium	*Pos*	vanadium	*Pos*
germanium	*Pos*	selenium	*Pos*
nickel	*Pos*	manganese	*Neg*
mercury	*Neg*	thulium	*Neg*

Tinkerbell is not full of the dental metal mercury, nor thulium, a lanthanide; he has no tooth fillings; nor was he drinking RO water (bringing thulium); this will speed his recovery. But each of the 7 natural metals are present, showing he is extremely over oxidized and toxic. His enzymes will already be out of commission in a far reaching way.

Metals in saliva, continued			
Fe_2O_3, ferrite	Pos	Fe_3O_4, magnetite	Neg
Fe3 +	Pos	Fe2 +	Pos
iridium	Pos	iridium dodecacarbonyl	Neg
south	Pos	north	Neg

A critically important metal, iron, is mostly in plain ferrite (Fe_2O_3) form instead of magnetite form (Fe_3O_4). This changed his magnetic polarization to south instead of north. His body's normal solution to this over-oxidation problem is iridium dodecacarbonyl, but it is exhausted, having only oxidized iridium instead of the reduced carbonyl form. Fortunately, he still has some reduced iron in the form of ions, Fe 2 +. This means he could still recover, with the correct magnetic or chemical treatment.

Cancer tests in saliva			
OPT	*Pos	DNA (excess)	Pos
Fasciolopsis buski	Pos	tumor nucleus	*Pos
Clostridium bacteria	*Pos	SV 40 virus	*Pos

The malignancy-causing parasite, the malignancy-causing bacteria and cancer virus are all present.

Free-floating tissue cells in saliva			
hypothalamus	Pos	pituitary cells	Pos
pancreas	Pos	cerebellum	Neg
pineal cells	Neg	bone cells	Neg
kidney cells	Neg	lung cells	Neg
cerebrum	Neg	pons cells	Neg

The same three organs are setting their cells free to float away in the body fluids of Tinkerbell, as for people with cancer.

Duplex and triplet test in saliva	
duplexes of hypothalamus and pituitary	Pos
triplets of hypothalamus, pituitary and pancreas with pancreas attached to pituitary	Pos

triplets of hypothalamus, pituitary and pancreas, with pancreas attached to hypothalamus	Neg

We see the same "law" is at work to make the **cat** tumor nucleus, the same as in people; the fusion of the pancreas cells is to the pituitary cells.

Complement C$_3$ test in saliva (a slash means touching)			
hypothalamus / C$_3$[*1]	Neg	duplex / C$_3$	Neg
tumor nucleus / C$_3$	Neg	C$_3$, free	Neg

There is no C$_3$, either free or in combination with its usual targets. There may still be some attached to food phenolic allergens or bacteria or parasites that were not tested, but not at these critical items, free cells.

Stem cell factor tests in saliva	
in hypothalamus[*2], organ of the brain, SCF is	Pos
in hypothalamus cells[*3], floating about, SCF is	Pos
in pituitary cells, floating about, SCF is	Neg
in pituitary, organ of the brain, SCF is	Neg
in pancreas cells, floating about, SCF is	Neg
in pancreas organ, SCF is	Neg

It appears that stem cell factor is found only in the hypothalamus of the brain, and in the free-floating cells as well, similar to people.

[*1] Testers, place the C3 test bottle so it touches the hypothalamus slide or bottle.

[*2] Place hypothalamus test bottle or slide beside (touching) the saliva bottle. This identifies the hypothalamus <u>organ</u> as **Tinkerbell's**. Place SCF on opposite plate.

[*3] Place hypothalamus test bottle on opposite plate to saliva. These are free-floating. Any organ found in the saliva or lymph would be free-floating. Attach SCF to the hypothalamus. If this union exists, it too would be found in the saliva and resonate there.

Stem cell factor tests, continued	
in tumor nucleus (triplet), SCF is	*Pos*
in duplexes, the hypothalamus end, SCF[4] is	*Pos*
in duplexes, the pituitary end, SCF is	*Neg*
in triplets (tumor nucleus), the hypothalamus end, SCF is	*Pos*
in triplets, the pituitary portion, SCF is	*Neg*
in triplets, the pancreas portion, SCF is	*Neg*

In triplets (tumor nucleus) the hypothalamus end keeps its SCF. It is not present in the pituitary or pancreas portions. It does not "flow" into these portions.

SV 40 virus invasion tests	
in saliva, SV 40 virus[5]	*Pos*
in free hypothalamus cells, SV 40 virus	*Neg*
in free pituitary cells, SV 40 virus	*Neg*
in free pancreas cells, SV 40 virus	*Pos*

It appears the pancreas got infected with the SV 40 virus. The SV 40 virus is both free as well as infecting the free pancreas cells, but not the free pituitary or free hypothalamus cells, at least not yet.

SV 40 virus invasion tests, continued	
in triplets, the hypothalamus is	*Neg* for SV 40
in triplets, the pituitary is	*Neg* for SV 40
in triplets, the pancreas portion is	*Pos* for SV 40

In the virus-invaded tumor nucleus (triplet) the SV 40 stays in the pancreas end and does not enter the hypothalamus or pituitary portions.

---

[4] Attach SCF to the hypothalamus end of the duplex and test, then move it to the pituitary portion and test again. Test the hypothalamus, pituitary, pancreas portions of the triplet the same way. Make the duplex with 2 slides; make the triplet with 3 slides (or bottles).

[5] Place saliva on one plate, SV 40 on other plate; test. Then place hypothalamus on other plate instead of SV 40 and touch it with SV 40; test. Then change hypothalamus to pituitary or pancreas, and repeat tests.

SCF invasion tests[6], continued	
in virus invaded triplets, hypothalamus portion is	*Pos* for SCF
in virus invaded triplets, pituitary portion is	*Neg* for SCF
in virus invaded triplets, pancreas portion is	*Pos* for SCF

Now we see SCF has entered the pancreas portion of the tumor nucleus.

Remember that the uninvaded triplets did not have SCF anywhere except in the hypothalamus cells and organ. After invasion by SV 40 virus, SCF appears in the pancreas part, too.

How did it get there? The clue is, first, in the free SV 40 virus, seen everywhere in the saliva, lymph and blood. It has been spreading throughout the body, easily, this way.

Secondly, there is SCF being made by the hypothalamus organ and its free cells throughout the body.

After invasion of the body by SV 40 virus, these two meet. SCF gets attached to the SV 40 virus so that SCF gets pulled along wherever the virus goes.

As the SV 40 virus enters the free pancreas cells it pulls SCF along with it into the pancreas cell. Now this powerful growing force, SCF, will be in the pancreas end of the tumor nucleus, exactly that end that will fuse to a body organ. When the tumor nucleus fuses itself to a body organ it is the pancreas end that fuses, so the SV 40 virus, along with its captive SCF, can slip into the new organ cells. A passageway was created that let the virus in, pulling its captured growing force with it.

The body organ cells must burst into growth with all the vigor of SCF, and HGH to follow. The polarization is to southerly wherever SCF goes but it is not perfectly clear which comes first. SCF is now in the body organ. One of these (SCF or south polarization) switches on DNA. This switch is not to make new proteins but to double itself and make a new cell. Now bcl-2 is turned on; ribonucleotide reductase is turned on,

---

[6] Place triplet opposite to saliva. Test each portion of the triplet with SCF touching it.

thiourea is turned on (only if Clostridium is present); cell division will happen, no more regular cell productivity. These two procedures are incompatible. Genes being used to double themselves cannot, at the same time, be transcribed (used to make a protein for metabolism).

The same things would be happening if this was just a wound instead of a tumor nucleus fusion event. The trauma of a wound changes the local polarization to south because the iron has been oxidized to Fe_2O_3. This invites SCF to come and heal it. SCF arrives with its south polarization. It means the whole area will become south polarized (possibly because water is diamagnetic). DNA, bcl-2, ribonucleotide reductase genes get busy. Soon cell division gets started to fill in the wound. How can we tell the difference between such simple healing and a tumor nucleus growth? In a wound many cells are given the signal to digest themselves—apoptosis. In a tumor they are not. In fact, apoptosis is blocked. A wound is a very busy place, with apoptosis everywhere[7].

In this way the growing force, usually safely locked up in the hypothalamus cells, escapes from the free-floating cells, only to be caught by passing SV 40 viruses and delivered to the pancreas cells of the tumor nucleus. When the tumor nucleus fuses to an organ, a powerful injection is given to the organ cells, an explosion of growth.

Tests at hypothalamus[8]	
PGE2	*Pos*
chlorogenic acid	*Pos*
Strongyloides	*Pos*
linolenic acid (oil)	*Pos*
potatoes	*Pos*

[7] Testers, search for phosphatidyl serine, the signal that starts apoptosis. A growing tumor does not have it.

[8] Place hypothalamus beside (touching) the saliva sample. Place PGE2 on opposite plate. Test.

Prostaglandin E2 (PGE2) is made by cells when an allergy is present. Regardless of which food allergy it is, or where it is, PGE2 is made. This test tells us the hypothalamus has an allergy. Many things are present; which one is causing the allergy?[*9]

We could expect chlorogenic acid, but is that all? The heterodyning principle can be used to find others. Strongyloides parasites are present, too. They are possibly responsible for it all. But stop for a moment. Strongyloides require potatoes. Has this cat been fed potatoes? Surely not! The substance in potatoes is not identified yet. It could be any substance found in the nightshade family. Cat food should be searched for it next.

From all these tests we can see that tumors start the same way in **Tinkerbell** as in people.

We can starve Strongyloides or kill Strongyloides and zap Strongyloides. For **Tinkerbell** we will do all of these, so no one method needs to be too powerful.

Strongyloides need the essential oil, linolenic acid to trigger their viruses. And they need a common food, potatoes. **Tinkerbell** needs the essential oil herself, too, as people do, but we are not starved in a few days as the parasites are. In **Tinkerbell** there is linolenic acid spilled all about, as it is in

---

[*9] Subtractions and additions are done (by heterodyning) on different plates. If cat's saliva is on the Right plate, with hypothalamus touching it, the chlorogenic acid sample will resonate with it if placed on the Left plate. PGE2 will resonate if it replaces chlorogenic. Now, if chlorogenic is "subtracted" from the saliva by placing it on the Right plate, PGE2 will be gone (not resonate). It implies that chlorogenic acid was a cause of PGE2 production. The subtracted item, chlorogenic, should be placed within an inch from the other bottles on the R plate, to give an "in series" construction, and therefore, subtraction. If it is placed at the most distant corner, we do not necessarily see this subtraction effect. In this case, there is still another cause of PGE2 production. Leave the first cause at the corner and search for new causes the same way. This time place the second cause at the same corner touching the first cause. If again the result is nullified, continue searching for more causes. When all causes found are put in series at the distant corner, the result with PGE2 are finally gone.

people with cancer. **Tinkerbell** ate too much of it because it was built into his "chow", which was made of plant materials, not his native food at all! We will return him to meat only. We will digest the linolenic oil "spills" in his lymph and organs using digestive enzymes. It will be gone in days. He should stay on his native food for which his digestive juices were designed. The first part of his cure should be return to meat, without linolenic acid, namely not with supplemental oil concentrates. Obviously, the meat-animals did not fully digest them either.

Strongyloides can be killed by levamisole, but the dose should be decided by a veterinarian.

Zapping kills very many larval stages of parasites and helps the white blood cells eat them. Soon it is all clear at the hypothalamus; no more PGE2, no more laminin, no more hypothalamus cells are being freed. If only the cancer already started could be undone as easily.

Tests at pituitary gland		
PGE2	Pos	There is an allergic reaction here, too.
laminin	Pos	sticky glue invites fusions
phloridzin	Pos	This is the food antigen causing allergy here.
Clonorchis	Pos	This is the parasite responsible.
oats	Pos	This is Clonorchis' essential food.

Again, a situation like a human cancer patient's is seen for **Tinkerbell** at the pituitary gland. The pituitary is exploding its cells in an allergic reaction to phloridzin. Clonorchis, the human liver fluke, is quite at home in a **cat's** pituitary as long as it has plenty of oats to feed its stages and itself.

We can stop feeding the parasites by not feeding oats to a cat. Then they will be gone in days, to search for oats, no doubt. It seems they are not killed, but simply leave, since there are no detox-illness after-effects. We can digest the remaining grain deposits with digestive enzymes, the same way as for linolenic acid. We can kill the liver fluke itself with the green

Black Walnut hull recipe. And zap it, too. But these have side-effects and must be watched closely for a cat.

Tests at pancreas		
PGE2	Pos	allergic reaction here
laminin	Pos	sticky glue invites fusions
gallic acid	Pos	this allergen, sprayed on grain or put in oils, is in his food
Eurytrema	Pos	pancreatic fluke is present
limonene	Pos	the fluke's essential food

PGE2 is also being made by the pancreas, in the allergic reaction to gallic acid.

But gallic acid has another role. It also is the trigger for SV 40 virus. The SV 40 virus comes with these flukes, but it is not always expressed. It requires a trigger just as our common Herpes I virus requires a trigger to be activated from its latent state. The SV 40 trigger is everywhere for **cat**, as for humans, in our grains and oils—it is gallic acid. Limonene is the essential food factor for Eurytrema. **Tinkerbell** has been eating lemons!

Tests for gallic acid		
in saliva	free gallic acid	Pos
	free complement C_3	Neg
	gallic acid / C_3 (gallic acid touching C_3)	Pos
in lymph[*]	free gallic acid	*Pos
	free complement C_3	Neg
	gallic acid / C_3 (gallic acid touching C_3)	Pos
in blood	free gallic acid	Neg
	free complement C_3	Pos
	gallic acid / C_3	Pos

Tinkerbell is loaded with gallic acid, some of it free to do its harm, some of it attached to C_3, a terrible waste of C_3. The saliva and lymph are already depleted of it. The blood is kept cleaner in **cat** as it is in us, and still has C_3.

---

[*] Testers, place the lymph bottle beside saliva.

Tinkerbell's gallic acid comes from vegetable foods, like ours. Although a few foods contain it naturally, the greatest amount comes from grains sprayed with it and oils to which it is added. **Cats** were never meant to eat vegetable foods. It would be easy, and natural, to return them to their native food, meat. This would pull a link out of the chain that leads to cancer for them, too.

The critical virus, SV 40, arrives with Eurytrema, the pancreatic fluke, in latent form (tucked away between the fluke's genes). **Tinkerbell** is hosting many more pancreatic flukes than a **cat** without cancer because his immunity has been destroyed by laundry bleach. Yet, flukes, like any living thing, can only live and thrive where the right foods are supplied, in this case limonene. This, too, is present in large amounts in his chow, coming from vegetable foods. It will be an easy matter to starve the flukes, stop triggering the virus and stop all the food allergies by going back to a meat diet. Flukes starve in days. Without all these, no more SV 40 viruses can come into the circulation. But those already established are hiding inside bacteria and inside **cat's** cancer cells. Both bacteria and cancer cells have become invincible (immortalized) due to many oncoviruses inside them. They were herded in by SV 40 virus. This is what is making him sick to the point that everybody gives up, as it is for humans. We will kill them all by restoring immunity.

These are **Tinkerbell's** bacteria. But a cat's common viruses were not tested. The bacteria come from his own intestinal tract, mainly salmonellas and E. coli, similar to humans.

Bacteria test in saliva			
mumps virus	Neg	Bacillus cereus	Neg
salmonella paratyphi	Neg	Staphylococcus aureus	Neg
salmonella enteriditis	Neg	Streptococcus pneumoniae	Neg
salmonella typhimurium	Pos	Streptococcus G	Neg
Shigella dysenteriae	Neg	Escherishia coli (E. coli)	Pos

Bacteria test in saliva			
Shigella sonnei	Neg		

He does not have as many (only 2) bacteria invading his body as a human cancer patient. He does not have mumps throughout his body, either. Both are advantages a **cat** has over people with cancer. It will make the task of curing him easier.

Oncovirus test in saliva			
MYC	Neg	Adenovirus	Pos
FOS	Neg	JUN	Neg
RAS	Neg	SRC	Neg
NEU	Neg	SV 40	Pos
CMV	Pos		

We might have expected SRC to be *Positive* since it comes from Strongyloides and **Tinkerbell** has a lot of Strongyloides and plenty of linolenic acid, too. But the oncovirus trigger is lauric acid, a different fat. He did not have SRC; in fact, he is missing the most serious oncoviruses for people, except for SV 40.

"Immortalized" bacteria, invaded by oncovirus	
Salmonella typhimurium / SV 40	Pos
Salmonella typhimurium / CMV	Neg
Salmonella typhimurium / Adenovirus	Neg

Only SV 40 are infecting Salmonella typhimurium directly, that is, without help.

"Immortalized" bacteria, invaded by oncovirus (continued)	
Salmonella typhimurium / SV 40 / CMV	Pos
Salmonella typhimurium / SV 40 / Adenovirus	Pos

But when all 3 viruses are present SV 40 can "sky lift" or transport the other two as well. This is how the oncoviruses become so numerous. They are sheltered inside bacteria and the bacteria will enter **cat's** tumor cells and even the immune cells. Now the tumor cells and even WBCs will appear to have mutations.

"Immortalized" bacteria, invaded by oncovirus (continued)	
E. coli / SV 40	Pos
E. coli / CMV	Neg
E. coli / Adenovirus	Neg
E. coli / SV 40 / CMV	Pos
E. coli / SV 40 / Adenovirus	Pos
E. coli / SV 40 / CMV / Adenovirus	Pos

Cat has a smaller set of oncoviruses and bacteria than human cancer patients. With a few treatments both by mouth and by enema, of turmeric powder and Lugol's iodine solution they should all be gone, even inside tumor cells.

A check of **Tinkerbell's** immune cells (WBCs) will show us their involvement.

White blood cell test* in saliva	
E. coli	Neg
Salmonella typhimurium	Neg
Adenovirus	Neg
SV 40	Neg
CMV	Neg

With so many bacteria and viruses swarming about, why are none seen inside the white blood cells?

White blood cell test, continued	
PCBs	Neg
heavy metals	Neg
benzene	Neg
asbestos	Neg
azo dyes	Pos

---

* Testers, place WBC test sample, real or a copy, beside saliva. Real WBCs can be made (see Syncrometer® Science Laboratory Manual).

Tinkerbell's saliva is full of all these immunity destroyers, arriving with the laundry bleach he was accustomed to drinking. Why are they not in the WBCs?

The WBCs have refused to eat anything except the dyes. And the dyes may have penetrated forcibly, as dyes were intended to do. Only zapping and homeographic drops can take the dyes out quickly enough to save him. He is obviously a very, very sick cat. Supplements such as vitamin B_2 and coenzyme Q10 can remove <u>free</u> dyes and be helpful, but once inside the immune cells the supplements don't have access. Ultimately, all these methods deliver the dyes to the kidney white blood cells.

Here they must be processed by the white blood cell's own enzymes to release them into the urine. Will he be able to do this?

White blood cell test, continued	
organic germanium	Neg
selenite form of selenium	Neg
organic vitamin C (rose hips)	Neg

His immune cells are totally empty of these vital elements just like human cancer victims! He needs these first!…and needs them immediately!…by IV if available! If not, we can use the same supplements as for humans: hydrangea powder, rose hips, selenite, with extra synthetic vitamin C and Ge-132. We must find a way to get them into his body; there is no time to lose.

Which dyes are responsible?

Dye test at saliva	
Fast Red RC salt	Pos
Fast Green	Pos
Sudan Black B	Neg
Fast Blue	Neg
Fast Garnet	Pos
DAB	Neg
Fast Red Violet	Neg

These are some of the same dyes used to color human foods. They also pollute his drinking water, through the laundry bleach and water softener salts being added to it.

Tinkerbell's story is quite like the human story of cancer.

Seeing the complexity of **cats'** cancer we will not expect miracles unless we do the right thing, and in time. We should expect "detoxification-illness", too. It should be constantly tested, or just assumed. Prions are the most dangerous because they block neurotransmission. Added to the insulating effect of wheel bearing grease the loss of innervation to large parts of the body would appear like sleep or coma. This must be recognized to prevent the belief that cat is dying.

Flu viruses appear as a result of killing the largest fluke (Fasciolopsis buski). Prions come from the Salmonella bacteria that are also escaping.

Tinkerbell's saliva shows he was in the middle of a bad detoxification-illness already, before we began any treatment. His body did it in it's own mysterious way. But his immune cells could not eat and destroy the detox pathogens without our help.

The best help is by IV, while feeding his immune cells and taking away all the allergies and other causes of illness. He will recover, as long as he eats and expels. It takes about 4 days to detoxify enough to see recovery begin. Ask your vet about the dose of the homeopathic flu remedy, Oscillococcinum. My suggestion is ¼ tube. Keep cat warm.

Summary:

1. We must quickly snatch away the toxic water and give clean water as nature intended, rain if it is clean.

2. We must free the white blood cells of dyes. This will enable them to kill the virus-infected bacteria and the bacteria and viruses themselves. The viruses are giving the cancer cells their immortality. And we must <u>feed</u> the white blood cells constantly, so they can work constantly.

3. We must feed **cat** only that food which she can digest and even help this temporarily with lipase and pancreatin enzymes. Give digestive enzymes throughout the day. Mix capsules with water; give by dropper. Never again feed vegetable food. Having deposits of undigested food strewn about the body invites those parasites that require it, our "everyday" parasites. Never again feed vegetable oil. Different oils feed an assortment of round worms, including filaria, and act as triggers that activate their latent viruses. There is a small amount of essential oils in animals; that will be enough. More could be gained by improving digestion.

At Tinkerbell's saliva	
Flu	*Pos*
prion protein	*Pos*
salmonella bacteria	*Pos*

4. For a sick cat, we should distinguish between detoxification-illness (Flu, Salmonellas and Prions) and other illness (E. coli and viruses). Feed by IV and by dropper for 4 or 5 days till recovery is on its way.

5. We must stop the over oxidizing effect of laundry bleach water and water softener forever and even the chlorination itself. Never give chlorine again. Stop the over oxidizing effect of heavy metals in commercial cat foods. Cook for **cat**.

6. We must not, accidentally, feed cat more heavy metals from her own dishes. They are of the most serious sort: thallium, mercury, strontium, aluminum, lead. Strontium is required by CMV virus. Aluminum is required by EBV virus. Tinkerbell has CMV, like so many people in USA. Strontium is so pervasive, it is even in the distilled water, making filtering

necessary for him. Test water and dishes with a conductivity indicator.

7. We must help **cat** kill her parasites until her own immune system can take over again. The green Black Walnut hull tincture, cloves and wormwood, plus levamisole, all in very tiny doses works best.

Levamisole kills Strongyloides, Ascaris and filaria worms. Find it at a horse shop where large animal medicines are. Cut large tablets to approximately 100 mg chunks. Then divide further. Grind fine in plastic bag with glass jar. Stir into water and give by dropper. This is to remove ferritin coating on white blood cells due to asbestos. Ask vet to check dose for your **cat**. If not found, use 10 mg, added to enema or by dropper once a day.

You have kept your promise to your pet. You have done all you could. If you succeed could you withhold this from her **cat** cousins? Vets are extraordinarily sensitive persons. Let him or her know. This is also the solution for other feline diseases.

Dog Cancer

Luke

Luke was a big, big dog. Age and arthritis were taking their toll, although he was still moving about and his tail wagged as he begged for "out" at the kitchen door. He had a tumor the size of a fist hanging from his neck. Each day he ate less, drank less, slept more, hurt more. Many trips to the vet did nothing to change that one feared conclusion. Leila thought about it all day long at work. "Should I have him put to sleep before he starts to suffer?" She had raised him from a puppy, 12 years ago. The bond was too strong to let him go.

She had tested her water, by Syncrometer® a year ago, just before Luke came down with this lump at his throat. It was fine—no laundry bleach, no water softener. Now his drool (saliva), though, had PCBs, benzene, asbestos, heavy metals and dyes, the exact recipe for cancer. It must be his dry dog food, Leila thought, and switched him to home cooked ground meat and liver.

She fed him the parasite program without hiding anything; he loved it. He got his Lugol's; that was easy, too. But his lump did not loosen or shrink. Getting IVs seemed too burdensome. Time passed.

Suddenly, he did not want to get up. His eyes half-closed. Leila helped him to his favorite spot under a shady tree and went to work, sending out samples of water, feed and saliva for testing.

The water had NSF-bleach now but she recalled that her water pipes from the city had been worked on most of the previous year. Nobody had thought much about it. Would the workmen have used regular laundry bleach, she asked?

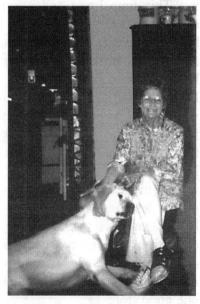

It was not "his time" and not "meant to be". It was abuse of the potable water and water-for-food-contact laws that took Luke from Leila

Fig. 107 Leila and Luke

Most certainly, I answered. No workman would want to deal with the hazard of 12% bleach (twice as strong as the laundry varieties) in difficult circumstances of underground trenches. Generously sloshing about the high quality NSF-bleach would go against the grain of expense-conscious supervisors, too. And anyway, if "bleach was bleach", wouldn't you rather pick up a couple of gallons as you needed it, rather than head for the pool store to get a 4-pack to stand around in the bed of your pickup truck? It loses potency with time. And hazardous chemicals in such large amounts are a constant worry.

This time Luke's saliva was full of laundry bleach and dyes, asbestos, PCBs, benzene and heavy metals. Nothing had been cleaned up in half a year in spite of the home cooking. And in spite of the "good" bleach coming to her kitchen faucet.

Leila now suspected the meat. Every kind of meat he had eaten was full of these same things. It was meant for humans. She saw the "Beef Blood" it was dipped in. Its very name disguised its' real intent, to keep the meat looking red. It tested *Positive* for laundry bleach and all the dyes in my collection. She quickly bought different meats from all the markets for miles around to find one good store. Only turkey giblets and beef bones for soup were free of dyes. She quickly cooked some during her lunch hour, and got the

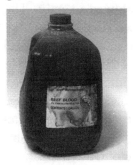

In reality beef blood is a red dye mixture, keeping meat looking deceptively red.

Fig. 108 Beef blood or hoax?

supplements ready. At 5 p.m. she zoomed home, with drops, zapper and all. Her neighbor met her. It was all over. Time had run out[*].

Frankie

Frankie was a big dog, too. He lived in an affluent sector of town, which served him badly. Better to lap water from ponds and ditches in a farm setting than the sparkling faucets that bring laundry bleach. But he was stuck, as we all are. He

---

[*] Special thanks to Leila who wanted to know the real cause of Luke's failure to recover. She found the beef blood, to educate us all, a fitting tribute to true love.

471

was old, and arthritic, just lying around and moving himself from kitchen rug to front porch to "out", and back again. His lump was hanging from the ribs, somewhat floppy, but not loose. It was the size of a fist. The vet, very sincerely, told Susan that all treatments would be a waste. There was nothing…but Susan got to work. His water was changed to a laundermat's from the Hispanic-Black part of town where no water softener was added and the water regulations were followed exactly. The Syncrometer® said it had NSF-bleach. Two drops of Lugol's were added to each bowl of his water. No new bowls or special plates were used.

His expensive Health Food Store chows were changed to Health Food Store ground round—ground before Susan's eyes. It had not been dipped in "Beef Blood" and had only NSF-bleach remnants. After Syncrometer® testing, Susan went back for pounds more. She made round meatballs and put most of them in the freezer.

Immediately she fixed one up for Frankie. It had ¼ tsp. green Black Walnut hull tincture in the middle. He swallowed it whole. Another, small one had 3 drops of straight Lugol's solution in the middle. A third one had ½ capsule wormwood. This was breakfast. He drank nothing and went to sleep. He didn't want to go for a walk with Susan, otherwise his favorite activity. At suppertime he went "out" briefly. When he came in he sniffed the cupboards for his favorite chow. His pleading half-closed eyes brought tears to Susan's eyes. Could she deny him his only pleasure in these last days? She went to the refrigerator and split open a meatball. It got ½ capsule cloves in one spot, 2 drops Lugol's in another, and ½ capsule wormwood in another. He took it standing and flopped down on his rug. Susan's daughter came and zapped him. Then he wanted "out" again. He was barely dragging his hind legs along, but she gave him no arthritis medicine till it could be tested for laundry bleach and water softener pollution. He hid under the porch steps a while then vomited and had diarrhea. Would he ever take another meatball? Susan cleaned him up.

Next morning Susan did exactly the same thing. This day she gave a capsule of vitamin C, too, in a separate meatball. Frankie stood now to take his meatballs in single gulps. He slept all day. He drank his "doctored" water, with 2 drops Lugol's in the bowl, without noticing the smell or taste. That evening he started working at his fur, gnawing and licking his rib region. He started to get up and bark several times at the front doorbell when it chimed, but felt too wobbly, too full of pain to meet the stranger. There was no pain medicine for him. He must lie still.

The third morning Susan and her daughter felt terribly sorry for him. They asked if they could break his mono-diet. They thought each day could be his last. He seemed to have taken a turn for the worse. He staggered as he walked. His eyes teared and he panted as if he was hot. Just "steer the ship; you're the natural doctor; he counts on your wisdom" was my answer. Susan did exactly the same thing. The water was from an east end gas station now. He didn't mind drinking it with Lugol's. He took all his meatballs and slept. But in the evening he wanted to go for a walk. Susan felt his lump, it seemed to be dangling. He wasn't dragging his legs so much.

Days 4 and 5 saw more tiny improvements.

On day 6 he suddenly jumped into the car to go shopping with her. Later, he went for a short walk, without much pain, it seemed. He wasn't missing his chow (a good time to throw it all in the garbage cans). His lump had come free from the ribs and was getting smaller. He was obviously digesting it or having the WBCs remove it.

That final downturn must have been detox-illness!

At that point I was not getting status reports anymore.

One half year later he was back on arthritis pills, but the tumor had disappeared and Susan felt it was divine intervention. She had her companion back and I could fade into the background.

Summary:

Notice that for Frankie nothing heroic was done. No IV's, no homeography or medicines, no enemas. He was strong enough to heal himself with just a little help for his immune system—real help, not a pill or potion, not <u>giving</u> anything, in fact. Only taking away! Taking away his toxic water and food.

Frankie was zapped, once a day, through his front paws and his back paws. Soon after, he would run a bit or try jumping. Was zapping essential? We cannot know.

If your dog has cancer, be sure to get these basics done that were done for Frankie. Clean, native food and water. If you can give more, like **Tinkerbell's** program, do that. If you are failing, make your promise to dogdom and turn yourself into a natural doctor. Leave nothing undone. Use "dog doses", twice as much of everything on **Tinkerbell's** program.

If you don't succeed, you did your best. That is your reward.

If you did succeed and your dog had been marked by the vet for his eternal sleep-shot, remember your promise and tell your vet. Show him or her what you did. Dogdom will thank you forever.

CHAPTER 18

ZAPPERS

Being able to kill your bacteria and other invaders with electricity seems like a panacea, especially when you can do it all in three, seven-minute sessions. But killing things that your body should have been able to kill itself, or things that should not have gotten into the body in the first place, should make us think: "Why did this happen to me? Could I have prevented this?" Prevention is infinitely better than treatment, and is the true goal for us all. Nevertheless, zappers are a superb <u>help</u> when the complete picture is kept in mind. This means respect for the immune system, understanding our extreme dependence on it for survival of our species.

The evolution of the zapper from the earlier frequency generator is described in *The Cure For All Diseases*. The advantage of not needing to know the frequency of the pathogens you wish to kill makes it exceptionally useful.

No matter what frequency your zapper is set at (within reason), it kills large and small invaders: flukes, roundworms, mites, bacteria, viruses and fungi. It kills them all at once, in seven minutes, even at 5 volts. But the current does have to reach them and there are certain hard-to-reach places: for instance the eyes, the appendix, the testes, the inner ear bones and most of the contents of the intestine.

How does it work? I suppose that a *Positive* voltage applied anywhere on the body attracts *Negatively* charged things such as bacteria. Perhaps the battery voltage tugs at them, pulling them out of their locations in the cell doorways (called *conductance channels*). But doorways can be *Negatively* charged too. Does the voltage tug at them so they disgorge any bacteria stuck in them? Perhaps it just closes these doorways. How would the *Positive* voltage act to kill a large parasite like a fluke? These questions cannot be answered yet, although the evidence is clear: a sudden release of parasite eggs into the blood, bits of parasite in the white blood cells, and later, the appearance of mold just where the flukes had been. Killing action is also suggested when a large fluke can no longer be heard on the Syncrometer® in seven minutes. Only further research will find more facts.

Another earlier question has a clear answer, now. Is the killing effect due to immune system stimulation? The answer is "*Yes*". The empowering effect on white blood cells is seen when they suddenly possess parts of the fluke and bacteria, when minutes before zapping they did not.

Other fascinating possibilities are that the intermittent *Positive* voltage interferes with electron flow in some key metabolic route, or straightens out the ATP molecule disallowing its breakdown. Such biological questions could be answered by studying the effects of *Positive* electrical pulses on pathogens in a laboratory.

The most important question, of course, is whether there is a harmful effect on you. I have seen no effects on blood pressure, mental alertness, or body temperature. It has never produced pain, although it has often stopped pain instantly. This does not by itself prove safety. Even knowing that the voltage comes from a small 9-volt battery does not rigorously prove safety although it is reassuring. The fact that thousands of zappers are in use suggests safety, too. And finding that one of its mechanisms is through the immune system, makes it even more appealing. Viruses and bacteria disappear in three minutes; tapeworm stages, flukes, roundworms in five; and mites in seven. People who are not ill need not go beyond this time, although no bad effects have been seen at any length of treatment.

The first seven-minute zapping is followed by an intermission, lasting 20 to 30 minutes. During this time, bacteria and viruses are released from the dying parasites and start to invade you instead. Such releases form the basis of "detoxification-illness", which must be controlled and counteracted. Each parasite has its own bacterial and viral escapees.

The second seven-minute session is intended to kill these newly released viruses and bacteria. If you omit it, you could catch a cold, sore throat or something else immediately. In fact, if you do, you know you killed some serious parasites. Again, viruses are released, this time from the dying bacteria. The third session kills the last viruses released.

A fourth and fifth session may be very beneficial, too, especially when we see bits of protein called "prion protein" streaming from killed Salmonella bacteria. But not enough experiments are completed to be sure that everyone needs extra sessions. Remember, cancer patients will be plate-zapping for 20-minute sessions anyway. So, the need for more regular zapping sessions is not yet indicated.

Do Not Zap if you are Pregnant or Wearing a Pacemaker.

These situations have not been explored yet. Don't do these experiments yourself. Children as young as eight months <u>have</u> been zapped with no noticeable ill effects. For them, you should weigh the possible benefits against the unknown risks.

That is all there is to it. Almost all. The zapping current is most effective for the blood and lymph, two rather salty (conductive) fluids. But it does not reach deep into the eyeball or testicle or bowel contents. It does not reach into your gallstones, or into your living cells where Herpes virus lies latent or Candida fungus extends its fingers. To reach deeper, the herbal parasite program (page 79) and homeography should be added to the zapper treatment.

Cancer victims have many nerve endings covered with motor oil and wheel bearing grease, that bring PCBs and benzene with them. You cannot pass enough electricity through your hands or wrists due to these insulators, nor will it penetrate the tumor effectively.

To reach specific organs electrically, with a significant effect, you will need to do plate-zapping (see page 488) and use foot electrodes. You merely need to put a sample of similar organ tissue on the zapping plate.

For cancer victims, copper pipe electrodes are placed under the feet just in front of the heels. The choice of copper is important because it is the most conductive metal, besides silver. The pressure of your feet on the pipes helps the current penetrate. Hand pressure is hard to keep up. A flat electrode provides too little surface for contact and produces too little pressure under the foot.

Blood and lymph are still the most important locations to zap. These are reachable by regular zapping (without a plate). Using foot electrodes helps greatly, for both plate-zapping and regular zapping.

In earlier books a circuit was described that produced a totally *Positive* electrical field at all times, called "*Positive* offset". But many zappers were built with small substitutions when the exact components were not available. This often brought the resulting electrical field too close to *Negative* so that brief excursions into the *Negative* field were inevitable. Even very brief "*Negative* spikes" are undesirable. For this reason the circuit given here has an additional component, a *Positive* offset resistor. With this addition, it is easy for the builder to measure the *Positive* offset on an oscilloscope. It will be ¼ volt. **Anyone purchasing a zapper should ask for this measurement. The consumer should also request <u>copper</u> electrodes of <u>tubular</u> design and plates of correct dimension (3¼ to 3½ inches <u>square</u>) and composition (aluminum).**

Although wrist straps are convenient, not enough research has been done to accurately compare effectiveness with the tubular design of electrodes. A very ill person should use the copper tube electrodes, of correct dimension, correctly placed and not risk poor conductance.

Zapping once a day is now a common routine for many persons. The elderly seem to be keeping more alert for their years. For many it is a daily pain-reliever, fatigue-lifter, or mystery-helper. For the ill, zapping all day, continuously, for a month or more has often brought significant improvement. Only further research can shed light on how all this happens.

Just as amazing as its action is the simplicity of the circuit design. Even a complete novice could build one.

Building a Zapper

You will be given two ways to build a zapper: the **shoebox** way and the **breadboard** way. The breadboard way for a 1000 Hz (1 kHz) zapper is on page 493.

Both have ¼ volt *Positive* offset. You will be able to test your zapper (or any commercially made one) for its *Positive* offset feature simply by observing it on an oscilloscope.

Hints for absolute novices: Don't let unusual vocabulary deter you. A "lead" is just a piece of wire used to make connections. When you remove a component from its package, label it with a piece of tape. A serrated kitchen knife works best, as does a large safety pin. Practice using the micro clips. If the metal ends are L-shaped bend them into a U with the long-nose pliers so they grab better. Chips and chip holders (wire wrap sockets) are very fragile. It is wise to purchase an extra one of each in case you break the connections. The "555" timer is a widely used component; if you can't locate this one, try another electronics shop.

The Shoebox Way

This circuit has been improved since the one given in earlier books.

A resistor has been added that gives every pulse an added *Positive* offset of ¼ volt. You no longer need to operate your zapper so daringly close to a *Negative* voltage.

Parts List for 30 kHz Zapper Circuit
Shoebox Way

Item	Radio Shack Catalog Number
Shoebox	
9 volt battery	
9 volt battery snap connector	270-324 (set of 5, you need 1)
on-off toggle switch	275-624A micro mini toggle switch
If not available, choose any toggle switch with holes in the contact points or Radio Shack 275-612	
1 KΩ resistor, brown-black-red-gold	271-312(500 piece assortment) use 2
3.9 KΩ resistor, orange-white-red-gold	Use 2 from the 500 piece assortment
39 KΩ resistor, orange-white-orange-gold	From 500 piece assortment
low-current red LED	276-044
.0047 uF capacitor	272-130 (set of 2, you need 1)
.01 uF capacitor	272-131 (set of 2, you need 1)
555 CMOS timer chip (TLC 555)	276-1718 (you may wish to buy a spare)
8 pin wire-wrapping socket for the chip	900-7242
If only 16 pin sockets are available, cut one in half OR leave half empty.	
short (12") alligator clip leads	any electronics shop, get 10
If not available, use 14" length from Radio Shack, 278-1156	
Micro clip jumper wires	278-017 (you need 2 packages of 2)
If not available, use mini-clip jumper wires 278-016	
2 bolts, about $^1/_8$" diameter, 2" long, with 4 nuts and 4 washers	hardware store
2 copper pipes, ¾" diameter, 4" long	hardware store
sharp knife, pin, long-nose pliers, tape, 4 twist ties or rubber bands	

To build your zapper you may take this list of components to any electronics store (Radio Shack part numbers are given for convenience). You may also order a kit, see *Sources*.

Assembling the Zapper

1. You will be using the lid of the shoebox to mount the components. Save the box base to enclose the finished project.

2. Pierce two holes near the ends of the lid. Enlarge the holes with a pen or pencil until the bolts would fit through. Mount the bolts from the outside about half way through the holes so there is a washer and nut

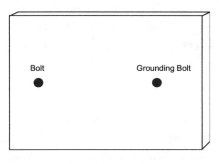

holding it in place on both sides. Tighten. Label one hole "grounding bolt" on the inside and outside.

3. Mount the 555 chip in the wire wrap socket. Find the "top end" of the chip by searching the outside surface carefully for a cookie-shaped bite taken out of it or an imprinted dot. Align the chip with the socket and very gently squeeze the pins of the chip into the socket until they click in place.

4. Make 8 pinholes to fit the wire wrap socket. Enlarge them slightly with a sharp pencil. Mount it from the outside. Write in the numbers of the pins (connections) on both the outside and inside, starting with number one, near the

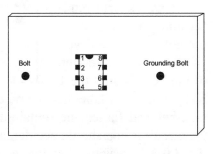

"cookie bite", as seen from outside. After number 4, cross over to number 5 and continue. Number 8 will be across from number 1.

5. Pierce two holes ½ inch apart very near to pins 5, 6, 7, and 8. They should be less than $^1/_8$ inch away. (Or, one end of each component can <u>share</u> a hole with the 555 chip.) Mount the .01 uF capacitor near pin 5 on the outside. On the inside connect pin 5 to one end of this capacitor by simply twisting them together. Loop the capacitor wire around the pin first; then twist with the long-nose pliers until you have made a tight connection. Bend the other wire from the capacitor flat against

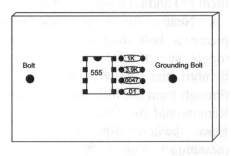

the inside of the shoebox lid. Label it .01 on the outside and inside. Mount the .0047 uF capacitor near pin 6. On the inside twist the capacitor wire around the pin. Flatten the wire from the other end and label it .0047. Mount the 3.9 KΩ resistor near pin 7, connecting it on the inside to the pin. Flatten the wire on the other end and label it 3.9 K. Mount the 1 KΩ resistor and connect it similarly to pin 8 and label it 1 K.

6. Pierce two holes ½ inch apart next to pin 3 (again, you can share the hole for pin 3 if you wish), in the direction of the bolt. Mount the 1

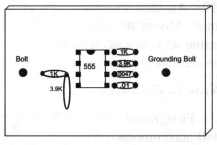

KΩ resistor and label inside and outside. Twist the connections together and flatten the remaining wire. This resistor protects the circuit if you should accidentally short the terminals. Mount the 3.9 KΩ resistor downward. One end can go in the same hole as the 1 KΩ resistor near pin 3. Twist that end around pin 3 which already has the 1 KΩ resistor attached to it. Flatten the far end. Label.

7. Next to the 3.9 KΩ resistor pierce two holes ¼ inch apart for the LED. Notice that the LED has a *Positive* and *Negative* connection. The longer wire is the anode (*Positive*). The flattened side of the red dome marks the *Negative* wire. Mount the LED from the outside and bend back the wires, labeling them (+) and (-) on the inside.

8. Near the top pierce a hole for the toggle switch. Enlarge it until the shaft fits through from the inside. Remove nut and washer from switch before mounting. You may need to trim away some

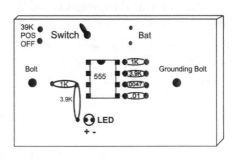

paper with a serrated knife before replacing washer and nut on the outside. Tighten.

9. Next to the switch pierce two holes for the wires from the battery snap connector and poke them through from the outside. Do not attach the battery yet.

10. An inch away from the switch pierce two holes ¼ inch apart. Mount the 39 KΩ resistor from the outside and label it inside and outside as "39 K, *Positive* offset." Flatten the wires on the inside.

Now to Connect Everything

First, make slits at each corner of the lid with a knife. They will accommodate extra loops of wire that you get from using the clip leads to make connections. After each connection gently tuck away the excess wire through the most convenient slit.

1. Twist the free ends of the two capacitors (.01 and .0047) together. Connect this to the grounding bolt using an alligator clip.

2. Bend the top ends of pin 2 and pin 6 (which already has a connection) inward towards each other in an L shape. Catch

them both together with a alligator clip and attach the other end of the alligator clip to the free end of the 3.9 KΩ resistor by pin 7.

3. Using an alligator clip connect pin 7 to the free end of the 1 KΩ resistor attached to pin 8.

4. Using three micro clips connect pin 8 to one end of the switch, pin 4 to the same end of the switch, and one end of the offset resistor to the same end of the switch. (Put one hook inside the hole and the other hooks around the whole connection. Check to make sure they are securely connected.) Connect the free end of the offset resistor to the bolt using an alligator clip.

5. Use an alligator clip to connect the free end of the 1 KΩ resistor (by pin 3) to the bolt. It is the output resistor.

6. Twist the free end of the 3.9 KΩ resistor by pin 3 around the plus end of the LED. Connect the minus end of the LED to the grounding bolt using an alligator clip.

7. Connect pin number 1 on the chip to the grounding bolt with an alligator clip.

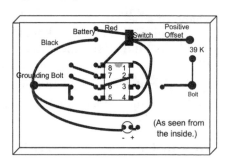

8. Attach an alligator clip to the outside of one of the bolts. Attach the other end to a handhold (copper pipe). Do the same for the other bolt and handhold.

9. Connect the minus end of the battery snap connector (black wire) to the grounding bolt with an alligator clip.

10. Connect the plus end of the battery snap connector (red wire) to the free end of the switch using a micro clip lead. Attach the battery <u>very carefully</u>. Before attaching the battery to its snap connector, cover one terminal with tape. After snapping in one terminal, remove the tape to attach the other terminal. This is to prevent accidental touching of terminals in a backwards direction. If the LED lights up you know the

switch is ON. If it does not, flip the switch and see if the LED lights. Label the switch clearly. If you cannot get the LED to light in either switch position, double-check all of your connections, and make sure you have a fresh battery. Even if it does light up, check every connection again.

11. Finally tie up the bunches of wire pushed through the slits in the corners with twist-ties or rubber bands and replace the lid on the box. Slip a couple of rubber bands around the box to keep it securely shut. For safer storage, place it inside a larger box.

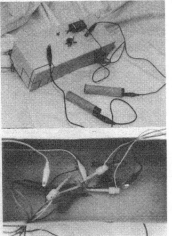

Fig. 109 Zapper under construction

Note: Having gained this much experience, you may prefer to build your next zapper on a piece of cardboard folded in the shape of a bench, ⌐⌐, and able to fit <u>inside</u> a shoebox for more protection.

Could you build this zapper the breadboard way? Yes, see page 493, and use the 30 kHz parts list.

• Optional: measure the frequency of your zapper by connecting an oscilloscope or frequency counter to the handholds. Any electronics shop can do this. It should read between 20 and 40 kHz. The shop can also read the voltage (peak to peak) and the amount of *Positive* offset (on the .5 volt-per-division scale). The voltage output should be about 8 volts.

• **Note**: a voltmeter will only read 4 to 5 volts because it displays an <u>average</u> voltage.

• Optional: observe the square wave pulses without holding on to the handholds. They begin to rise from a base voltage of about ¼ volt. This is the "*Positive* offset". The tops and bottoms of each pulse are flat, each lasting about the same time (50%) called the duty cycle. The rise and fall of each pulse is vertical, without a spike in the *Negative* direction (down). When you grasp the handholds (called "under load") the peak-to-peak voltage drops considerably, and the shape has rounded instead of square corners for each pulse. This is a reflection on your body's capacitance; it is normal.

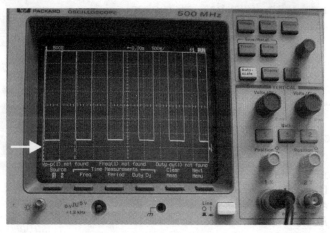

At a range of .5 volts per division, it is easy to see the offset. Before the unit is turned on, the zero line is found at arrow on left side of screen. (Also see arrow at right side). Turning it on shows the elevated bottom edge of each pulse. Also, no spikes go below the zero line into the *Negative* field at any time.

Fig. 110 Zapper output with ¼ volt Positive offset

• Optional: measure the current that flows through you when you are getting zapped. You will need a 1 KΩ carbon resistor and oscilloscope. Connect the grounding bolt on the zapper to one end of the resistor. Connect the other end of the resistor to a handhold. (Adding this resistor to the circuit decreases the current slightly, but not significantly.) The other handhold is attached to the other bolt. Connect the scope ground wire to one end of the resistor. Connect the scope probe to the other end of the resistor. Turn the zapper ON and grasp the handholds. Read the voltage on the scope. It will read about 3.5 volts. Calculate current by dividing voltage by resistance. 3.5 volts divided by 1 KΩ is 3.5 ma (milliamperes) of current.

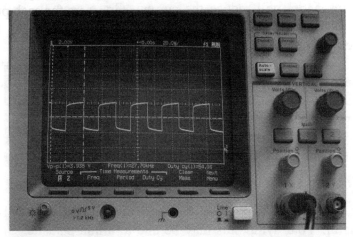

Duty cycle, voltage and frequency are less important than absence of *Negative* spikes and presence of the extra ¼ volt *Positive* offset.

Fig. 111 Zapper output under load shows effect of body capacitance

If Someone Else Builds your Zapper

Parts List

R1	1 K
R2	3.9 K
R3	1 K
R4	3.9 K
R5	39 K
C1	.01 μf
C2	.0047μf
U3	MC1455
LED red	2 ma LED

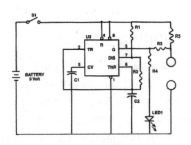

Give this to an electronics person to build in a project box.

Fig. 112 Zapper schematic

487

Using The Zapper

1. Wrap handholds in <u>one</u> layer of wet paper towel before using. More will reduce the current. Grasp securely and turn the switch on to zap. Keep a bottle of water handy to keep them wet.

2. Zap for seven minutes, let go of the handholds, turn off the zapper, and rest for 20 minutes. Then seven minutes on, 20 minutes rest, and a final seven minutes on. This is the routine for regular zapping.

3. For plate-zapping, stay connected for 20 minutes at any one tissue location, and move on to others after that.

Testing the Zapper

Trying the zapper on an illness to see "if it works" is not useful. Your symptoms may be due to a non-parasite. Or you may reinfect within hours of zapping. The best way to test your device is to find a few invaders that you currently have. (This is described in the *Syncrometer*® *Science Laboratory Manual*). This gives you an exact starting point. Then zap yourself. After the triple zapping, none of these invaders should be present. If they do survive, especially the larger ones like Fasciola flukes, they are undoubtedly saturated by an insulating substance such as PCBs, Freon or benzene. For this reason, plate-zapping is chosen.

Plate-Zapping

By passing the zapper current through a capacitor plate in the same manner as the Syncrometer® current, a similar effect can be observed. The item placed on the plate <u>directs</u> or invites the current; in fact, nothing else will be zapped. My interpretation is that the capacitor plate on the resonance box has a "standing wave" relationship to an identical capacitance in your body (actually, a capacitance-inductance unit), making the resistance between them essentially zero. For this reason the dimensions and composition of the capacitor plates are important. Nearly all the current will go to this location in your body. The standing wave relationship can be seen for the Syncrometer® where the addition of two picofarads capacitance to the plate destroys resonance, but the further addition of two microhenrys inductance restores it again.

Making a Plate-Zapper

I have experimented and gotten good results from two configurations. One uses two sardine can lids to form a single plate. The second uses two pieces of aluminum as separate plates. The advantage of the first configuration is that it is easy to make from items around your home. The advantage of the second configuration is you can do two locations at once. Theoretically, a three-plate, or four-plate, or fifty-plate configuration would increase efficiency even more, but it would also bring a proportional increase in detoxification-illness.

> **Only make plate-zappers as described below.** Other shapes, sizes and compositions have either not been tested or not been found useful.

Single Plate-Zapper

The easiest plate-zapper to build uses sardine can lids (not other cans). After careful washing and unrolling to make the surface as flat as possible, you mount them on the lids of empty vitamin bottles (the kind with plastic caps). Make a nail hole near the center of each lid and bottle cap. Find sheet metal screws to fit the holes. Tighten the can plates to the lids just enough to be still movable by finger touch.

Place your two lids so they overlap slightly. They are held together tightly by the grip of an alligator clip lead, making a single plate out of it. Fasten the other end of the alligator clip to the bolt of your homemade zapper (***Positive*** side). Now attach a second alligator clip lead from this plate to a copper pipe. A third alligator clip lead goes from your zapper grounding bolt to the second copper pipe as usual.

The two can lids must be very securely connected at all times. Use copper pipes for best contact to your body. The high frequency and single layer of wet paper prevent the copper from penetrating your skin.

Double Plate-Zapper

Get two $^1/_{32}$ inch (1 mm) thick aluminum plates. They should be 3¼ to 3½ inch (8 to 9 cm) square. Drill a hole in the center of each one and mount on a cardboard or plastic box with bolts. Place them about 2-3 inches (5-8 cm) apart.

Run a lead from the *Positive* output of your zapper to <u>each</u> of the plates (two leads altogether, clip them directly onto the edge of each plate). Then run a lead from <u>each</u> plate to a single copper pipe. There is a lead from the *Negative* output of the zapper to the second copper pipe as

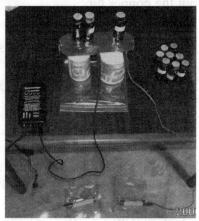

Using a homemade or purchased zapper, connect the *Positive* output to your sardine can plate. From there another lead goes to a foot electrode (copper pipe). The *Negative* output goes to the other foot. One location and a few bacteria are on the plate.

Fig. 113 Homemade plate-zapper

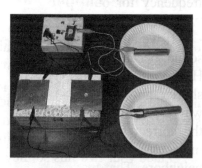

Fig. 114 Double plate-zapper

usual. You will need five alligator clip leads altogether.

Plate-Zapping Tips

Because you should use your feet to zap, you may wish to put the copper tubes on the floor. The tubes should be wrapped with only <u>one</u> layer of wet paper towel. To protect your floor, shove paper plates inside plastic bags underneath the tubes.

With plate-zapping, a 9 volt battery will wear out even quicker than for other arrangements. Of course, your body is benefiting from this greater energy input by converting it, in some way, for itself. You need to check the battery voltage after every zap at first. If the battery voltage ends up at 8.9 or lower, you will have to repeat the last zap. Start each zap at no less than 9.4 v. Expect to drain about .4 volts from the battery for each zap using this dual plate arrangement. Get rechargeable batteries, a battery charger, and a voltmeter all of which will save you money and delays.

For detailed instructions see the *Plate-Zapping Schedule* on page 94.

The Zappicator

Attaching a zapper to a loudspeaker brings the electric pulses to the magnet that makes the speaker's paper cone vibrate. The paper cone vibrates the air at the same frequency. We can hear this if the electric pulses are at the correct frequency for our ears, which is from 20 Hz to 20,000 Hz (vibrations per second).

If we attach a zapper to a speaker we would not hear any sound, because the zapper outputs a frequency of about 30,000 Hz (too high), although the vibrations continue. Each pulse is shorter now and might reach the molecules themselves, the way a passing train can rattle the dishes in your cupboard. If the correct frequency is found you could "rattle" a specific molecule and perhaps destroy it without harming the neighbors. That was the theory. But experiments showed that the incoming pulses had to be totally *Positive* (100%) and the circular magnet around the speaker had to be producing a north pole magnetic field to have such an effect. Moreover, if an

491

actual current was running through the loudspeaker, the whole phenomenon vanished!

I experimented with other frequencies, hoping to find one that not only destroyed bacteria and viruses, but "bad molecules" like phenolics in food. I found 1,000 Hz worked well, which surprised me because I expected a much higher frequency.

I could not understand the physics involved, but there were no exceptions. Only the single lead attachment worked, from the (+) output of the zapper to the (+) end of the speaker. If the (-) end was used at all, this unusual chemistry does not occur. The loudspeaker must be acting as if it were an antenna, suggesting that resonance is involved in finding and destroying the "bad molecules." Fortunately I did not find evidence that "good molecules" like vitamins and organic minerals were affected. They let the pulses pass through unnoticed, like open gates letting through the traffic. But "bad molecules," like food allergens, PCBs, benzene and phenol were destroyed. In fact, phenol appeared after benzene disappeared. After this, wood alcohol appeared as if phenol molecules had broken in half. With longer zappication even this wood alcohol disappeared, producing formaldehyde, and this broke down further to formic acid. Some significant "chemistry" is going on during zappication.

Zappicating food is so beneficial you are encouraged to build this device. The circuit is just like the zapper, but with a few component changes to lower the frequency to 1000±5 Hz.

There will be no sound because no current is flowing. But a very tiny voltage and the 1 kHz frequency are affecting all the food that touches the plate or touches other food that is touching the plate. That is easy to see on a frequency counter.

The zappicator circuit will also have the *Positive* offset feature, namely, a special resistor to produce a ¼ volt offset, so no *Negative* voltage could ever be delivered accidentally. It will produce a frequency of 1000 Hz, instead of 30,000.

Building the Zappicator

The zappicator has two parts:
- a speaker box (with one or two loudspeakers) where food is placed and
- a 1 kHz zapper to supply power to the box

First we will build the 1 kHz zapper. We will build it on a breadboard to avoid the tangle of wires, clip leads, and the soldering of other methods.

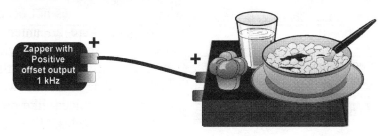

Fig. 115 Zappicator with speaker box and 1 kHz zapper

The Breadboard Way

Instructions for making a 1 kHz zapper:

Parts List for Zappicator Circuit	
Item	**Radio Shack Catalog Number**
9 volt battery	
9 volt battery snap connector	270-324 (set of 5, you need 1)
on-off toggle switch	275-624A micro-mini toggle switch
if not available, choose any toggle switch with holes in the terminals, OR Radio Shack 275-612	
1 KΩ resistor, brown-black-red-gold (2)	271-312 (500 piece assortment)
2.2 KΩ resistor, red-red-red-gold	use one in the assortment
4.4 KΩ resistor	use one of the 4.7 KΩ resistors in the assortment (yellow-violet-red-gold)

493

Parts List for Zappicator Circuit	
144 KΩ resistor	use two of the 270 KΩ resistors in the assortment (red-violet-yellow-gold)
39 KΩ resistor (for *Positive* offset) orange-white-orange-gold	use one in the assortment
low-current red LED 2 ma	276-044
.0047 uF capacitor (2)	272-130 (set of two)
555 CMOS timer chip (TLC 555)	276-1718 (you might want to buy a spare)
alligator clip leads (2)	any electronics shop
or use Radio Shack 278-1156 (set of 10)	
breadboard	276-175 (called Experimenter Socket)
breadboard wires	276-173
2 copper pipes, ¾ inch diameter, 4 inches long	plumbing store
long nose pliers, scotch tape, wire stripper	

The total cost, as of 2004, was about $29.00 not including the copper pipes.

A breadboard is a plastic pad with holes in it. If you look closely at the Radio Shack "Experimenter Socket," you can see the rows are lettered A through J, while the two outermost rows are X and Y. The columns are numbered 1 through 23. Any other breadboard will work, too. The components connect by contacting a metal board under the holes. Here are some tips for the novice builder:

If the end of a wire is not bare, use a sharp knife to scrape off about ¼ inch (1 cm) of the plastic insulation. When stripping wire, if you accidentally cut some of the

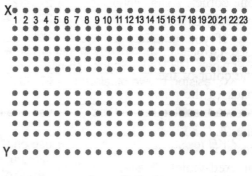

breadboard

wire strands off, then cut them all off and start fresh. Hopefully you will succeed before you run out of wire!

If the wire is solid, great, but if it is stranded then twist it with your fingers to help keep the strands together.

When you push a wire (either solid or stranded) into a hole in the breadboard, you should feel it go in securely. If you tug the wire gently it should not come free. If you turn the breadboard upside down and shake it, nothing should fall out. Sometimes (especially with stranded wire which is flexible), the wire will bend instead of going in. Just straighten it out and try again. Hold the wire as close to the end as possible to prevent bending, or grab it with long nose pliers.

You don't need to know this, but if you are wondering how the rest of the breadboard works, holes A1 through E1 are connected internally, A2-E2 are connected to themselves, A3-E3, and so forth. Also F1-J1, F2-J2, etc. Finally, X1-X23 and Y1-Y23 are already connected internally. To connect different rows or across the center groove, jumpers are used, of different lengths, called breadboard wires.

The resistors, capacitors, and LED have long, bare wires. Don't let them touch each other; check each one before attaching the battery. You can cut them shorter if you wish. (You can buy wire cutters, but you can also just use household scissors although cutting wire may dull the scissors.)

The resistors and capacitors have no orientation so can go in any way. But the 555 chip does, it has a small circle or dot in one corner. Also, the LED has a flat side on its rim (hard to see but easy to feel) that tells you which way it goes.

If you bought the Radio Shack resistor assortment you may be wondering how you tell them apart! The answer is by the color of the bands on the cylinder. There is a chart on the back of the package, but to make it easy, the 1 KΩ resistor is brown-black-red-gold; the 2.2 KΩ resistor is red-red-red-gold; the 4.7 KΩ resistor is yellow-violet-red-gold; the 39 KΩ resistor is orange-white-orange-gold and the 270 KΩ resistors are red-violet-yellow-gold. All the resistors in the assortment end with a gold band, so when reading the colors, start at the non-gold end.

The 555 timer chip is sensitive to static electricity. A good way to make sure you are not charged with static electricity is to touch a metal cold water pipe or faucet before handling the chip.

Although you are working with bare wires and electricity, there is little chance of harming yourself. During assembly the battery is not connected. Even while you are using the zapper, there are no voltages higher than the nine volts of the battery in this circuit. Still, take care not to come in contact with the components while the battery is connected in order not to make a spark or damage a component.

Plug in all the components as shown in the pictures.

Attach the battery last. Do this very carefully to avoid accidentally contacting its terminals backwards. Cover one battery terminal with tape first. Then snap in the free terminal. Remove tape and snap in the other terminal.

If you have a voltmeter and wish to check the output you will find it measures approximately 4.5 V. That is because the zapper is switching between nine volts and zero volts about 1000 times per second. The average of nine and zero is 4.5 V.

Step-by-Step Assembly

1. Examine the 555 timer chip. Find the dot or "cookie bite" at one end. This starts the numbering system for the legs, called "pins". The pin nearest to the dot is #1. Count them all. Find the 8th row on the breadboard and insert the chip across the "aisle" or groove as shown. Ease the chip in gently. If the pins refuse to go in evenly on both sides you may ease it out again with your fingernail and press the pins a bit closer together. The chip should lie flat against the breadboard when in place. Each pin connects to the row of 5 dots it is in. Identify the row of dots for each pin.

2. Insert the red wire of the battery snap connector. This will bring *Positive* (+) electricity to the whole row of 23 dots, called X, at the edge of the board.

3. Insert the black wire of the battery snap connector. This connects all the dots on the other edge, called Y, to the *Negative* (-) side of the battery. This is also called "ground". Do not attach the battery yet.

4. Insert the jumper (red) that will bring the (+) electricity to pin 8.

5. Insert the jumper that connects pin 1 to ground. Jiggle the jumpers till they go in smoothly or try a different one. Also try bending the wires slightly inward for easier fitting. You have now completed *Diagram A*.

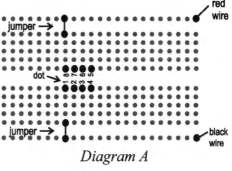

Diagram A

6. Connect pin 8 to pin 7 through a 1 KΩ resistor (brown-black-red-gold). Since this is a very short distance the ends of the resistor will seem too long. Bend one end over and down to make a "hairpin". Then cut both ends about ½ inch (1 cm) from the end of the resistor; then insert.

7. Connect the row of dots at pin 7 to pin 6 through a 270 KΩ resistor (red-violet-yellow-gold). Again, bend one end of the resistor in a hairpin; cut the other end off to make them even. Insert. Repeat with a second 270 KΩ resistor right beside it. This "parallel" configuration reduces the resistance to half, namely, 135 KΩ. This value is close enough to 144 KΩ as required on the parts list. This value works as well.

8. Next, you need to connect pin 2 on the 555 chip to pin 6. To do this, choose a jumper (green) that can take you away from the crowded conditions at pin 6, all the way to row 15 from row 10.

9. Then jump from here across the aisle (orange). From here jump to the row of dots at pin 2 (blue). Now pin 6 is connected to pin 2. You have completed *Diagram B*. (Some of your previous connections are omitted for clarity.)

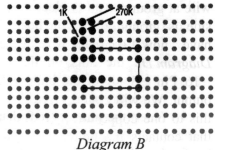

Diagram B

10. Connect pin 6 to another outlying row, such as row 17, through a capacitor, .0047 μF. Push the end at pin 6 in first; then bend the other end slightly inward to insert easily.

11. Insert the other capacitor, also .0047 μF, between pin 5 and the same row. After solid insertion straighten out the wires and make sure no wires are touching other wires inappropriately. If any insertion is especially difficult, use long nose pliers to grasp a wire near its end for firmer pushing.

12. Connect the outlying ends of the capacitors (row 17) to ground using a jumper that crosses the aisle (white).

13. Pin 4 also gets energized by the battery. Connect pin 4 to an outlying row (row 3) with a jumper (gray). Connect the same row to the (+) side of the battery with a jumper. You have now completed *Diagram C*.

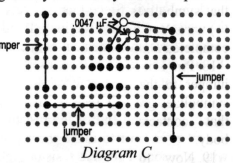

Diagram C

14. Now to connect the LED. Connect pin 3 to an unused row, such as 14, through a 2.2 KΩ resistor (red-red-red-gold). Find the flat side of the red dome on the LED. The flat side has the shorter wire.

15. Insert the longer wire of the LED at row 14, the shorter wire at ground. The flat side is grounded. You have now completed *Diagram D.*

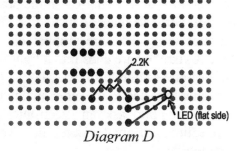

16. Pin 3 is the output. We will connect this to one copper pipe that contacts the body, but we will do this

Diagram D

through an output resistor. Connect pin 3 to an outlying row, such as 2, through a resistor of 1000 Ω (brown-black-red-gold). This resistor protects the circuit if you accidentally short the two copper pipes as you hold them.

17. Connect an extra long jumper at row 2; it must reach to the outside of the box that will hold your zapper. Choose a light color that symbolizes the hot (+) wire. You have now completed *Diagram E.*

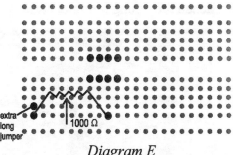

Diagram E

18. Pin 1 is already grounded. Connect another extra long jumper to the ground row, using a dark color (green) that symbolizes ground. This will connect to the other copper pipe that contacts the body.

19. Now to add the offset resistor. Connect the 39 KΩ resistor between the battery and the output at row 2. This completes *Diagram F.*

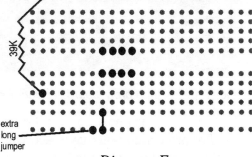

Diagram F

499

20. To include a switch, pull out the red wire of the battery snap connector from its seat in the breadboard. Cut the red wire in half. Strip ½ inch of insulation from each newly cut end. Practice using the wire stripper on a different piece of wire first. Twist the bare ends into a tight form. Insert one end in the hole of one switch terminal. Make a tight connection. Connect the other bare end to the other switch terminal.

If possible, ask an electronics shop to solder these 2 connections for greater durability. Reinsert the red wire in the breadboard.

21. Connect the battery, but do this VERY CAREFULLY. Remember to cover one battery terminal with tape until the other terminal is safely seated in its holder. Then remove tape and seat the other terminal. You could destroy the chip if you touched the wrong terminals briefly.

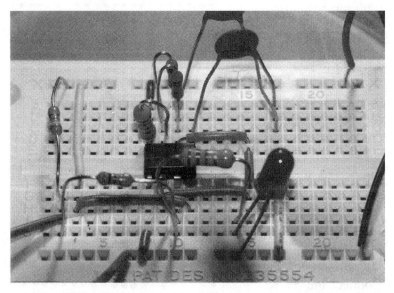

Fig. 116 Finished breadboard zapper (1 kHz) for zappicating foods

22. The LED may now light. If it does not, throw the switch.
23. For protection you may place your zapper inside a plastic container with lid. Mount the switch and battery on the outside for convenience.

Troubleshooting

If the LED still doesn't light, it may be in backwards. Disconnect the battery, tape over one terminal, turn the LED around, and reconnect the battery. Being in backwards does not harm the LED. If it still does not light, or flickers, suspect the switch connections. Remove the switch or solder it.

If the battery gets hot, disconnect it immediately! Check that there are no bare wires touching each other. Double-check that your wiring matches the picture. You may have drained the battery a lot, so replace it with a new one.

If everything looks perfect, but the LED still doesn't light, you may have a defective component. That's why the Parts List advises getting a spare 555 timer chip. The 555 is the most likely component to fail. Disconnect the battery and try swapping chips (pay attention to which corner has the circle). None of the rest of the components are likely to fail, but you can try swapping them if you like.

Make sure your battery is fresh. Use a battery tester.

Seeing the Output

An oscilloscope shows you a high-speed picture of how the voltage changes. You can actually "see" the zapper go from zero to nine volts and back repeatedly. And you can calculate the frequency to make sure it is about 1000 hertz (low-frequency) or 30,000 hertz (regular zapper).

Oscilloscopes are expensive, so rather than buy one, it is better to ask your local television or VCR repair shop if they would use their oscilloscope to check your zapper quickly. Here is how the zapper output typically looks. When your zapper is turned on, the bottom flat lines of each pulse should be ¼ volt above (more *Positive*) the zero line. To see the offset more clearly, change to .5 volts per division, see page 486.

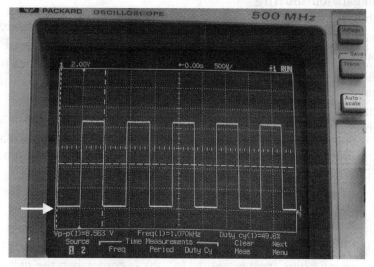

The *Positive* offset is visible just above the zero line.

Fig. 117 Output as seen at 2 volts per division range

Making the Zappicator Food Box

Get these supplies:

• zapper with a 1 kHz output, like you just made

• plastic carton, such as a cottage cheese or food container, or a plastic project box

• 4 ohm or 8 ohm loudspeaker, 2" or 2½" (5-7 cm) diameter, with a north pole face

• one alligator-to-banana clip lead (a piece of insulated wire with an alligator clip at one end and a banana clip at the other) to fit your zapper. Whatever fits is acceptable.

• compass

• roll of tape, sharp knife

Many loudspeakers on the market are south pole. Be careful. Take your compass with you as you shop; the compass' north should be attracted to the face (see picture). A field strength of 10 to 20 gauss is preferred. This means the

502

magnet on the speaker should be able to lift a loose chain of six paper clips. The current and watt ratings given for the speaker are not important. Some loudspeakers have "collars", or domes, or are encased, or shielded. Do not choose them. They do not work.

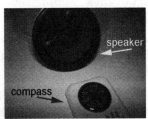

Fig. 118 Choose speaker with north pole face

The magnetic field is not necessarily stable either.

Dropping the speaker or overheating it could change the polarity. Check yours before use with a compass once a week.

Assemble the zappicator food box parts.

1. Find the (+) and (−) sign on the loudspeaker. You will be attaching a lead (wire) to the plus side.

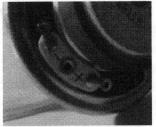

2. Cut a hole, about ½ inch square in the side of the plastic carton for the lead to pass through.

Fig. 119 Find the (+) sign on speaker

3. Attach the loudspeaker to the bottom of the carton, inside, taping it down securely, or using hot glue around the edge of the cone.

4. Push the alligator clip lead through the hole and attach it securely to the (+) connection on the speaker. Attach nothing to the *Negative* terminal.

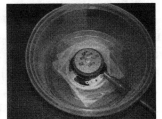

5. Find the (+) terminal of your 1 kHz zapper. You must be sure of this. If you did not build it and if it is not marked, take it to an

Fig. 120 Attach loudspeaker inside the carton

electronics shop; the clerk can check this for you in a minute. Label it. Connect the free end of the clip lead to the (+) terminal of the zapper. If you need to use two leads to connect your speaker (+) terminal to your zapper (+) terminal, do so. Attach nothing to the *Negative* terminal.

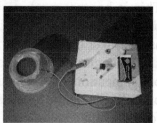

Fig. 121 Connect speaker to (+) output of zapper

6. Turn carton over to give you a flat surface for food placement. Place food, packaged food, beverage container, or filled plate on the top of the carton. It may hang over the edge. Turn zapper on for specified time.

Using the Zappicator Food Box

Metal objects, like cans, placed on the zappicator will become magnetized by zappicating, showing a south pole at the base and north pole at the top. Numerous poles are induced, not necessarily stable. The food inside the container shows the same polarity as the part of the container that is touching it (not opposite). For better quality food you should empty the can first and zappicate in a non-metal container. *All the canned food in the market place is half north and half south from the effect of the earth's magnetic field. This could be its worst feature.*

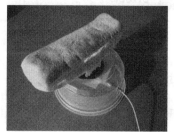

Glass jars should have their metal lids removed before zappicating. This gives all the food a north polarization like the polarity of the speaker.

Fig. 122 Place food on top of carton

Otherwise the metal lid becomes polarized so that half the entire can becomes north and the other half south.

Foods and beverages become north polarized, although they may have started out south or without any polarization.

504

This is because water is **diamagnetic** and takes on the same polarity as the field nearest to it instead of the opposite polarity as iron-like(tin can) metals do.

Changing your food to north polarized is an extra benefit of zappication. The other goals are to disable parasite eggs and other living things as well as changing harmful molecules, like food phenolics to harmless forms (isomers).

Attaching an ordinary zapper with output of about 30,000 Hz to a loudspeaker is almost as useful as using a 1000 Hz zapper. Be sure to disconnect the (-) output. Again, some phenolics and other "bad" molecules are destroyed, leaving the "good" ones intact. Both food and water are given a north polarization, which is beneficial.

Use the same instructions for mounting the loudspeaker. Attach a 30 kHz zapper the same way as for the zappicator.

In this chapter you learned to:

Make a zapper in a cardboard box or on a plastic "breadboard."

Make a 30 kHz zapper or a 1 kHz zapper.

Use a 30 kHz zapper with 1 or 2 plates for better effect.

Use a 1 kHz zapper with a speaker for better effect ("food zappicator").

CHAPTER 19

RECIPES — For an Immune Depressed Society

Read old recipe books for the fun and savings of making your own safe food even though it does take more time! Kitchen help would be welcome. Throw away the grinders, blenders, juicers, choppers; they contaminate all your food with plastic and heavy metals. Home cooking without these will bring flavor back...maybe even the children back...to the table. Children can often taste chromium, copper, strontium, chlorine, malonic acid in food, especially after getting tooth fillings or sealant. Avoid the recipes that have processed (cans and packages) ingredients. When cooking from scratch you can hardly go wrong nutritionally. But it needs to be safe and sanitary.

The importance of this book is the emphasis on higher standards of food sanitation and safety. Sanitation from parasite eggs and bacteria or viruses; safety from the five immunity-destroyers: asbestos, benzene, PCBs, metals and dyes.

To make food sanitary and safe I have recommended three chemical methods and two electrical methods. They are not equal. Choose carefully to suit your needs.

> But isn't this just too much? Especially for a healthy person? Too much caution, care and cleanliness? Is all this really necessary? Isn't a little dirt good for you? These are comments that we sometimes hear.

It is years of using the Syncrometer® and listening to the sick that provides the answer.

Yes! It is necessary. It is long overdue. We are wading in filth—our own, our animals', and others'—that cause mutations and feed our bacteria and viruses. We are wading in toxins: metals, solvents, and dyes. But it "looks" clean and safe enough to us and we might think, "With a glossy floor and gleaming glasses on the table, what could go wrong? Surely it can't be so significant."

Let us take a trip back in time.

A Medieval Weekend

Imagine you have just landed in a medieval town in the year 1250. The family, your ancestors, has invited you to dinner and to spend the night. You hide your car in the woods, to not attract attention, and walk ½ mile along the wide path to their home. You pass many people, all walking, leading animals, stepping over manure deposits, carrying water in buckets which are set down on the ground to rest arms, carrying milk from the neighbors in open pails, carrying bundles of firewood and a hefty stick to fend off dogs.

You arrive just before supper. The table is half set and the milk already poured. Flies are in each glass (screens weren't invented until later). You want most to wash your hands and get a glass of water, but you change your mind. A sick person in the bedroom next to the kitchen is said to have the plague. So all you want is to wash, not drink. But there is no water for washing; only a water bucket for drinking. One dipper hangs over the rim for all to share. The washbasin is being used in the bedroom. You decide against even washing your hands.

Your relatives are very friendly, eager to hug and kiss every square inch of you. You wipe your mouth as often as possible, discreetly.

For supper you get rye bread and milk (freshly carried), a piece of meat roasted marvelously (your relatives are upper class) and for desert a hunk of cheese, delicious cheddar. You look around for cutlery. There isn't any. It's all fingers, hands and slurping. You make do. You wipe hands inside your shirt. Flies find you tasty now.

After supper you try to find some water; there must be a town supply. You walk to find it and do. It's a gathering place…for pigs and cows and sheep and dogs and you! You beg for some from the person at the rope but the people think you're <u>wasting</u> it on your hands and face. You dry up on your clothes feeling embarrassed. Now it's time to find a toilet. But there is none. The very young children go in a potty where mother cleans them up. Mother uses water from the basin, which is being shared next door. The older children and adults fend for themselves in a community shack. Finally you're forced. You try to look casual, just in case there was a choice. There isn't. Some giggling kids are peeking in through the cracks getting a look at the newcomer. But there is no more waiting. It's diarrhea! What? Salmonella already? Then it strikes you. There's no paper. What are others doing? Nothing. And it's an indelicate subject; you can't talk about it when you already know the answer. There's no grass, no leaves, no hay, no anything. Paper wasn't invented.

You would like to wash your hands and bottom in your own urine; that seems logical; and then rinse them in your own spit—but nobody else seems to be doing that. They merely wipe their hands on their clothes and go about their chores.

You finally emerge and get ready for bed, unwashed. So does everybody. The flies are settling down but the mosquitoes are starting up, through all the open windows. The buzz makes a faint chorus. You hide everything including your face till you are semi-choked.

You sleep in your underwear and put out the candle as quickly as possible to stop attracting insects.

The next morning you see the darkened corners of the bedroom. You wonder if there are bedbugs and whether you got bitten.

Everybody is getting ready to go to work, and to the village school, and to the fields. But Mother stays in the house to visit with you. She laughs and tries to cheer you up with a little song as she washes dishes (which cleans her hands from the sick bed) and sweeps the floor.

This is your chance to talk. What would you say? Would you say, "My dear great-great-great-great-great-grandmother, you are doing wonderfully well. The children are beautiful and your husband is so helpful. I hope your son gets well." "Oh, yes, it's in God's hands," she says. That seems to bring as much relief as giving an antibiotic.

Would you tell her about germs? The importance of washing hands? Paper or something in the toilet? Wash water in the toilet? Separate water glasses (about six or seven for her to wash each day)? Flies?

Probably not; it would be too difficult to explain or put into practice. You get in your car and vanish. You're home again.

There's No Place Like Home

Everything looks and feels different.

You notice it when anybody doesn't wash hands after toileting. You notice when anybody doesn't wash hands before eating because you know where those hands have been. You notice when dirty hands are fingering the food which will soon be served.

You see a thousand counterparts of your medieval relatives. Even in the room next to the kitchen is a grown child with "chronic fatigue" on the couch. And in another room beside the kitchen the sounds and smells of bowel elimination are taken for granted. It seems rather close to food preparation but it's an indelicate subject so is never discussed. Stains of pet "messes" are in the carpet. Smells of pesticide and laundry soap and fast food are everywhere. The cats jump on the kitchen counter to check into any food left out "for them." The dog runs about licking everybody on the face and getting into their popcorn as they lie in front of the TV.

We have not learned. Not in 800 years. Despite knowing that sanitation eliminated plagues and epidemics of the past! Despite being able to actually see our tiny but mighty enemies through a microscope! We must change. We must clean up.

Clean out. Sanitize. Or give our loved ones to whatever plague comes next.

Half the Story

Sanitation is only half of the current challenge. The other half is toxicity. Brought by our dishes, our water, our food, our artificial teeth, our cosmetics and the very act of sanitizing in such mindless ways as laundry bleach in our drinking water, pesticide on absorptive food, and isopropyl alcohol in mouthwash.

When disease was killing our species in medieval times, sanitation helped to rescue us.

When toxicity began to kill our species 100 years ago it brought new kinds of illness. What will rescue us this time?

This time we have two plagues: infectious disease and toxicity disease. If our very sanitation procedures cause our toxicity-illnesses, can we be rescued at all?

Let us take a trip to the future to see if solutions were found.

A Future Weekend

Discouraged by the absence of progress in 800 years you decide to visit the future instead. You buckle up in a space suit for a space ship going to 2200 A.D.

You land without having eaten much, excreted much, breathed much or heard or seen much, except TV. All this was convenient for the travel company, which could give you a suspended-metabolism shot instead.

You dock on the 30th floor of the tallest building on this human-inhabited planet called Di Dah and check twice to make sure you'll remember the parking spot. You had read about its history—all 200 years of it and always wanted to meet your future relations. Di Dah, pronounced like hurrah!, stands for the letter A in Morse Code, the first human-colonized planet.

People are walking about, to work, to school, to restaurants, to games and theatres, free of bulky space suits, but in baggy suits instead. A plastic tarp overhead keeps the air in, manufactured constantly to a controlled pressure. The weather is controlled by moving artificial clouds about electrically. Excrement and excretion are disinfected in each home now and piped directly to the hydroponic gardens and fisheries and even to a pond, under development, fondly called "the ocean". It reminds you of a book you read where human "leavings" were always sold to a farmer. It is treated here as valuable since not much of either is produced. In fact, the people don't eat at all, they only sip or drink everything. Their teeth are all replaced with implants at an early age, "preventively", they say, or just end up missing, for the poor.

You go to visit your future great, great, great grandchildren, with 3 children of their own. The parents, your relatives, are wearing baggy suits, front and back, which seem to have no exits. But the young children are running about free from baggy clothes and still with teeth, though very small. You decide not to ask questions but just to observe and smile, letting your joy at seeing them come first. Then you're hungry and you're happy to see there is a table.

The mother seats you and buzzes everyone else in the family. Nobody sets the table. A robot steps out of the closet to take your order. You select from a page of food pictures. The robot procures it from shelves, opens, dumps, heats in a microwave and serves it. Each entrée pours.

Milk comes from a mixing device, still called "The Cow". You select cream content, vitamin content, and additions or some other beverage.

Some entries are labeled "yellow vegetables", others "greens", yet others "starches", and others "proteins". Vitamins and minerals are simply ordered up, too. Everything tastes good, certainly edible, if not exactly delicious.

You can select food by weight—not its weight, though…your weight. If you don't want to absorb any of it, you just enter zero. Your great, great, great grandchildren plugged in 25%. But you decide to forgo that "luxury". The children enjoy mixing everything together for a grand drinking spree—a "slurp-up"…as they called it. Even a grain or two of something solid that wasn't smooth started a fuss. You did wonder how their teeth could grow with so little use, but decided that bad genes were probably the real cause, and best not mentioned.

You downed your lobster, fries, and lettuce, in salt-free, MSG-free, vitamin-packed entrees and started punching in for chocolate-caramel-strawberry desserts, to follow the family pattern.

Little Teena left the table and was reminded by the robot to brush her teeth. Yes, she called out, but jumped in your lap instead to look at your teeth. What a disgusting marvel, her mind seemed to say.

"How come you still have teeth, she asked?"

"It's not nice to ask personal questions" the mother reminded her.

Teena grinned. "I'll be losing mine when I'm 12", she said. "I'm 8 now and I've already lost 6", she said with a smirk. "Don't boast, now, Teena" her father said gently.

The robot reminded her again and she dashed upstairs.

Her older brother had been checking me out carefully, too. Admittedly, I was trying not to stare into his mouth.

Supper was over and everybody dispersed to their computer or TV. The time given to each was carefully disciplined by the proud parents. I watched the robot clear everything into the dishwasher, shredder, or compactor and managed to sneak a bit of solid food I had leftover from earth in my pocket.

I looked out the window, trying to see anything that flew or crawled. Of course not, silly, I told myself.

The mother made a special entrée selection for a sick child in the room next to the kitchen.

Paul, age 14, was hooked up to a dialysis machine, and a respirator, as he lay on the couch. He could plug in for a medicine to lower temperature, raise a neurotransmitter for better mood, or reduce blood sugar. Wow! That's not really being sick, I thought. But he was not allowed to leave this little "sick room", so it must have been serious enough. Right after

513

Paul, his younger brother Eddie, age 12, was hooked up. O my, two sick children, I thought; how sad for the family.

But nobody was sad, not even the parents. In fact they didn't mention it. They just showed me the linens and towels and the bathroom I would be sharing with Teena. She giggled to overhear that.

I headed for bed at the earliest opportunity, hoping to secretly chomp further on my dried breakfast roll. It was exceptionally quiet in the apartment and even next door. I could see everybody had put earphones on. Occasionally they spoke by intercom to get help with homework. But then it came to me…

Nobody is brushing their teeth except Teena. In fact, nobody is using a bathroom either, except Teena. Nobody was flushing. Could they be wearing their dialysis machines right with them—inside their baggy clothes?

Quietly, before bed, the parents went to the family "debulking" room, and changed whatever needed to be changed and threw the rest down a "biological waste" chute. No toilets needed!

But surely there's a shower, I hoped. A shower would be so nice to warm up on. After all the debulking was done, the robot called out "shower time". What a relief. But I respectfully waited for my hosts to get family chores done first. Soon everybody arrived in one grand shower stall, all together. I felt out of place, not joining in. What about sex, I thought. These kids are too old for total nudity. Everybody threw their clothes in a heap—for the robot. And underneath their clothes was not underwear. It was a proudly displayed barrel-of-sorts: the new model dialyzer, they said. So much better for the whole family, they explained. They could cuddle and play, throw water and wrestle each other—all, except get the carefully taped DO-ALL Brand device off.

Paul was too sick though, and had to stay downstairs. His special germs could contaminate the new devices and the new gene-inhibitor for him was not fully researched and developed yet. Lots of kids were dying, the TV blatted out upstairs, unless they took a handy new drug. Eddie could still shower.

I noticed I had not gone to the bathroom I shared with Teena. Not for the bowels nor for the bladder. "What's the matter with me?", I worried. Am I already getting the "DO-ALL" disease…in one day?

I went to bed as dry as a bone. Now others were taking their sleeping pills and insulin. "Do they have diabetes too?", I wondered. I politely declined their gracious offers. Thank you, thank you, I said, as the mother pushed a few "sleepers" into my hand, "just in case, in the middle of the night, you know how hard it is to be awake". She tucked in her family and then sat down to do her own things for a half hour: a bit of crocheting, from a new magazine that kept her somewhat satisfied as she struggled along on her own eternal path.

Next morning, everybody went to work, or school, except Paul. They said their cheery goodbyes to me, as I smiled my appreciation for their hospitality.

You can leave messages with the robot, they said, in case you need anything.

I sat down to keep Paul company for my last half hour on planet Di Dah. I wondered now if it was named for Diabetes and Dialysis, not Morse code mythology as the history books said. He shoved his earphones on like any earthling child. I turned to the robot. What could I say as a parting message? You don't have to have DD on this planet? You could be preventing it. You need to get back to nature, at least real food and water. You should remember your origins as earthlings. You should be finding a cure. Should be…should…

I left this message with the robot: "My dear, dear family, thank you for everything, your wonderful hospitality. Your family is so special to me and I'll tell my family all about you. Some day please visit me, too. I love you, I love you, I love you…much more than you can know". Then I struck out the last bit, it might sound condescending.

I smiled goodbye at Paul and left. Back in my spaceship people were quickly gobbling some real food they had left onboard and scrambled into their space suits.

Soon we were back on good green earth. I was so longing for it, I could have eaten a handful. At my house the TV news was talking about another breakthrough, a new quicker treatment for diabetes, by self-injecting or self-medicating with an automatic control. No talk of cure. Or prevention. That stood out clearly now.

As I got dressed for work, my child pushed on his earphones to go to school. On the street, early morning runners weren't listening to birds or the wind either. They had earphones on, too.

At 11 a.m. my children would be given their medicine by the school nurse. I didn't know what it was. I quietly decided to study it. Was anybody preventing it or trying to cure? All the children that I knew were taking medicine. Nobody talked about toxicity or sanitation or about cure or prevention. Was it a forgotten concept?

I ate my good chewy food and drank real water, though I realized my children did not. Theirs was chlorinated, colored, vitamined, and made to sparkle or fizz. Then, joy of joys, the bathroom called! It was the bowel and bladder. They were still real. We are still blessed, I said to myself. We must start to work to keep our blessings.

Food Sanitizers

The Ancient Ways

Washing, cooking, baking, pickling, drying, frying! These are the time-honored ways to make food edible and sanitary. They did an excellent job in times when toxicity did not play a big role. These ways showed many advantages: preserving food for winter, softening food for babies and the elderly, making food safe from parasites and disease germs even though they might have been called "evil vapors" at that time.

New Ways

Now we have grilling and microwaving. It is a huge experiment in overheating food. It should be watched closely. Each of these heats the food higher than before. This denatures the food more so more minerals are oxidized to toxic metals. These metals feed our pathogens. It is happening on a gigantic scale.

None of these methods is a solution for our immunodepressed society. Lugol's solution, ozonation, sonication, zappicating and HCl are my suggested improvements.

Lugol's Rinse

Lugol's iodine has been used for decades by travelers to foreign lands to wash their fruit and vegetables. We never thought our food in the United States could be so filthy it required iodine treatment. But it is by far the most efficient "sterilizer" no matter what the level of filth. When animal refuse is used as fertilizer or produce is grown in distant countries where different diseases abound, I would feel much safer with my trusty iodine bottle always handy. Whether I am cooking or eating I can always sanitize most food in minutes.

- Lugol's iodine solution (see *Recipes*, page 554)
- water

Fill a sink or a bowl with a measured amount of water. Draw a line here, so future treatments do not require measuring again. **Add one drop Lugol's per quart (or liter) of water.** Dip lettuce, spinach and any other produce so everything is well wetted for one minute or more. Rinsing is optional. (Eating traces of iodine is not harmful, but iodine is powerful so do not add it directly to the food on your plate or your beverages; it would destroy some food value and eventually become toxic.) Do not save the water for later use—it will lose its potency. If you wash so many vegetables that you can no longer see the color of the iodine it has lost its effectiveness. Add another drop.

Keep Lugol's out of reach of children. Keep it in small (½ oz.) dropper bottles as further protection against accidental overdose.

If your Lugol's was not made from scratch, it will probably have wood alcohol or isopropyl alcohol pollution. Be sure to order the dry compounds, not a ready made solution. Your local pharmacist would be glad to help. You will only need diet scales, plastic spoon and cup.

Cautionary Note:

Lugol's iodine can "crawl" out of its bottle even when it is tightly closed! It can stain the sink and counter top. If this happens use vitamin C immediately to make it colorless, then wipe away.

Ozonation

Ozone can kill bacteria and viruses in food and beverages with surprising speed. In less than 10 minutes all the food in your refrigerator could be sterilized. You simply place it all in a plastic bag so the ozone can build up a slight pressure. This pressure will push it to the bottom of a quart container, right through a stick of butter, and right through meat. Of course the containers or packaging should be open to allow the ozone to enter.

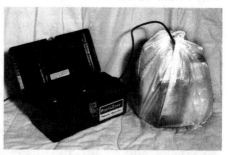

Plastic shopping bag holds groceries and ozonator hose. Ozonating semi-sterilizes and destroys many toxins.

Fig. 123 Ozonating food

The advantage of ozone, besides speed, is that it turns into oxygen and water, leaving no toxicity behind.

Another advantage is that it can do oxidizing chemistry, although this takes more than 10 minutes. The Syncrometer® shows that the estrogens in dairy products (estrone, estriole and estradiol) are destroyed in 15 minutes. Azo dyes sprayed on meats can be destroyed in 15 to 20 minutes. And many phenolic food substances can be destroyed in 15 minutes as well.

Ozone has great penetrating power which Lugol's does not. Lugol's has great attaching ability so surfaces are immediately sterilized. Lugol's does not penetrate. Each property has special value.

> Persons who are allergic to iodine should not use Lugol's. Such allergies develop after a large dose of it has been injected as part of a kidney or thyroid scan. The doctor will warn you about it afterwards. If you are unsure, you could call your doctor's office to check your record.

Sanitizing with ozone only takes 7 minutes. Safety from dyes and other chemicals, including chlorine, takes 10 to 20 minutes. But metals cannot be destroyed. They will always be metals, even though they become oxidized metals. Can motor oil, wheel bearing grease, and PCBs be ozonated? This has not yet been tried.

> Safety from heavy metals is not possible by ozonating them.

After turning off the ozonator, the packages and containers should be closed again. Ozonation continues, on its own, for about 10 more minutes, even while refrigerated.

Immunodepressed persons should ozonate all their food for its sanitizing effect. Excess ozone flavor can be blown away as the food is warmed later. Flavor changes can be compensated with spices and can be reduced by ozonating a shorter time. Do not ozonate supplements, medicines, or herbs.

HCl Food Sanitizer (5% USP)

- 1 drop per cup water

Immerse produce. Agitate food well. Let stand several minutes. No need to rinse; this is edible (but don't put it directly in your mouth).

To kill most bacteria and parasite eggs, and to destroy traces of benzene and PCBs, add several drops directly to any food. Stir the food with a non-metal (hardened plastic) utensil <u>while adding</u>. Although 1 drop per cup is enough for clear liquids, three drops is safer when particles are present or the food is solid. Do not exceed 15 drops per meal, not counting food preparation.

What a Sonicator Can Do

Ultrasonic cleaners have been in use many decades. They are used to clean scientific instruments, even glassware, to a level not possible any other way. Sonicators can be bought in the form of jewelry cleaners. When jewelry is being cleaned, even the oily film of fingerprints comes off. We will use an ordinary jewelry cleaner, of a good size, but with water for the immersion fluid, not a solvent.

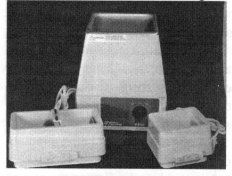

Fig. 124 Jewelry cleaners like these can remove PCBs

The food is placed in a plastic bag and lowered into the tank of water. The unit is turned on for five minutes.

Even PCB and benzene can be removed. In fact, these are chemically destroyed as well! The pounding action of water as a very fine tremor-activity evidently oxidizes the benzene, because the Syncrometer® detects its oxidation product, phenol, after five minutes. Another five minutes of sonication destroys even the phenol. Perhaps the same kind of action destroys PCBs because they "disappear", too. Asbestos also "disappears", presumably shattered. Food that is eaten after it is sonicated for benzene, PCBs and asbestos does not show up in the immune system; this is my guide to toxicity. It is no longer toxic.

But metals cannot be destroyed by sonication. They are elements; their form may be changed to an oxidized or hydrolyzed form, but this does not change the fact that a metal is present. Lanthanide metals are not destroyed either. Only hot water washes can remove these. Azo dyes as a group cannot be destroyed by sonication either. You must rely on hot water washing for these ultra-important immune system toxins.

You can rely on sonication to destroy parasites, their stages, and bacteria even if they are deeply imbedded in meats, bones, or inside cans or packages. Viruses and prions will disappear, too, evidently disrupted by the same shaking action.

Molds on food, together with mycotoxins, are also shaken off and destroyed.

Tiny bits of pituitary gland and hypothalamus that float in eggs and dairy foods are destroyed in 10 minutes, slightly longer than bacteria.

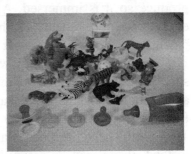

Long sonication can destroy some food phenolics but cannot be relied on.

Clean PCBs off plastic toys and baby things.

Large and small sonicators can be purchased from the

Fig. 125 PCB on plastic

Internet and from *Sources*; the 1½ gallon size is by far the most useful. A five-minute built-in timer is also a great time saver. Avoid the variety that strictly forbids touching the bottom of the tank.

Start with a general kitchen cleanup as soon as you get your sonicator. Clean up baby things first; babies are the most vulnerable. Shake all the PCBs off baby toys, baby bottles and nipples, even though they have already been used and washed. PCBs don't "go away" by washing, they only spread. Sonicate baby medicine, swabs, band-aids, toys. Sonicate your kitchen sponges, your toothbrush and comb, your dentures, and everything else that goes in your mouth (yes, even cigarettes).

Hot Water Washes

Produce has been sprayed a number of times. More laundry bleach with its 5 immune destroyers gets stuck each time. Along with these come asbestos shreds from the conveyor belt, and a waxy coating dried onto the produce with hot air blasts. The result is a coating of PCBs, benzene, asbestos, azo dyes, heavy metals, malonic acid, motor oil, wheel bearing grease, and often water softener salts with uranium.

Run the hottest water you can from your faucet into a large stainless steel bowl used only for this purpose. Add all the produce so it is immersed. After 1 minute, dump it all, rinse everything and repeat. If the fruit has small milky-white patches on it, throw it away; it is pesticide residue.

This will not clean up waxed produce. Do not purchase such food. Certain foods show deep penetration of chemicals and should have 3 hot washes with drying in between. Examples are potatoes, sweet potatoes, carrots, and tomatoes. They still need testing. Purchase from farmers' markets instead, if you can be assured it has not been sprayed against sprouting.

Dried produce needs 2 hot washes as well, such as beans, rice, grains, lentils.

It is convenient to sanitize your produce right after hot washing, using a few drops of Lugol's, HCl, or by ozonating.

So far, we have discussed ways to kill the living invaders in our food. They don't come separate from the nonliving things—the toxins—things that our ancestors did not have to worry about. Now they are always mixed. No single method can do everything. Zappicating food has been added to reduce toxicity, and to improve its biological value. It is a magnetic treatment.

Magnetic Polarization of Food

One of Nature's deepest mysteries is the influence of the earth's magnetic field on our bodies, on our health...perhaps on all living things. Fruit and vegetables, leaves and flowers, even nuts and grains are north polarized when they are freshly picked or purchased. Inside, where the seeds are, the polarization is southerly. But the soft parts begin to age and wilt and show deterioration within a week of being stored in the refrigerator. The northerly polarization is changing to southerly! It happens gradually. A large bunch of grapes will have some turned completely south in a few days, the wrinkled ones, while others are still completely north (the freshest looking ones). The seed does not change its polarization.

My conclusion is that we were meant to eat northerly polarized food, with just a little bit of southerly food in the form of seeds. Yet, most of the food we eat, even refrigerated food, has turned at least partly south. We are getting an overdose of south polarized food as well as water.

That is why I recommend zappicating our food, especially when we are sick.

Zappication

Water that is simply zapped gets electrical energy, just a voltage, impressed on it. We know, from bottle-copying, that water can hold very many frequencies of electrical energy. Food and our bodies are mainly water. Is it the same in food? Such research is badly needed.

Food that is simply put in a magnetic field has magnetic forces impressed on it. We can see that from making north and south polarized water.

Electrical energy even generates magnetic energy and vice versa, so we always receive a dose of both even when only one kind is applied. This, too, needs much more research in our bodies and food.

A third form of energy is physical, as our ears can sense when waves of air pressure reach them. Here we know that frequency is very important because it makes different sounds. Our ears can only hear sound when the frequency is under 20,000 Hz.

The zappicator combines all 3 kinds of energy and delivers them at the same frequency. The voltage from a zapper is attached to an electro magnet which exudes its own magnetic field while pushing a diaphragm back and forth to create a physical effect at the same frequency. What does that do to food? A few things have been noticed, so far:

1. It changes the angle of light that is passing through each molecule of food further to the left if an amino acid is zappicated. The d-amino acids are changed to l-amino acids this way. Remember, the body considers d-amino acids as allergens; it only uses l-forms itself. The food has been improved, not so allergenic, <u>before</u> you eat it. Of course, changes can come <u>after</u> you eat it. It could change back to a d-form in a southerly zone.

2. It changes the polarization of the food to north, if the north side of the magnet faces the food. Food has been made "fresher".

3. Most bacteria, viruses and parasite eggs can't be detected afterwards. Were their growing points disabled by being turned northerly? This could be temporary, if it is reversible, but still useful.

4. Benzene gets oxidized to phenol, at least at trace levels. PCBs disappear, no doubt slightly changed, an important step, nevertheless.

5. Phenolic food antigens disappear if the correct frequency is used. Many are affected between 1000 and 1010 Hz. Perhaps they were oxidized further. The body could choose to reduce them again or make something equally toxic, but the ability to make food less allergenic beckons again.

6. A zappicator placed on plastic teeth in your mouth, instead of food, stops seeping of plastic, dyes, or malonic acid

from them. Did it complete the polymerization process, or harden it all in some other way?

7. Placed on a cancerous lump on the skin, it seems to shrink in 24 hours. But much more improvement is needed in strength of magnet, and protection from stray south fields before you could experiment safely.

8. Finally, food seems to taste better. Maybe changing d- to l-amino acids or alpha to beta forms or L- to D-sugars can be tasted. These are all effects of zappication. Only more research can tell us.

Again, we must not demonize the opposite polarization. It is part of us, too, just as the seed belongs to the fruit. But much greater care is needed in handling south pole forces. Notice how nature has its south pole seed securely encased. Don't do south polarization experiments till you have gained much experience with northerly ones.

Research on food and water…finding what is good for us and what is bad, has barely begun. Food is fascinating, all the more when we're hungry. As a species we are very hungry. Perhaps we would only need half as much food if it was correctly polarized for our bodies, and at the same time give us much more energy than we have now. With these purposes in mind, make yourself a zappicator (page 493) but don't throw away the Ancient Ways yet. Don't rely solely on new ways.

Zappicate food 10 minutes. Zappicate eggs and dairy foods 15 minutes or more. Check the polarity of your zappicator with a compass once a week. Some magnets can change their polarity by being heated, dropped, or wetted. Best of all, test the results in your food with a Syncrometer®.

Selecting your Recipes

Get to know yourself. From your cancer location you can find your allergen. Use the *Food Table* on page 36 to find foods that don't have this allergen. Notice, that overall there are about 50 times as many *N's* as *P's*. But, once you find your culprit food, you might realize you were eating it much too often. Strengthen your resolve to kill all F. buski as fast as detox-symptoms will allow, to stop new allergies. And to get the nickel and Salmonella out of your body as soon as possible, too. Meanwhile find old cookbooks with recipes made from scratch.

A very good rule is not to eat the same food twice in a day or two days in a row. Have your refrigerator full of food, go shopping a lot, have help cooking; it is not a luxury when you have serious illness, <u>it is necessary</u>.

Kitchen Necessities

- several sets of stainless steel saucepans
- a blender, only if tested for metal seepage
- an ozonator
- a bread maker without Teflon coating
- stainless steel and HDPE♲ cutlery and utensils
- stainless steel bowls, meat platters, graters, funnels
- food grinder (use for less than 4 seconds at a time)
- dishes, glasses, cups and storage containers of HDPE♲ or high impact plastic that you have tested
- a conductivity indicator (see page 581).
- large and small zippered plastic bags without color or odor, nor laundry bleach disinfectant (have them tested)
- 2 filter pitchers with tested, and later boiled, charcoal. This is to get the last bit of strontium, ruthenium, and aluminum out of your water.

Test all items that will have food contact with the conductivity indicator before purchasing more.

To <u>cook</u>, use stainless steel only. To fry use stainless steel or iron skillet, not Teflon coated. To warm food, use boiling water so the temperature reaches boiling point, not higher. Higher temperatures oxidize our minerals to metal!

To store food, use HDPE♲ and stainless steel containers. Make temporary bowls and place settings from water jugs.

Going Shopping

Shop for kosher foods whenever possible. Search for these symbols: □, K, ☆. Shop for Asian imports. This still does not guarantee their safety. Don't shop for anything in glass bottles unless you can test for thallium. That is a major seeped metal from both amber and clear glass.

Organic produce has much less <u>dye</u> and <u>pesticide</u> pollution than regular produce, but only if the local water, used to spray on the shelf for freshness, is not the laundry bleach kind. Asbestos tufts adhering to the outside of foods is just as severe a problem, though. When I tested some farmers' market produce, it was free of asbestos. Search for <u>organic produce at farmers' markets</u>. Potatoes and sweet potatoes, not sprayed against sprouting or greased against wilting, would be a rare find. The others have malonic acid deep inside. Next best might be a small corner grocery store. Ask which day their produce arrives to get it fresh.

No foods are safe, though, unless cleaned up with hot washes and later sterilized. Do not buy a spray that removes spray, either; the one I tested had more solvents than the original sprayed food.

Dessert and Tea

Many recipes call for safe sweetener. Choose yours with the help of the *Food Table*. Also see page 36.

Citric Tangerine Dessert

- 2 tangerines
- 2 citric acid capsules
- 1 tsp. safe sweetener
- heavy whipping cream (*optional*)

Hot wash tangerines and save peels in freezer. They have health value. Place tangerines in zippered plastic bag or other non-seeping container. Add citric acid and sweetener. Mash and mix with stainless steel whip or roll over the bag with a glass jar. Top with cream.

Lettuce A'la Crème – A TV Snack

- the greenest head lettuce you can find, with many loose outer leaves
- 2 citric acid capsules
- ¼ cup heavy whipping cream
- sodium-potassium salt (*optional*)

Peel away many loose lettuce leaves to get away from sprays. Dip head in Lugol's water for 3 minutes. Add citric acid to whipping cream in a HDPE♻ bowl. Tear pieces of lettuce off the head (don't cut) and dip into the sour or salty cream.

Coconut - Tangerine Juice

- milk of one fresh coconut (give the meat away)
- 2 tangerines

At a certain time of year the new coconut crop is in. The meat is soft and the "milk" plentiful. If someone would crack and clean it for you, you could consume one a week. Until you are well you must have the "milk" only; the "meat" has too much plant oil for your digestion. Nevertheless, you will be getting both organic germanium and selenium. Peel the tangerines after 2 hot washes. Save the peels in the freezer for future flavoring. Pour the milk into a blender. Add the tangerines, seeds and all. Blend 4 seconds only. Immediately strain through steel strainer. Do not store this; drink immediately. *Optional:* To make a slurpee out of this, add a piece of frozen banana before blending.

Hydrangea Tea (as organic germanium)

- ½ cup hydrangea root, (c/s), organic
- 3 cups pure water
- stainless steel strainer

Soak the dried roots at least 4 hours to get the maximum goodness out of them. Then simmer for ½ hour at low heat in a stainless steel pan. Let cool and strain into a HDPE🔺 container for storage. Test for inorganic germanium, it should not be there. Several sips provides one dose of germanium for the *3-Week Program*. Add sweetener to taste.

Brazil Nut Split (as organic germanium, selenium)

- 1 whole nut in the shell
- sturdy nutcracker
- 1 frozen banana
- whipping cream, heavy, kosher, ozonated

Crack the nut when you are ready to use it. Choose a different nut if it is discolored or doesn't taste good after nibbling. Scrape away blemishes. Place frozen banana on stainless steel platter or HDPE🔺 dish. Dribble whipping cream over the banana. Before it freezes sprinkle ground Brazil nut over cream. Grind it by pounding in a plastic zippered bag or rolling it with a jar. All nuts have germanium and selenium, but eating more than one large nut a day challenges your digestion of linolenic acid.

Rose Hips Tea (as organic vitamin C)

- 1 tsp. rose hips, coarse ground, with seeds, organic
- 1 cup water
- sweetener or heavy whipping cream

Bring water to a boil in stainless steel saucepan. Add rose hips, cover, and remove from heat. When cool pour into safe cup and drink right away. This can replace one dose of the capsules plus vitamin C capsules in the program. You may add sweetener or whipping cream to taste.

Banana Split (as organic vitamin C)

- 1 frozen banana
- 2 tbsp. heavy whipping cream
- 1 tsp. rose hips, coarse ground

Place banana in HDPE⬦ bowl. While frozen, pour on the whipping cream. Before this freezes, sprinkle on the rose hips. Add sweetener if desired. You may add nuts to rose hips.

Santa Split

- 1 large or 2 small frozen bananas
- ¼ cup heavy whipping cream, kosher
- 1 tsp. anise seed, stored in freezer

Place banana in HDPE⬦ bowl. While frozen, pour on whipping cream. Before it freezes, sprinkle on anise seed. **Variations**: 1 tsp. frozen tangerine peel. It is easy to decorate with these spices to form a snowman.

Lettuce - Nut Salad

Use Romaine lettuce or Bok Choy. These need sanitizing after removing outer leaves. A 5 minute dip in Lugol's water or the routine ozonation is enough.

- lettuce, 1 head
- 1 Brazil nut or 4 Hazel nuts
- ¼ cup heavy whipping cream
- 2 capsules citric acid
- sodium-potassium salt (*optional*)

Tear the lettuce into tiny pieces. Add citric acid to cream in a HDPE⚠ bowl. Pour over the lettuce. Sprinkle on the pounded or ground nuts (grind or pound nuts by hand or with a jar or a can rolled over the nuts in a zippered bag).

Barley Water

This is an ancient "medicine". It has organic manganese.
• whole barley

Add 4 times as much water as barley and let stand at least 4 hours. Decant and drink. Cooking changes it to plain manganese metal that feeds Shigella.

Tapioca - Barley Pudding

Put into a 2 quart pan.
• 1½ cups water
• ⅓ cup small tapioca pearls (see *Sources*)
• 1½ teaspoons whole barley (grind first for 3 seconds)

Soak the above for one hour, then add:
• 1 ⅓ cups water
• 2 cups heavy whipping cream, tested, ozonated
• ½ to ⅔ cup safe sweetener (*optional*)
• ¼ to ⅓ cup pure maple syrup (*optional*)
• ¼ tsp. salt (*optional*)

Bring to a boil and let boil for only one minute, stirring constantly with a stainless steel spoon. *Optional*: Add contents of two nutmeg capsules and a tsp. of the spice mix below. Serve warm or cold. Makes approximately eight 4 oz. servings. *Note*: For thinner consistency use ½ cup more water.
Spice Mix
• 1 tsp. coriander seeds
• 1 tsp. cardamom seeds
• 1 tsp. anise seeds

Grind 3 seconds; then let grinder blades cool and grind another 3 seconds. Store in freezer to keep potency.

Spice Mix Straight

These spices (above) can be chewed whole; no grinding needed if your teeth are up to it. Adding sweetener or whipping cream makes it a dessert to be nibbled on for hours. A few detox-symptoms next day will be a real reward.

Burdock Tea

This is called an herb, but it is too delicious and flavorful for this simple label.

- 2 tbsp. burdock root, organic, (c/s)
- 1¼ cups water

Bring water to boil in stainless steel saucepan. Add burdock and turn down heat to simmer, covered. Simmer for about 20 min. Cool. While it is cooling, it will turn sweetish, and the grounds will settle. Then you can pour it off without a strainer. It is so good straight, nothing needs to be added. Even the "grounds" are good, spooned up with syrup. Do not make herb teas in the microwave. Some organic germanium would get destroyed and phenolics that should be destroyed would escape. Burdock fights E. coli.

Eucalyptus Tea

This tea is too flavorful to be considered an herbal tea, provided you can pick it off the tree! Most important…it does not need to be tested for thallium or other pesticide. There are several varieties. Gather:

- 5 long leaves or 10 short-variety leaves
- 2 inches of twig (that holds the leaves)
- a marble size piece of bark, if available

Rinse under faucet and place in stainless steel pan. Add 2 ¼ cups water. Bring to a boil, covered. Then turn down heat to simmer for 10 minutes. Cool. Notice the beautiful red color it develops and delicious aroma. You may add whipping cream. During a cold or cough, sip it throughout the day for 2 days (if it lasts that long). It is the only herb, besides oregano (oil) that I have found can kill Clostridium bacteria.

There are many other herbs used to improve health, discussed in this book. Make these as teas, adding whatever makes them enjoyable. Do not combine them unless they are traditionally combined. They could destroy each other. You need the extra liquid, besides, to stimulate more urine flow.

About Eggs

In earlier books I gave egg recipes, knowing they had malvin and gallic acid allergens, and knowing they had hypothalamus and pituitary cells afloat in them. I thought they could be made safe with special treatments. But since then I have found the MYC virus, the SV 40 virus and sometimes even OPT itself in eggs. It makes no sense to eat them anymore. Not all eggs have all of these. It probably depends on the animal waste and soy products in their feed. Free-range chickens could present a different picture. But without testing by Syncrometer®, it seems to me to be quite unwise to eat either chickens or eggs. Eggs in Mexico were free of the contaminants found in USA eggs, but should still be tested for allergens.

About Milk

When cows were free and roamed in meadows of grass and flowers, they produced a moderate amount of milk, a moderate amount of manure and money and a large amount of health in growing children.

But now they are fed quite unnatural food (soybeans, yeast culture, carbohydrates) to increase milk production. These processed concentrates and even the water at the dairy, now give her daily doses of laundry bleach. In fact, dairymen are encouraged to pour <u>extra</u> bleach into their water trough, and it is not the NSF kind. Now cows are becoming immunodepressed, like humans, getting recurrent mastitis and necessitating lots of antibiotics. They, too, develop increased parasitism. We would expect many "Flu" attacks as a cow's body manages to kill its own flukes. But cows also get more than their share of digestion problems, so that allergies would be expected. PGE2 from allergy attacks would trigger prions to emerge from her Salmonella bacteria. She could be expected to get prion protein attacks, periods of dizziness, loss of appetite or staggering. Cows with chronic Salmonella could develop chronic prion disease, which could explain BSE. Lowered productivity as a goal(!) for cows seems like an intelligent

solution, so all these trends can be reversed while it is still possible.

With a heavily parasitized cow we would expect to see Bacillus cereus and tyramine in her milk. And we always do, even in cheese and all other dairy products. Nutmeg kills these bacteria.

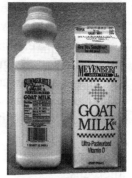

Switching to goat milk by sick people is another intelligent solution, to reduce allergens obtained from cow's milk.

Fig. 126 Popular varieties of goat milk

Even goat milk provides more lactose than can be quickly digested. We use only heavy whipping cream on the program and even this will get treated with lactase enzyme to remove the tiny bit left in it. After you are well, goat milk, limited to 1 cup a day, would be a boon to your nutrition.

Plain Goat Milk

There is no way of knowing whether a dairy is using laundry bleach to sanitize equipment or NSF-bleach, or steam, or old fashioned Lugol's iodine. For this reason you should send a sample to a Syncrometer® tester before becoming a milk consumer.

C - Milk

- milk
- vitamin C powder
- nutmeg

Cold milk can absorb a lot of vitamin C without curdling or affecting the flavor. Try ½ tsp. vitamin C and a pinch of nutmeg in a HDPE⬢ "glass" of ice cold goat milk.

Buttermilk - C

Mix equal amounts of heavy whipping cream and ultra pasteurized goat milk. Stir in 1½ tsp. vitamin C powder per 8 oz. glass. Add $^1/_8$ capsule of nutmeg powder, zappicate. If it does not form flakes readily, add ¼ tsp. citric acid per glass. **Citric acid kills Salmonella bacteria.**

Raw Certified Milk

Undoubtedly, fresh goat milk is the most nutritious food in existence for a young, sickly or allergic child. But don't use it unless you can find which disinfectant is being used at the farm. Have <u>your</u> milk streamed straight into a HDPE⬢ water jug. Cut away the part across from the handle to make this easy for the milker. Or purchase a milking bucket designated only for your child—test it yourself for seeping metal. Supply the strainer and strainer holder yourself, too, selected for <u>no conductivity of their soak waters</u>. Do not use plastic or throw-away strainers. Make your own from a paper towel or double cheese cloth, squeezed clean under the hot faucet. Then dip in Lugol's water and place in strainer or funnel. Make your own funnel from another HDPE⚠ jug.

After straining into a fresh jug add 1 drop Lugol's and 1 drop HCl to each cup (without measuring) while stirring. The Lugol's should be made from scratch, not bought ready made.

Except for this special circumstance Lugol's should not be added directly to food.

5-Minute Raspberry Ice Cream

Why buy ready made ice cream when homemade is twice as delicious?

- 1 pint heavy whipping cream previously treated with ¼ capsule lactase enzyme for several hours and ozonated
- 1 carton raspberries from a farmers' market, disinfected with a drop of Lugol's in a cup of water, then <u>frozen</u>
- ½ cup safe sweetener
- wheat germ (freshly opened, nitrogen packed)
- nuts (optional)

Dump frozen raspberries into blender. Pour whipping cream and sweetener over them. Blend for 4 seconds (only). Pour it all into a stainless steel bowl, already chilled in freezer. Don't clean the blades. Quickly sprinkle wheat germ or ground nuts over the top. Cover with close fitting zippered bag and place in freezer. Prepare it a day ahead. Try using other frozen fruit like blueberries, peaches, strawberries. Raspberries have a special anti-cancer factor, **ellagic** acid, as do Brazil nuts. Freeze many pints.

Pear Slush

- 1 large pear
- 1 tbsp. safe sweetener
- $^1/_8$ tsp. citric acid
- 1 tbsp. water

Double hot wash the pear. Peel and cut away the stem and flower end, leaving no blemishes. Place in blender with sweetener, water, citric acid, seeds and all (pear seeds are powerful virus killers). Blend 4 seconds (only). Scoop into chilled stainless steel sherbet servers and freeze inside a large zippered bag. Serve frozen. **Variations**: Add topping of pounded or rolled nuts and whipping cream. *Note*: Use any other raw fruit desired, but always add the citric acid.

Complete Meal Drinks

When a meal is missed weight is lost and the body is stressed. During dental work, especially, weight is easily lost that cannot be regained. Every effort should be made to keep up the usual calorie intake. You can make a drinkable "meal" that needs no preparation, and provides the fat, protein, and carbohydrate essential for life. The principles are:

(1) no vegetable oil to avoid triggering oncoviruses

(2) no eggs or milk

• ½ cup heavy whipping cream

• ½ cup water or barley water

• 1 tbsp. safe sweetener

• 5 capsules mixed amino acids (read label for phenylalanine or tryptophane presence in case you must avoid these). This is the protein source. **Variations**: ½ capsule nutmeg, 1 tsp. clove tea, 1 tsp. hydrangea tea, or any other spice, ground nuts.

Stir all together. The whipping cream should already have been treated (overnight) with ¼ capsule lactase per pint, then ozonated. Take lipase-containing digestive enzymes with this. Change the spice at each meal.

CALORIES: 477

Salt

Plain Salt

Use <u>pure</u> salt only (see *Sources*), like for laboratory use. Grocery store salt and sea salt as well as other kinds of salt have processing contaminants, not to mention aluminum additives, and often have Ascaris eggs and mold.

Two To One Sodium - Potassium Salt

- 2 cups pure salt
- 1 cup potassium chloride

Mix. Store in tightly closed HDPE jar with barley added to absorb moisture. Label. Use in a saltshaker. If you don't mind the taste, a one-to-one mixture is even more beneficial.

B - C Salt

This is the easy way to get vitamin B_2 and vitamin C into all your food:

- ½ cup pure salt or sodium-potassium salt
- 1 capsule vitamin B_2
- ½ tsp. vitamin C (ascorbic acid) powder (also try 1 tsp.)

Shake together in HDPE bottle or non-seeping jar. Zappicate. When using this salt in cooking, wait until the end to add it, to preserve its vitamin power.

Sweetening

All granulated forms of all sugar varieties I purchased at USA grocery stores or health food stores had asbestos fibers and D-mannitol in them!

Organic sugar from Paraguay and Mexican sugars did not have asbestos.

Sucrose purchased from a chemical supply company did not have asbestos, nor D-mannitol or other pollutants.

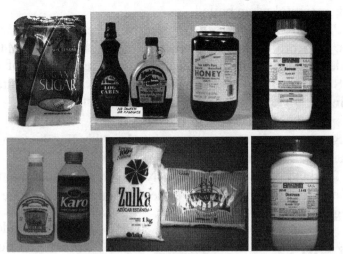

Organic sugar from Paraguay, maple syrup, locally produced honey, sucrose (crystal N.F. grade), agave syrup, dark Karo syrup, two Mexican sugars, and dextrose.

Fig. 127 Safer sweetening

Honey had asbestos fibers except when locally produced. Clover honey routinely had coumarin allergen. Orange blossom honey had many allergens.

All honey has fructose, normally a desirable form of sugar if not overdone. But fructose is the antigen for RBCs and should be *avoided in blood cancers* and *liver failure*.

Honey should be tested for strontium, beryllium, vanadium and chromium, air pollutants that land on flowers.

Maple syrup very frequently has gallic acid. Boiling 1 minute destroys it. Very many varieties have ASA; test yours.

Dextrose is a "powdered sugar" variety. It is usually made from corn and carries corn antigen as well as air pollutants strontium and beryllium with it. Dextrose is the sugar used in IV solutions. They should be tested for strontium, beryllium and corn antigen..

Agave syrup often has caffeic acid and cinnamic acid, but boiling destroys both. However, it also has fructose which yields mannitol when boiled.

Plain fruit juices can be used as sweeteners. But when Yeast is a problem even plain and natural sugars should be avoided. *Always avoid in breast and skin cancers.*

Sorghum mold is a fungus that grows in many of our organs; it gives us tiny red "blood blisters" and I believe it is responsible for strokes in the elderly.

Sonication destroys asbestos; it also kills Sorghum mold, present in all natural sweeteners.

The land of sweets is obviously strewn with land mines. If you are living dangerously, at least minimize each one by changing the variety at every meal.

Spreads

Real Butter

Use butter for baking and all other purposes, not oil. Find undyed, organic, kosher butter. Ozonate the whole pound for 10 minutes after opening each quarter; then plop it into a bowl of cold water for 5 minutes to draw out metals. Turn after 5 minutes for another treatment, since it floats.

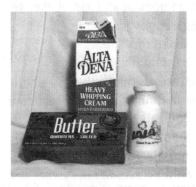

No wrong bleach in this food. Lala is Mexican cream. The glass bottle does not seep, either!

Fig. 128 Safe butter and cream

It is fortunate if you can still find a butter without laundry bleach disinfectant. Choose several for testing by Syncrometer®.

If you can't test, ozonate it, boil it, or do both (if you are very sick). Never eat fake butter, as in margarine. Nickel is used as a catalyst to make it!

Do not use special grease-sprays, they contain silicones which accumulate in tumors.

If you are stuck on an airplane or stranded, put one drop Lugol's on your real butter, mix it well. Put another tiny drop on each other food you are served, as well as in the water. This is the second exception when you may put Lugol's in a food.

Homemade Butter

- 1 pint heavy whipping cream, already treated with lactase, and ozonated.

Pour it into a polyethylene jar or one you tested and found not to seep. Cover with zippered plastic bag before using the lid. (Do not use stretchable wraps; they leach furiously). Leave enough empty space in the jar to shake the cream.

Shake for 5 minutes. Soon the cream feels "thick". It gets thicker and thicker until suddenly it all separates into butter and buttermilk. Keep shaking a few more minutes till a solid ball of butter is formed.

Pour off the buttermilk. Don't consume this. Throw it out. It contains the extracted dyes, asbestos and heavy metals that may have been in the cream.

Add very cold water and shake again to "wash" the butter until the water remains clear. Finally, sculpt the butter and place on a safe serving dish or in a HDPE♲ jar. Makes about ¼ pound.

Preserves

- 1 cup fruit
- 1 tbsp. water
- ¼ tsp. citric acid
- sweetening

Soak fruit twice for one minute in very hot water to remove dye, asbestos and malonic acid. Peel if possible. Heat to boiling in water, stirring with stainless steel spoon. When done, add half as much sweetening as there is fruit and bring to boil again. Cool. Zappicate.

Fruit is often unevenly ripened. This changes its nature. I suspect this is the reason that bad chemicals like phloridzin and chlorogenic acid appear in them. Save such fruit for cooking, as in jams or jellies because this destroys these phenolics.

Dressings

Queen of Hearts Dressing (takes all supplements)

Fruit juices are easily made into dressings for many purposes, over vegetables, over rice, and even over a pile of vitamins dumped from their capsules.

- 1 cup fruit juice
- ½ tsp. (or more) citric acid powder
- 1 tbsp. sweetening
- 2 tbsp. thickener (rose hips, hydrangea powder, vitamins)
- extra spice (thyme, turmeric, fennel, nutmeg, oregano)

The first concern is ripeness of the fruit. Always boil the fruit juice first. Add citric acid. The citric acid provides tartness equivalent to lemon juice and at the same time destroys traces of leftover caffeic acid while killing Salmonella bacteria. The second concern is D-mannitol from the sweetening. It develops into Nerve Growth Factor (NGF), a neurological allergen. Test for this. A third concern is spice potency. Bulk powders <u>always</u> lose potency unless kept in <u>freezer</u> as soon as purchased. Capsules are largely protected.

Add juice to thickener in small amounts, while stirring, to make a paste first. Then add the remainder to the thickness desired. The thickener can be any assortment of dry supplements that needs to "go down" at that meal. By keeping the fruit juice and citric acid mixture always handy and varied, any pile of vitamin powders can be consumed the easy way: on top of a lettuce salad.

Finally, add sweetening, citric acid, and spice to taste, rotating them, to avoid allergies.

Tomato Sauce

Choose perfect cherry tomatoes because they do not produce malvin and are often unsprayed. Sterilize with Lugol's water or ozonate.

- 2 cups whole tomatoes
- ½ cup water
- ¼ tsp. sodium-potassium salt
- 1 tsp. oregano leaves, organic, or fresh (garden)

Purchased oregano needs testing for thallium and other spray residues. Bring all ingredients to a hard boil for 2 or 3 minutes in a stainless steel saucepan. Empty this into a polyethylene container as soon as cool enough. Keep refrigerated or frozen. Keep oregano frozen, too. You can use a manual "food mill" to separate peels, seeds, etc. (see *Sources*).

Sour Cream - C

- 2 cups heavy whipping cream, already treated
- ¼ tsp. citric acid
- ¼ tsp. vitamin C powder
- pinch of pure salt

Stir until smooth. Refrigerate two hours before serving.

Baked Goods

Bake cookies, cakes and pies from scratch, using unprocessed ingredients. Do not use paper cupcake cups, the wax coating has benzene. Do not use aluminum baking pans, bowls, measuring spoons, or foil wrapping. Do not use

543

stretchable plastic film. Do not use plastic or wood utensils; use stainless steel. Use aluminum-free baking powder, pure salt, and butter instead of oils.

Cereals

Barley is the best choice, because it does not have menadione, even when stale. Other cereal grains should be nitrogen packed to avoid developing menadione. Store in freezer after opening. Do not ozonate, to avoid oxidation.

Choose only the coarse-ground varieties to avoid nickel and chromium contamination from the grinding blades. Don't risk this with breast cancer.

Corn is a poor choice because it picks up air pollutants like strontium, beryllium, vanadium, chromium, each of which feeds an important pathogen.

Maria's Best Pancakes

- 32 ounces of Bob's Red Mill rice flour
- 1 stick of butter *(Trader Joe's salted, turquoise package)*
- 2 eggs
- ½ tbsp. vitamin C
- 1 tsp. salt
- 1 tbsp. baking soda
- ²/₃ to ¾ cup of heavy cream *(Lala crema Pura de Vaca brand in Mexico)*
- raisins *(Fairfield)*
- 24½ oz. water *(depending on consistency)*

Combine all ingredients (except water) in large bowl. Mix together then add water to desired consistency.

Fish and Seafood Recipes

Since all varieties of fish and seafood had Fast Garnet dye and "shrimp" antigen (*the cause of lymphomas and lymph node metastases*) these recipes have been omitted. But you may fish it yourself and eat it within 6 hours. Don't use "household" laundry bleach to clean up, nor buy fish at a fish market.

Beans, Dried Peas, Lentils, and Garbanzos

In the uncooked state, these have no onion chemicals. But if they are cooked at too high a temperature many onion sulfides are made. They must not be heated higher than boiling water. This excludes steaming, frying, pressure cooking, microwaving. When they are warmed up later, they must again not be heated higher than boiling water. Valuable, nutritionally, as they are, I consider them too hazardous for cancer patients.

Meats

Sanitation of meats is quick and easy now that sonication and ozonation are available to penetrate deep into the interior. Safety from laundry bleach treatment can be found by testing with a Syncrometer®. But the extra dye used everywhere now and unsaturated oils dispersed in the meat create almost unsolvable problems. USA animals have been fed unsaturated oils, gallate-sprayed grains and given laundry bleached water to drink, like their owners.

Heightened parasitism is seen in chickens and beef. The animals seem sickly, judging by frequent antibiotic use (read the ads in animal feed stores), and not fit for consumption even by a healthy person. Four kinds of free-range raised (vegetarian) animals did not show these weaknesses:

(1) free-range, organic turkey
(2) free-range lamb
(3) free-range beef
(4) buffalo

Bone Marrow - Beef Broth

Buying long bones cut into short pieces where the bone marrow can be gotten out brings you **lactoferrin**, much needed in anemia and bone marrow disease (blood cancers). It is one of the few "meats" that is not dyed in the USA. But you should ozonate it anyway.

Part of the fat in the bone marrow of regular beef will be the unsaturated oils, linolenic and linoleic acid. You should avoid these if you have respiratory diseases because they are the triggers for some of these viruses. Stick to the free-range varieties or wait till your coughing is gone.

- 3 or 4 beef bones, cut to expose the bone marrow
- ½ lb. of an inexpensive cut of beef, including sinews, gristle, cartilage
- 1 bay leaf, tested
- sodium-potassium salt (to taste)
- HCl, 5 drops

Treat bones and meat in original package in sonicator, or ozonate for 10 minutes. Place meat in large stainless steel pan. Save bones for later addition. Cover with cold water. Bring to boil. Remove and discard foam that develops at first during cooking, using stainless steel or HDPE🏠 spoon.

Now switch to HDPE🏠 spoon (stainless steel will stain with HCl drops). Add other ingredients and cook till done (about 1 hour). Add bones and cook five minutes more. Cool. Eat some bone marrow as soon as cool enough. (If it is absolutely delectable, eat the whole thing and make more in a few days.) Pour off the broth into HDPE🏠 container. Drink one cup a day. Refrigerate. If fat solidifies at the top, do not throw this away. It belongs with the broth. Reheat it daily so it can be mixed. **Variations**: Make a cream soup out of leftovers: choose a vegetable, seasoning herb, like thyme, and lastly add cream.

Vegetables and Fruits

Most are sprayed with combinations of wax, dye, pesticide (thallium!), antisprouter, antimold, etc. Azo dyes (Fast Green and Fast Garnet) are present in most sprays, as are heavy metals and malonic acid. They penetrate the food deeply. But double soaking in hot water for one minute each time removes it. Even organic pears, plums and oranges must be double soaked this way. Peeling is not sufficient. Potatoes and yams will not come clean, though. Thallium pesticide and malonic acid penetrate too deeply to come out. If you have leg pain (caused by thallium), or effusions, shop only at a farmers' market and test even these.

Ozonate produce to destroy leftover traces of dyes.

Parasite Killer Recipes

Detox-Tea

Prion protein is present in all of us, repeatedly, as our bodies kill Salmonella bacteria. Our WBCs eat prions promptly. But if our WBCs do not have enough germanium, selenite, and vitamin C, the prions are not killed but escape and enter the brain and nerves. Light headedness and disorientation is felt. That contributes to detox-illness. You can kill them in hours with:

- 1 tsp. fennel seed (freshly ground)
- 1 tsp. sage, organic, (freshly ground)
- 3 heaping tsp. birch bark
- 1 tbsp. sweetener
- 3 cups water

All herbs should be tested for thallium and laundry bleach. Thallium pesticide is often used in foreign countries.

Birch bark is the strongest prion killer and could be used alone. Make birch bark tea by adding to boiling water and then simmering for 5 minutes. Add other ingredients to the birch bark tea. Set to cool. Drink 1 to 3 cups a day. **Variation**: Reishi mushroom, unboiled, instead of birch bark. Make fennel-sage tea. Let cool, add 1 tsp. Reishi, also called Ganoderma.

Parasite Punch

By killing parasites in different ways you reach them in different places. Note how vulnerable they are, when common herbs can kill them. You do not need all of these. Each herb kills some.

- 1 tsp. hydrangea powder
- 1 tsp. cloves (freshly ground)
- 1 tsp. nutmeg powder
- 3 drops wintergreen oil
- 3 drops sage oil, Clary
- 3 drops peppermint oil
- 3 drops juniper oil
- 3 drops frankincense
- 3 drops coriander oil
- 3 drops cardamom oil
- 6 oz. tea made from Pau d' Arco bark, cooled
- 6 oz. tea made from mullein leaf, organic, cooled
- ¼ cup water or heavy whipping cream
- 10 capsules wormwood (200-300 mg per capsule)

Test all items for thallium and laundry bleach. Leave out untested items and those that are allergenic to your cancer.

Place the powders in a tall HDPE♲ "glass", except wormwood. Add the drops of herbal oils. Then add the liquids, while stirring, to make an enjoyable beverage. Add heavy whipping cream and sweetener to taste. Zappicate each item or the final beverage. Wormwood is bitter. You might prefer to leave it in capsules.

All oils can be substituted with 1 tsp. powder of the same herb. All powders can be emptied from capsules; they will be fresher than bulk supplies. Use only coarse ground varieties. Add more water if you use more powder.

If you are missing some ingredients, simply leave them out. Add them later when you do have them.

Drink this once a day for one week within 15 minutes (not while driving). Then cut the dosages in half and later in quarters when you are much healthier. Leave out anything you don't tolerate well. Expect detox-illness and minor symptoms, letting you know it works.

Pau D'Arco has several other names, including Lapacho and Taheebo.

If some of these herbs are already being taken in different ways, omit them here.

Buski Tea

- 1 tsp. anise seeds
- 1 tsp. coriander seeds
- 1 tsp. fennel seeds
- 2 cups pure water
- ½ tsp. whole cloves
- 4 capsules nutmeg
- 1 cup barley water
- sweetener

Make barley water recipe first and refrigerate. Add seeds to pure water and simmer 10 minutes (longer times lose activity). Add cloves and remove from heat. When cool, add cold barley water and nutmeg and sweetener. Refrigerate. Strain 1 cup to drink and put back solids. Next day, repeat. On 3rd and 4th day, eat the solids, with extra sweetener if desired. This tea reaches leftover Fasciolopis in "unreachable" places like eye muscles, jawbone, spine, so expect minor pain here and protect yourself from detox-illness. If no detox is felt, take the 4 cups closer together until you can feel the effects.

Be sure all spices are tested; store them in freezer.

Spice Tea

- ½ tsp. whole cloves or 6 capsules
- 1 tsp. anise seed
- 1 tsp. turmeric powder
- 1 tsp. coriander seed
- 1 tsp. cardamom seed

- 1 tsp. fennel seed or 6 capsules
- ¾ tsp. nutmeg, ground
- 2½ cups barley water
- 1 cup pure water

Combine anise, coriander, cardamom and other seeds in grinder and grind 4 seconds or by hand. Add to boiling water and remove from heat. Add cloves or empty capsules. Add turmeric. Add cold barley water.

Strain one cupful through stainless steel strainer and return the solids to the saucepan; refrigerate.

Add a safe sweetening to the cup of tea. Sip over 1 hour. This is one day's portion. Next day, strain another cupful and sip as before; do not reboil.

Finally, you may eat the solids, one-half the first day and the remainder on the next day.

This tea can activate the liver to produce a green bowel movement. Even "gallstones" may appear. You may add other spices or hide supplements in this tea. It kills a variety of parasites, bacteria and viruses. Protect yourself from detox-illness. Test all spices beforehand.

Buski Bait

This is the strongest (raw) version of the spice recipes. You will need strong teeth to match your will. Take detox protection and feed your WBCs all day, too.

- ¼ tsp. whole cloves
- 1 tsp. anise seed
- 1 tsp. coriander seed
- 1 tsp. cardamom seed
- 1 tsp. fennel seed
- 2 capsules nutmeg
- 1 - 6 capsules turmeric
- sweetener
- 1 tsp. uncooked barley (ground)
- wormwood capsules

- 2 tsp. Black Walnut tincture (optional)

Grind the seeds and cloves together for 4 seconds (only) or by hand. Dump into safe jar. Add remaining powders, except wormwood, and enough straight sweetener to make a paste. Nibble it all raw, bit by bit till gone—it could take 6 hours. Take 9 wormwood capsules several times during this period, chasing it down with 2 tsp. BWT each time.

Keep a flashlight and plastic cup and fork handy on the toilet tank to capture what you might suspect, and Lugol's drops to sterilize it. Take detox protection.

Six Fresh Seeds

- 6 large apricots OR 6 peaches OR nectarines (in order of effectiveness)

Let them completely ripen if you have time.

After two hot washes, remove the pits, saving the fruit to cook thoroughly for other uses.

To crack open pits: find a rock or piece of cement brick. Slide it into a zippered plastic bag. Position it in your sink over the drain. Or, if you are near a cement sidewalk, slip the 6 pits into a double zippered plastic bag. Procure a heavy hammer. After cracking the pits, remove the seeds and place in grinder. If you are very sick choose the larger seeds, at least the size of your thumbnail. Adding the following is optional:

- ¼ tsp. nutmeg
- ¼ tsp. ground barley
- 3 tsp. shredded coconut or flakes

Grind 1 tbsp. whole barley first for 4 seconds (only) in coffee grinder and store in freezer. Grind all ingredients together for 3 seconds only. Eat it all within one hour. The raw barley provides the drying effect that keeps fresh seeds from clogging the grinder and brings organic manganese.

It may be thought that amygdalin or "laetrile" is the active ingredient, but there is no evidence for this. Clinical trials got stalled decades ago after finding it promising against cancer. Amygdalin keeps its potency but the active ingredient in this recipe does not.

Apricot kernels in health food stores have lost their potency, in spite of refrigeration, so you must prepare your own. Do not crack these pits ahead of time nor store seeds, although you may store pits. The Syncrometer® finds that the active ingredient is <u>already a part of our metabolism</u>, somewhat like a vitamin, and in similarly small amounts. It is not yet identified, chemically. Sick organs have none. The correct amount is essential for us but large amounts are toxic, somewhat like trace elements and hormones. I have not seen any side-effects. Nevertheless, do not take more. Six Fresh Seeds can single handedly kill SV 40, Fasciolopsis buski, the tumor nucleus, and prions, as well as destroy many phenolics. The dose is one set of 6 kernels daily for 5 days; then take 5 days off and repeat the cycle till you are much better. Note: Only the apricot kernels are essential; you may grind by pounding. See old warning on page 248.

Green Black Walnut Hull Tincture (homemade)

- your largest stainless steel (not aluminum, ceramic, plastic, enamel, or Teflon) cooking pot
- Black Walnuts, in the hull, each one still at least 50% green, enough to fill the pot to the top
- grain alcohol, about 50% strength, enough to cover the walnuts
- distilled, unfiltered, unchlorinated bottled water in 1 gallon jugs with zero conductivity seen with the indicator
- vitamin C powder (capsules are fine)
- 2 ounce amber glass bottles and HDPE♳ bottles
- HDPE♳ jugs, as used for vinegar or water

The Black Walnut tree produces large green balls in fall. The walnut is inside, but we will use the whole ball, uncracked, since the active ingredient is in the green outer hull.

Wash the walnuts carefully with water that does not have laundry bleach disinfectant. Put them in the pot and cover completely with the alcohol. Sprinkle on 1 tsp. vitamin C. Cover with lid. Let set for three days. Add another tsp. vitamin C. Pour into HDPE♲ gallon jugs, using stainless steel funnel or homemade HDPE♲ funnel. Discard walnuts. The vitamin C helps to keep the color green, as does the non-chlorinated, unfiltered water. Potency is strong for several years if unopened, even if it darkens slightly. Pour as soon as possible into 2 oz. amber glass or HDPE♲ bottles. Freeze these after opening, to preserve green color.

When preparing the walnuts, wash only with cold tap water. Rinse with distilled, unfiltered water to remove all chlorine. You may need to use a brush on areas with dirt. If you are not going to use all of them in this batch, you may freeze them in a zippered plastic bag. Simply refrigerating them does not keep them from turning black and useless. The pot of soaking walnuts should not be refrigerated. Nor does the final tincture need refrigeration.

Exposure to air causes the tincture to darken and lose potency very quickly. To reduce air exposure, fill the pot as much as possible while still keeping a snug fitting lid. Even more importantly, the HDPE♲ jars or bottles you use to store your tincture should have as little air space as possible and should not be repeatedly opened before use. A large jar should be divided into the 2 oz. size bottles all at one time. Quality is better if poured originally into 2 oz. (1-serving) containers.

There are several ways to make a 50% grain alcohol solution. Some states have Everclear™, 95% alcohol. Mix this half and half with distilled, unfiltered, water. Other states have Everclear™, that is 76.5% alcohol. Mix this two parts Everclear™, to one part water. Do not use vodka or the flask-size Everclear™; it must be 750 ml or 1-liter. Smaller bottles have wood alcohol or isopropyl alcohol pollution.

This is the first time that purchased water is allowed in this very important recipe. A half-million lives of cancer patients

<u>could</u> be saved in a year. There is a lot at stake. You may buy distilled water in 1-gallon jugs if it passes these tests:

- Syncrometer® testing for PCBs, benzene, laundry bleach should be *Negative.*
- Heavy metals and sodium hypochlorite should be *Negative.* Any variety of chlorine bleach has hypochlorite.
- Thulium should be *Negative.*
- Azo dyes should be *Negative.*
- Malonic acid should be *Negative.*

Some varieties of bottled distilled water will pass this test. But if you can't test yourself and wish to make tincture, you can test the distilled water yourself with a chlorine test kit and a conductivity indicator (see *Sources*).

- Test for chlorine; there should be none.
- Test for conductivity; there should be none.

Now you have found the "good" distilled bottled water. It still has some very important metals that could be found by Syncrometer®, including strontium, aluminum, thulium, chromium, vanadium, ruthenium. These can be filtered out through a charcoal filter if you <u>boil</u> the activated charcoal first for 5 minutes (see page 587).

Any brand of bottled distilled water will not be the same in different sizes and in different parts of the country. Be sure to use only the size and source you have tested. You may also use rainwater stored in HDPE♲ water jugs and only filtered through washed paper, see page 153

Lugol's Iodine Solution

It is too dangerous to buy a commercially prepared solution for your internal use. It is certain to be polluted with isopropyl alcohol or wood alcohol. Make it yourself or ask your pharmacist to help you. You must <u>see the stock bottles</u>, not trust the pharmacist. The recipe to make 1 liter (quart) is:

- 44 gm (1½ ounces) iodine, granular, USP

- 88 gm (3 ounces) potassium iodide, granular, USP
- diet scales and plastic cup and spoon
- large HDPE⬢ bottle with screw cap (see *Sources*)

Dissolve the potassium iodide in about a cup of water in HDPE container. Then add the iodine crystals and wait till they are all dissolved. This could take ½ hour with frequent shaking. Then fill to the liter mark (quart) with pure water. (Draw a permanent line here.) Be careful to avoid laundry bleach water for preparation or you would pollute it yourself. Place a plastic zippered bag, not kitchen wrap, over the top; then close tightly before storing. Keep out of sight and reach of children.

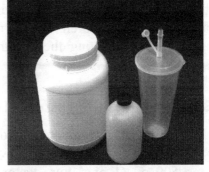

Suitable high density polyethylene containers can be found on Internet.

Fig. 129 Containers that do not seep

Do everything inside the kitchen sink. Wipe stains up promptly with vitamin C. The dropper bottle should be made of polyethylene with built in drop dispenser or a separate pipette (see page 444).

Lugol's Iodine Drops

- 6 drops Lugol's iodine solution
- ½ cup water

This specifically kills Salmonella bacteria in your body. It can be taken at any time. If taken at end of meals, it helps to sterilize the food just eaten so gives you double benefit. <u>Do not use if allergic to iodine</u> (see page 519). Do not add it to other beverages. Do not take with vitamins since these will become over oxidized. If the problem has not cleared up in two days, do the Lugol's-turmeric enema for several days. Lugol's gives the fastest relief for most food-related stomach distress; it takes about one hour.

White Iodine

- 88 gm (3 ounces) potassium iodide, granular, USP

Add potassium iodide to one quart/liter cold tap water. Potassium iodide dissolves well in water and stays clear; for this reason it is called "white iodine". Label clearly and keep out of reach of children. Do not use if allergic to iodine. It is useful for disinfecting the mouth but it is not as strong as Lugol's.

Benzoquinone (BQ) (for clinical use only)

- 500 mg benzoquinone powder (not hydroquinone). (One size 00 capsule filled with powder, by hand.)
- 500 ml (1 pint) pure water. The variety "for injection" often has laundry bleach contamination. Distilled water that shows no conductivity nor chlorination is much safer.

This should be made and supervised by a physician. Prepare 2 non-seeping HDPE🛆 bowls by cutting off the bottom ends of 2 water jugs of 1 gallon size. Pour 1 pint of water into each bowl. Empty the BQ capsule into one bowl, stirring with a non-seeping plastic spoon until completely dissolved (about one minute). Further dilute this as follows: ½ ml BQ solution, as prepared above, is added to a second pint of water in the second bowl. It may be drawn up with a HDPE🛆 pipette. All quantities can be approximated, since the final concentration should be one part per million but need not be exact. After the second dilution, the BQ solution must be used within 20 minutes. If there is further delay, the solution must be made up from the powder again. A dose of one cc (2 cc for persons over 100 lb.) is given in the muscle (IM) in the hip after cleaning skin with ethyl alcohol. This is 1 mcg. Give the shot slowly to reduce burning. Patients may exclaim over their improvement by the time the needle is out.

The BQ solution is thrown out when it is 20 minutes old. All containers are used only for this purpose. Before first use, they are rinsed with distilled water to remove any adhering antiseptic. It is only rinsed and drained after that—never chemically cleaned or brushed.

The Bowel Program

Bacteria are always at the root of bowel problems, such as pain, bloating and gassiness. They cannot be completely killed by zapping, because the high frequency current does not penetrate the bowel contents.

The worst bowel bacteria are the Salmonellas, Shigellas, and E. coli because they have the ability to grow in the rest of your body. One reason bowel bacteria are so hard to eradicate is that we are constantly re-infecting ourselves by keeping a supply on our hands and under our fingernails. The second reason is that the bacteria are themselves infected by oncoviruses that give them protection from your WBCs.

1. The first thing to do is improve sanitation. Use 70% (approx.) grain alcohol in a spray bottle at the bathroom sink. Or Lugol's iodine, one drop per cup water. Sterilize your hands after bathroom use and before meals by spraying or dipping them.

2. Second, take Lugol's solution, six drops in ½ cup water 4 to 6 times daily. This is specifically for Salmonella, which is responsible for at least half of all bowel distress.

3. Third, use turmeric (2 capsules, 3 times daily). This is the common spice, which I find helps against Shigella, as well as E. coli. Expect orange colored stool. Increase to 6 capsules (1 tsp.), 3 times daily for serious problems.

4. Fourth, use fennel (2 capsules, 3 times daily). Take turmeric and fennel, one after the other and 1 minute after Lugol's for fastest relief.

5. Fifth, take four digestive enzyme capsules all together, any variety.

6. Sixth, take 1 tsp. tincture or 2 capsules freeze-dried Black Walnut, preferably at bedtime.

7. Seventh, do a Lugol's-turmeric enema or a Lugol's-turmeric-fennel enema once a day as described on page 269.

8. Eighth, <u>if you are constipated</u>, take Cascara sagrada, an herb. Start with one capsule a day, use up to maximum on label. Take extra magnesium (300 mg magnesium oxide powder, two or three a day), and drink a cup of hot water (flavored is fine) upon rising in the morning. This will begin to regulate your elimination. Constipation is usually caused by *Clostridium botulinum*, which makes its own chemicals in your colon to inhibit the neurotransmitters there. These are the normal driving force for intestinal movement. Use betaine hydrochloride capsules, three with each meal, to keep Clostridium out of your colon. Constipation can also be caused by other bowel bacteria. Certain drugs, such as morphine or similar painkillers produce constipation as a side-effect. You must work hard to be sure you expel bowel contents at least once a day...if necessary, with an enema.

With this powerful approach, even a bad bacterial problem should clear up in <u>two</u> days. If it doesn't, you are feeding them their special requirements. They all require special heavy metals (see page 225). This is like fanning flames. Test all your dishes and cookware for seeping heavy metals with a conductivity indicator. Throw out all stored food in your refrigerator. It may have bacteria. Eat only ozonated or sonicated food. Keep your own hands sanitary. Keep fingernails short. <u>Do not put fingers in mouth</u>. Your tummy <u>can</u> feel flat, without gurgling, and your mood <u>can</u> be good. Remember, cancer is <u>not</u> the cause of your bowel problems. You ate polluted food and nurtured the bacteria.

It may take all the remedies listed. Afterwards, sanitize all your food, put HCl drops in all your food, and eat out of non-seeping dishes.

Moose Elm Drink - also known as - Slippery Elm

For sensitive stomachs when nothing wants to stay down, and for obstructions:

- 1 tbsp. moose elm (also called slippery elm) herb
- 1 cup cold water
- sweetener (*optional*)

Start by making a paste of the powder and a bit of water as if it were cocoa. Gradually add more water to consistency desired. Sweeten. Zappicate. This can be drunk hot or cold. Sip one cup a day. You may use heavy whipping cream, diluted with water or other beverage. Test the herb first for pollution.

Alginate/Intestinal Healer

For intestines or stomach that are sore from surgery or cancer.

- 1 tsp. sodium alginate powder
- 1 cup water

Boil together, stirring with stainless steel spoon. Simmer till dissolved. Add to soup, stew, moose elm drink, pudding or pie filling. Alginate is not digested—it merely forms a long ribbon of soothing gel that coats trouble spots and finds its way through the narrowest passageway to keep it open. Use 1 cup a day. It is quite tasty combined with Moose Elm. **Alternate recipe:** Soak alginate in water about 4 hours or overnight until completely dissolved and pourable, instead of boiling.

Lugol's Enema

Add ¼ tsp. (25 drops) of Lugol's iodine to 1 pint of very warm water; pour into Fleet™ bottles (giving yourself several doses), or enema apparatus (see *Sources*). Administer enema slowly and hold internally as long as possible. Cold water will cause spasms and inability to hold it. Prepare only a cup the first time; do not force yourself to hold more than is comfortable.

Black Walnut Hull Enema

Add 1 tsp. of Black Walnut Hull Extra-Strength, or homemade, to 1 pint of very warm water. Repeat as above.

Giving Yourself the Perfect Enema

Any drop you spill and everything you use to do the enema will <u>somehow</u> contaminate your bathroom. Yet you must leave it all perfectly sanitary for your own protection. So follow these instructions carefully.

Spread out a large plastic trash bag on top of a towel on the bathroom floor. Place a plastic zippered bag beside it. Set a chair nearby, too. The trash bag is for you to lie on. Lie on your back if you have nobody to help you.

The enema apparatus shown is best for larger volumes. It is easy to see through every part, to know what is happening.

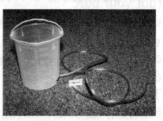

Test the apparatus first, in the bathroom sink to see how it works. Wipe away the grease that comes with it on the applicator; it is sure to be a petroleum product and be tainted with benzene.

Fig. 130 Enema container, tube, pinchcock

Place a dab of butter onto the zippered bag for the lubricant. Or place a wet bar of homemade soap on it. Also alcohol and paper towels.

After filling the container with the enema solution, run some through the tubing until the air is out of it and close the pinchcock. Place it on the trash bag.

Insert the applicator tube as far as you comfortably can. Then lift the container with one hand while opening the valve with the other. The higher you lift it, the faster it runs. Take as much time as you need to run it in. You may wish to set the container on the chair. Very warm liquid is easier to hold. Don't force yourself to hold it all. At any time you may close

560

the valve, withdraw the applicator, and place it on the paper towel.

If you cannot insert the tube, you will need to do a pre enema with just a Fleet bottle first (see page 269).

<u>Cleaning up the apparatus, the bathroom, and yourself:</u> This topic is seldom discussed, but very important. Notice that some bowel contents have entered the container by reflux action, which is unavoidable. Consider the whole apparatus contaminated. For this reason you must never, never use anybody else's apparatus, no matter how clean it looks.

First, wipe the applicator tube with toilet paper. Then fill the container and run it through the hose into the toilet. Repeat until it appears clean; this is appearance only; you must now sterilize it. Fill it with hot tap water and add Lugol's iodine (not your pure variety!) or povidone iodine (from a pharmacy) until intensely red in color. Place the tube to soak, rinsing the whole length of it with the iodine water. Empty both tube and container; then wipe the outside of the tube with paper. Do not dry the container. Store it all in a fresh plastic shopping bag. Throw away the bags and soap. Clean the sink with chlorine bleach (NSF variety, 5 or 6%). Then wash your hands with Lugol's water.

Organ Improvement Recipes

Kidney Cleanse

- ½ cup dried hydrangea root, organic, (c/s)
- ½ cup gravel root, organic, (c/s)
- ½ cup marshmallow root, organic, (c/s)
- 4 bunches of fresh parsley
- ginger capsules
- Uva Ursi capsules
- Black Cherry Concentrate, 8 oz., tested
- vitamin B_6, 250 mg
- magnesium oxide, 300 mg in powder form

All herbs should be tested for thallium and laundry bleach pollution. Organic varieties are less likely to have these. Do not ozonate them. Zappicate later.

Measure ¼ cup of each root (this is half your supply) and set them to soak, together, in 10 cups of water, using a stainless steel saucepan tested for seeping. After four hours or overnight, add 8 oz. black cherry concentrate, heat to boiling and simmer for 20 minutes. Drink ¼ cup as soon as it is cool enough. Pour the rest through a stainless steel strainer into a HDPE⚠ container. Refrigerate.

Find fresh parsley at a small neighborhood grocery store where the water has the correct disinfectant bleach. Give it 2 very hot washes. Boil the fresh parsley in 1 quart of water, or as much as needed to cover it, for <u>five</u> minutes (rolling boil). Drink ¼ cup when cool enough. Freeze 1 pint and refrigerate the rest. Throw away the parsley.

Dose: Each morning, pour together ¾ cup of the root mixture and ½ cup parsley water, into a safe cup. Drink this mixture in divided doses throughout the day. Refrigerate. <u>Do not drink it all at once</u> or you will get a stomachache and feel pressure in your bladder. If your stomach is very sensitive, start on half this dose.

Save the roots after the first boiling, storing them in the freezer. After 13 days when your supply runs low, boil the same roots a second time, but add only six cups water and simmer only 10 minutes. This will last another eight days, for a total of three weeks.

After three weeks, repeat with fresh herbs. You need to do the Kidney Cleanse for six weeks to get good results, longer for severe problems.

Also take:
- ginger capsules: 2 with each meal (6 a day)
- Uva Ursi capsules: 2 with each meal (6 a day)
- vitamin B_6 (250 mg): one a day
- magnesium oxide (300 mg): one a day

Ginger and Uva Ursi remove methyl malonate from the kidneys which clogs them. It is also the cause of kidney failure and cystic kidneys (see page 376). Take these supplements just before your meal to avoid burping. If you are already taking these supplements, omit them here. The boiled parsley combines with each one of the 5 malonic acid members that I call the M Family, and removes them.

Some notes on this recipe: this herbal tea, as well as the parsley, can easily spoil. Heat it to boiling every third day if it is being stored in the refrigerator; this resterilizes it. If you sterilize it in the morning you may take it to work without refrigerating it (use a HDPE♳ container or a zippered plastic bag inside a jar). Fold the bag over the edge to drink it.

When you order your herbs, be careful! Herb companies are not the same! These roots should have a strong fragrance. If the ones you buy are barely fragrant, they have lost their active ingredients; switch to a different supplier.

Liver Cleanse

This is particularly important in any disease-prevention program. Cleansing the liver of gallstones dramatically improves digestion, which is the basis of your whole health. You can expect your allergies to disappear, too, more with each cleanse you do! Incredibly, it also eliminates shoulder, upper arm, and upper back pain. You have more energy and increased sense of well being.

It is the job of the liver to make bile, 1 to 1½ quarts in a day! The liver is full of tubes (*biliary tubing*) that deliver the bile to one large tube (the *common bile duct*). The gallbladder is attached to the common bile duct and acts as a storage reservoir (see page 99). Eating fat or protein triggers the gallbladder to squeeze itself empty after about 20 minutes, and the stored bile finishes its trip down the common bile duct to the intestine.

<u>For many persons, including children, the biliary tubing is choked with gallstones</u>. Some develop allergies or hives but some have no symptoms. When the gallbladder is scanned or

x-rayed nothing is seen. Typically, they are not in the gallbladder. Not only that, most are too small and not calcified, a prerequisite for visibility on x-ray. There are over half a dozen varieties of gallstones, most of which have cholesterol crystals in them. They can be black, red, white, green or tan colored. The black ones are full of wheel bearing grease and motor oil, which turns to liquid in a warm place. The green ones get their color from being coated with bile. Notice in the picture how many have imbedded unidentified objects. Are they fluke remains? Notice how many are shaped like corks with longitudinal grooves below the tops. We can visualize the blocked bile ducts from such shapes. The ducts have been too weak to open for a long time. Weakness comes from interrupting the nerve impulses with the insulator-like automotive greases. Other stones are composites—made of many smaller ones—showing that they regrouped in the bile ducts some time after the last cleanse.

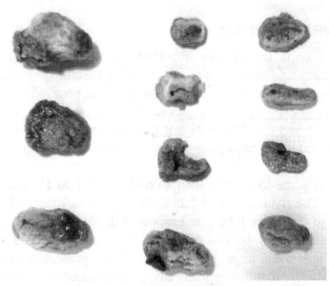

Fig. 131 These are gallstones

At the very center of each stone is found a clump of bacteria, according to scientists, suggesting a dead bit of parasite might have started the stone forming.

As the stones grow and become more numerous the backpressure on the liver causes it to make less bile. It is also thought to slow the flow of lymphatic fluid. Imagine the situation if your garden hose had marbles in it. Much less water would flow, which in turn would decrease the ability of the hose to squirt out the marbles. <u>With gallstones, much less cholesterol leaves the body, and cholesterol levels may rise.</u>

Emptying the liver bile ducts is the most powerful procedure that you can do to improve your body's health.

But it <u>should not</u> be done before the parasite program, and for <u>best results</u> should follow the kidney cleanse.

Gallstones, being sticky, can pick up all the bacteria, viruses and parasite eggs that are passing through the liver. In this way "nests" of infection are formed, forever supplying the body with fresh parasite eggs and bacteria. No stomach infection such as ulcers or intestinal bloating can be cured permanently without removing these gallstones from the liver.

Cleanse your liver twice a year.

Preparation:
• You can't clean a liver with living parasites in it. You won't get many stones, and you will feel quite sick. Zap daily the week before, or get through three weeks of parasite-killing before attempting a liver cleanse. If you are on maintenance parasite program, you are always ready to do the cleanse.
• Completing the kidney cleanse before cleansing the liver is also highly recommended. You want your kidneys, bladder and urinary tract in top working condition so they can efficiently remove any undesirable substances incidentally absorbed from the intestine as the bile is being excreted.

Choose a day like Saturday for the cleanse, since you will be able to rest the next day.

Take no pills or vitamins that you can do without; they could prevent success. Stop the parasite program and kidney herbs, too, the day before. Even stop zapping and taking drops.

Ingredients

Epsom salts	4 tablespoons
Olive oil	½ cup (light olive oil is easier to get down)
Fresh pink grapefruit (*for brain and spinal cord cancer use apple juice, with citric acid, see page 271*)	1 large or 2 small, enough to squeeze ½ cup juice (you may substitute a lemon, adding water or sweetener to make ½ cup liquid)
Ornithine	4 to 8, to be sure you can sleep. Don't skip this or you may have the worst night of your life!
Pint jar with lid	
Black Walnut tincture, any strength OR 2 freeze-dried capsules	10 to 20 drops, to kill parasites coming from the liver.

Double hot wash the grapefruit. Zappicate the oil to destroy traces of benzene and PCBs or add a few drops of HCl to the bottle and shake.

Eat a no-fat breakfast and lunch such as cooked cereal, fruit, fruit juice, bread and preserves or sweetening (no butter or milk). This allows the bile to build up and develop pressure in the liver. Higher pressure pushes out more stones. Limit the amount you eat to the minimum you can get by on. You will get more stones. The earlier you stop eating the better your results will be, too. In fact, stopping fat and protein the night before gets even better results.

2:00 PM. Do not eat or drink after 2 o'clock. If you break this rule you could feel quite ill later.

Get your Epsom salts ready. Mix 4 tbsp. in three cups water and pour this into a safe jar. This makes four servings, ¾ cup each. Set the jar in the refrigerator to get ice cold (this is for convenience and taste only).

6:00 PM. Drink one serving (¾ cup) of the ice-cold Epsom salts. If you did not prepare this ahead of time, mix 1 tbsp. in ¾ cup water now. You may add ¹/₈ tsp. vitamin C powder to improve the taste. You may also rinse your mouth.

Get the olive oil and grapefruit out to warm up.

8:00 PM. Repeat by drinking another ¾ cup of Epsom salts.

You haven't eaten since two o'clock, but you won't feel hungry. Get your bedtime chores done. The timing is critical for success.

9:45 PM. Pour ½ cup (measured) olive oil into the pint jar. Squeeze the grapefruit by hand into the measuring cup. Remove pulp with fork. You should have at least ½ cup. You may use lemonade. Add this to the olive oil. Also, add Black Walnut Tincture or have freeze-dried capsules ready instead. Close the jar tightly and shake hard until watery (only fresh citrus juice does this).

Now visit the bathroom one or more times, even if it makes you late for your ten o'clock drink. Don't be more than 15 minutes late. You will get fewer stones.

10:00 PM. Drink the potion you have mixed. Take 4 ornithine capsules with the first sips to make sure you will sleep through the night. Take eight if you already suffer from insomnia. Drinking through a large plastic straw helps it go down easier. You may use salad dressing, cinnamon, or straight sweetener to chase it down between sips. Take it to your bedside if you wish. Get it down within five minutes (15 minutes for very elderly or weak persons).

Lie down immediately. You might fail to get stones out if you don't. The sooner you lie down the more stones you will get out. Be ready for bed ahead of time. Don't clean up the kitchen. As soon as the drink is down walk to your bed and lie down flat on your back with your head up high on the pillow. Try to think about what is happening in the liver. Try to keep perfectly still for at least 20 minutes. You may feel a train of stones traveling along the bile ducts like marbles. There is no pain because the bile duct valves are open (thank you Epsom salts!). **Go to sleep**, you may fail to get stones out if you don't.

Next morning. Upon awakening take your third dose of Epsom salts. If you have indigestion or nausea wait until it is gone before drinking the Epsom salts. You may go back to bed. Don't take this potion before 6:00 am.

2 Hours Later. Take your fourth (the last) dose of Epsom salts. You may go back to bed again.

After 2 More Hours you may eat. Start with fruit juice. Half an hour later eat fruit. One hour later you may eat regular food but keep it light. During the day take the parasite killing herbs and zap. By supper you should feel recovered.

Alternative Schedule 1: Omit the first Epsom salts dose at 6 p.m. Take only one dose, waiting till 8 p.m. Change nothing else. Many people still get stones with one less dose. If you do not, do the full course next time.

Alternative Schedule 2: After taking the first dose of Epsom salts in the morning, wait two hours and take a second dose of the oil mixture and go back to bed. After 4 more hours take another dose of Epsom salts. This schedule can increase the number of stones you remove.

How well did you do? Expect diarrhea in the morning. This is desirable. Use a flashlight to look for gallstones in the toilet with the bowel movement. Look for the green kind since this is proof that they are genuine gallstones, not food residue. Only bile from the liver is pea green. The bowel movement sinks but gallstones float because of the cholesterol and automotive grease inside. Count them all roughly, whether tan or green. You will need to total 2000 stones before the liver is clean enough to rid you of allergies or bursitis or upper back pains permanently. The first cleanse may rid you of them for a few days, but as the stones from the rear travel forward, they give you the same symptoms again. You may repeat cleanses at two-week intervals. Never cleanse when you are ill.

Sometimes the bile ducts are full of cholesterol crystals that did not form into round stones. They appear as "chaff" floating on top of the toilet bowl water. It may be tan colored, harboring millions of tiny white crystals. Cleansing this chaff is just as important as purging stones.

How safe is the liver cleanse? It is very safe. My opinion is based on over 500 cases, including many persons in their seventies and eighties. None went to the hospital; none even reported pain. However it can make you feel quite ill for one or two days afterwards, although in every one of these cases the maintenance parasite program had been neglected. This is why the instructions direct you to complete the parasite and kidney cleanse programs first.

Warning: If you do change these recipes you might expect problems. The liver is quite sensitive to details. If you plan to make changes, be sure to seek the help of a therapist.

This procedure contradicts many modern medical viewpoints. Gallstones are thought to be formed in the gallbladder, not the liver. They are thought to be few, not thousands. They are not thought to be linked to pains other than gallbladder attacks. It is easy to understand why this is thought: by the time you have acute pain attacks, some stones <u>are</u> in the gallbladder, <u>are</u> big enough and sufficiently calcified to see on x-ray, and <u>have</u> caused inflammation there. When the gallbladder is removed the acute attacks are gone, but the bursitis and other pains and digestive problems remain.

The truth is self-evident. People who have had their gallbladder surgically removed still get plenty of green, bile-coated stones, and anyone who cares to dissect their stones can see that the concentric circles and crystals of cholesterol match textbook pictures of "gallstones" exactly.

Immunity Boosters

L-A Recipe

- 1 tsp. L-aspartic acid
- 1 tsp. L-lysine powder
- 1 $\frac{1}{3}$ cups water

Heat ingredients together, covered, till completely dissolved; it will be near boiling. Use a stainless steel pan and stirring spoon. If it develops a white crystalline precipitate at the bottom, it must be reheated to get it redissolved. Add enough water to keep it dissolved. Since it has no preservatives, you <u>must</u> reheat it to near boiling every fourth day to kill any growing bacteria.

Dose: take 1 teaspoon 4 times daily (or 2 tsp. twice a day). Take on an empty stomach, such as before meals. There are no side-effects.

L-G Recipe

- 1 tsp. L-glutamic acid powder (not glutamine)
- 1 tsp. L-lysine powder (you may open capsules)
- 1$\frac{1}{3}$ cups water

Prepare as for L-A. The dose depends on illness. For viral conditions it is higher: one tablespoon (not tsp.) 4 times daily (2 times daily if less ill). The regular dose is 1 tsp. 4 times daily.

Mechanism of L-G. These two amino acids combine chemically in hot water to make eight or more different dipeptides. Each is a form (isomer) of L-G. L-G travels to your thymus; this much can be observed electronically. Does it help T-cells survive? Does it do some other vital task? Today, 10 years after its discovery, some questions can be answered.

L-G is found normally present in at least ten kinds of white blood cells including lymphocytes, neutrophils, and even eosinophils. The CD4s and CD8s normally kill viruses but without L-G they do not. They seem to fill up on them or attack them but are not able to kill them. All CD4s and other white blood cells that do not have L-G present, have mercury and/or thallium stuck inside them. This is coming from amalgam deposits, located in very many places in the body. You have been robbed of your natural L-G making ability.

Fortunately, taking L-G as made in this recipe, helps the CD4s and others to expel their mercury and thallium. Perhaps it is the body's own heavy metal chelator. Now they can kill viruses again and get your body well. If more amalgam comes their way they again fill up on all 50 or so, metals. Most of them can be destroyed or detoxified somehow. Only mercury and thallium cannot, they remain stuck in the lymphocytes and other specialized white blood cells till they are given L-G.

Taking repeated doses of L-G can clean up the white blood cells repeatedly but this is only permanent after amalgam has been removed from the whole body. Nevertheless, this can be accomplished in about six weeks, provided there are no amalgam filled teeth still in your mouth.

As soon as L-G returns to the CD4s they manufacture **interleukin 2** again, another important immune chemical. When the CD8s get their L-G they begin killing vagrant tissue bits, tumor cells, and virus filled cells. And life is back to normal.

Dental Recipes

Hardening Dentures

Various kinds of dentures, including colored, can be hardened using this recipe. This means they will not seep acrylic acid, urethane, bisphenol-A, phthalates, metals, or dyes, to a detectable level. The hardening was tested with a Syncrometer® by soaking dentures of various kinds and colors in water for many hours and sampling the soak-water. If you will not be able to test, repeat this 3 times:

- Heat tap water in a saucepan till it just begins to steam. Turn off heat. Place dentures in water. Cover. Let stand ½ hour. Remove and rinse. Repeat with fresh water.

Your mouth should have no reaction, no redness, no burning, and no odd symptoms from wearing your dentures. If symptoms occur, repeat the hardening recipe. Also repeat after every visit to the dentist even for the most minor adjustments.

Dental Bleach

This is for use during dental work and for occasional denture cleaning. Do not use it as a regular mouthwash or as a daily denture soak. You would get too much chlorine.

The chemical name for bleach is **hypochlorite**. There are different grades. The grade used for laundry is not acceptable. Purchase "USP" or NSF quality from your local pool and spa store. Try to find the 5 or 6% strength you are used to. Also search the Internet for local NSF brands. If you can only find 12%, notice that it is twice as strong as you are used to! Take it to an expert chemist, like your pharmacist, to help you dilute it to 6% first. This means equal parts bleach and water.

Always add bleach to water instead of water to bleach. You will need 2 empty HDPE♲ gallon jugs with screw cap lids (not snap-on), like vinegar bottles. Check the bottom for those letters. Rinse and fill each empty jug halfway with pure

572

water first, then fill each one to the top with 12% bleach. Notice that you will get 2 gallons of 6% bleach this way, the strength you are used to.

Do not store any 12% bleach in your home—not even in the garage. It must all be changed into 6% as soon as you bring it home. Do not store the 6% bottles under your sink. Put them in your laundry room, on a very high shelf.

Although you will now be using an acceptable grade of 6% bleach this doesn't mean you can use any quantity you want. <u>Bleach is very caustic</u>. It must be diluted before you can use it without harm. <u>Please follow these directions carefully</u>.

- 1 tsp. (5 ml) bleach, USP grade (5-6% hypochlorite)
- 1 pint water (500 ml)

Use a HDPE⚠ pint bottle (see *Sources*). Fill with pure water.

Use a plastic teaspoon to measure and mix. The result is .05% hypochlorite. This is only a quarter as strong as the .2% solution recommended by Bunyan, but is strong enough.

Keep out of reach of children. If accidentally swallowed, give milk to drink and see a doctor at once.

Hardening Toothbrushes and Other Small Plastic Things

Buy a new toothbrush. Many new styles and brightly colored brushes have come into the marketplace. They seep large amounts of plasticizer and dyes! They are especially dangerous to children and sick persons. Harden them by dropping into steaming hot water for ½ hour, the same way as hardening dentures.

Oregano Oil Tooth Powder

- 5 tsp. baking soda
- 5 drops oregano oil

Place ingredients in zippered plastic bag. Squish the mixture in the bag till well mixed. Store in HDPE♳ closed jar or keep in original bag. Zappicate the final product. This is about a 2-month supply. Brushing daily will keep clostridium bacteria at undetectable levels. Dip dry toothbrush in powder. Oregano oil straight in your mouth could make you jump with burning sensation although it does not harm you. If you accidentally get too much, chew bread and keep your tongue at the roof of your mouth.

Immediately after dental work your mouth is too sore to brush. In fact, it is unwise to use a brush at this time. Simply **rub** your teeth after flossing. Wind a strip of paper towel around your finger. Dampen with a few drops of water and dip into the powder.

Denture Cleaner

- Dentures that acquire gray or fine-lined discoloration are growing clostridium bacteria! Kill them by brushing with Dental Bleach and letting them stand without rinsing until the discoloration is gone.
- Soak in Dental Bleach overnight.
- Sonicate once a week.

Don't keep partials or dentures in your mouth at night.

Denture Adhesive

- 1 rounded tsp. sodium alginate
- 1 cup water
- 2 tsp. grain alcohol (any concentration), tested for laundry bleach, isopropyl alcohol, wood alcohol

Let mixture stand in water 4 or more hours till completely dissolved. To make it stronger, add more alginate and wait longer. Keep notes on your favorite concentration.

Body Care Recipes

Take care of your personal needs using <u>only homemade recipes</u>. There are many more in earlier books by this author.

Use borax for all cleaning purposes: laundry (see instructions on box), dishes (use in granular form to scour), dishwasher, 2 tsp. plus 1½ tsp. citric acid as the rinse. Also use it to shampoo and for personal soap. It inhibits bacteria, leaving a residue that deters them.

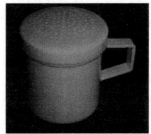

Fig. 132 Salt shaker makes elegant borax dispenser

Borax Liquid Soap

- an empty 1 gallon plastic jug
- $^1/_8$ cup borax powder
- funnel
- homemade liquid soaps

Pour the borax into the jug, fill with <u>very hot</u> tap water. Shake a few times. Let settle. In a few minutes you can pour off the clear part into dispenser bottles. This is the soap! It will not suds or bubble, but it should feel slippery between your fingers. If it does not, add another spoonful. The most common mistakes are not using hot enough water and pouring crumbs into your dispenser bottles.

For dishes in the sink, add liquid soap to your borax soap. For really greasy dishes use homemade lye soap. This is much too strong for regular use on your skin, though. Find gentler recipes in earlier books.

Shampoo: Pour a heaping tbsp. borax into a plastic container and enough <u>very hot</u> water to dissolve. There should be no crumbs left at the bottom. If there are, add more water. Scoop it up over your hair by hand. Rub it in lightly. By the time all your hair is wetted, it will already be squeaky clean.

Massage scalp, too. Borax removes dandruff bacteria. To rinse, use <u>citric acid</u> (see *Sources*). Remove traces of benzene from citric acid by microwaving the entire box for 1 minute first. Ascorbic acid, lemon juice or vinegar are not strong enough to rinse out borax. Put 1 teaspoon citric acid in a plastic container like a cottage cheese carton. Add about 1 cup of water to it after you are in the shower. Leave rinse in hair for one

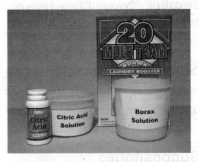

Make a bottle of borax liquid to fill your soap dispensers and shampoo bottle. Use citric acid to rinse and condition.

Fig. 133 Borax and citric acid for the shower

minute while showering your body; then rinse out lightly. After rinsing, your hair should already feel silky. If it does not, make more rinse while you are in the shower.

Baking Soda Shampoo

- 1 tbsp. baking soda (remove traces of benzene by microwaving the whole box for two minutes
- 1 cup <u>very hot</u> water

Place both in a plastic container and stir with your fingers until dissolved. This is the soap. To <u>shampoo</u> scoop it up over your hair by hand; if you pour it, too much runs off. This time rinsing with ascorbic acid (1 tsp. to 1 cup water) or vinegar (equal parts vinegar and water) works. Leave rinse in hair one minute. To add sheen to hair, wash a whole lemon twice in hot water; then press lemon against hair.

Deodorant

Sweating removes toxins from the body. It should be encouraged. A cancer patient should use <u>no</u> chemicals to retard sweating. Sweating in the armpits undoubtedly protects the breast. Wash with borax water alone. After you are well, you could use a homemade recipe described in earlier books.

Shaving Supplies

Switch to an electric shaver to avoid all chemicals. But don't spray chemical lubricant into the shaver!

Suppositories

Coconut oil poured into pen caps and cooled can be used as suppositories. Test first for malonic acid. Add ground herbs or supplements you wish to insert.

Skin Lotion

After finding major air pollutants in all corn products, it seems wiser to switch to a different starch. Beryllium, strontium, vanadium, and chromium are now present in large amounts, causing multiple chemical sensitivities. Even one capsule using cornstarch can set off a delayed reaction.

- 3 tsp. pure arrowroot starch (see *Sources*)
- 1 cup water

Test starch for laundry bleach. Boil starch and water until clear, about one minute. Cool. Pour into dispenser bottle. Keep refrigerated. Use arrowroot starch dry on rashes, fungus, moist or irritated areas and to prevent chafe. Adding magnesium oxide or zinc oxide makes it even drier.

Massage Oil

Instead of using <u>any</u> oil, which brings malonic acid and other pollutants , make yourself an arrowroot solution:

- 4 tsp. arrowroot starch
- 1 cup water

Boil starch and water until clear, about one minute. For a lighter effect use 2 tsp. cornstarch instead of 4. **Variations**: Add a vitamin E capsule, 400 units, add vitamin C, 1000 mg.; add a vitamin A plus zinc capsule. These additions may heal skin lesions faster. Keep refrigerated.

Lipstick

A stick of raw red beet cut like a "French fry" is more convenient and useful than any recipe. Store in plastic bag in refrigerator. Use also on cheeks for rosier complexion.

SAMPLING, TESTING AND HARDENING

How to Test your Water

Only water that is disinfected with laundry-type bleaches have oil and grease in them and the correlation is 100%. The difference between these kinds of waters is easy to see with the naked eye if they are carefully prepared. I will describe 3 ways to find which water has laundry bleach disinfectant.

The Theory

The principle underlying these methods is that oil rises in water. The top portion of the water will then have more oil and grease than the bottom. The top portion will have less electrical conductivity because electricity travels less well through oil than water. A conductivity meter or a handmade device could be used to compare the conductivity at the top and bottom of a water sample. On the other hand, oil detection paper could be dipped into the surface. Only very oily water could be detected this way, though, such as water from Africa. Thirdly, a flashlight could detect oil if there is a film on the surface and if the beam makes the correct angle to see it. These methods do not identify the oils chemically, but they are more reliable than laboratory methods, for simply finding them present.

There are no quantitative aspects to consider. If <u>any</u> oil is seen in a water sample it has laundry bleach in it. And you can infer the presence of PCBs, benzene, and the other toxins.

Making a Water Sample to Test

If your water department adds liquid laundry bleach once a week you can expect the pollution level of its whitening agents and surface tension reducers (meant for laundry), namely metals and dyes, to be highest one day of the week. If you only took one water sample and it was 6 days past the adding time, you might not detect the low level of grease or PCBs in your water. To be sure that you catch the grease and oil, you should sample for 7 days in a row and add them all together. Make at least 2 samples a day, more would be better. A 1½- or 2-gallon wastebasket would be fine. Wide, deep containers are excellent, because most of the water is far away from the sides so the oil can reach the top. Rinse your container several times in the water you are testing first. Then, twice each day pour about ½ cup cold and ½ cup hot water from your kitchen faucet into your container. This makes 14 cups total, almost a gallon. Keep the container on the kitchen counter where you can watch it and protect it from any vibration.

Do not carry the container anywhere, once you have started to collect; do not disturb it. Do not use a lid or tight-fitting cover. Even a tiny disturbance that merely vibrates the water upsets the ultra thin layer of oil that is trying to form a film at the top. If you disturb the container the film will tear and move to the sides. It will stick there and attract more oil to the sides. Just below the water's edge the sides will later feel greasy. Cover the container with a piece of paper to keep out the dust. Keep a flashlight nearby and wait.

You may make 2 containers full of water samples in case you accidentally disturb one.

The Wait and See Way

The grease is slowly rising, some of it sticking to the sides. The wider the pail the less sticks to the sides and more will reach the top. After 3 weeks you could start to search for tiny grease granules afloat on the surface.

It may take 2 to 3 months for enough to rise to be visible. A glass jar lets more grease reach the surface than a plastic one. In a tall bottle, it may have risen too high to test *Positive* by Syncrometer®. Shaking the bottle makes it test *Positive* again. Any shipment for testing should be glass, but unless shaken at the point of use, the results will be variable.

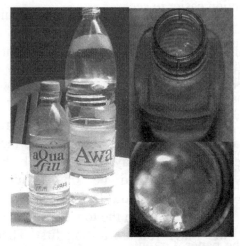

Unopened water bottles from Africa develop oil slicks at the surface in 3 to 6 weeks, if left undisturbed.

Fig. 134 African bottled water

Drop a short hair from your head or piece of fish line onto the surface of the water to mark it for easier searching with a flashlight. Find the hair and you will have found the surface. The hair should be rinsed and dried first and cut to only a 2 inch (5 cm) length. Shine your flashlight from many angles and heights till you can see the hair and the entire surface of water. Look for a thin film on the surface occurring in small swirls and patches. Clean water is perfectly clear.

If the water has been disturbed start over. It will never reach the surface after it has stuck to the sides. Be patient. Keep the water at least 3 months.

Take a photo of the film and pail; describe it carefully in written notes. Be prepared to repeat this water test if you or someone else believes there is a flaw in it.

The Oil Detection Test Paper Way

The theory: Oil attracts oil. Oil will "wet" an oily paper surface but not a perfectly clean dry surface. Test papers are made for this purpose. They are colored to make the "wetting" action easier to see.

The method: Cut a short strip of oil detection paper (see *Sources*). You may put a small drop of your water onto the paper or dip the paper. Neither way is perfect. Try both. A plastic pipette will hold the oil

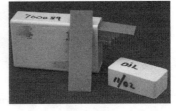

Fig. 135 Oil detection paper

on its own surface and not release it to the paper. A glass dropper may not pick any grease up. A strip that is stuck into the water may release a lot of the oil it gathered, on its way out. But if oil is plentiful, all these objections might not matter. Allow several hours to see repeated evidence of oil penetrating the paper. Granules of grease may remain as granules instead of penetrating the test paper as oil would. This method was meant for higher quantities of oil, such as I find in African waters.

The Conductivity Way

There are a variety of conductivity indicators on the market. By collecting the water in a large container with a spigot at the bottom you can compare top with bottom water more easily.

An inexpensive device is available that has a very short gap (.5 to 1 mm.) between two wires that connect to a battery and tiny LED light. When current is flowing the LED lights up. When the two wires are stuck into clean tap water, considerable electricity will flow. You can adjust the gap to be more or less sensitive. Water with oil in it is less conductive, so the light will be dimmer. Compare the top and bottom layers of water that has stood over a month. Draw it from the bottom to compare with the top. Water that is flowing cannot show you the conductivity differences.

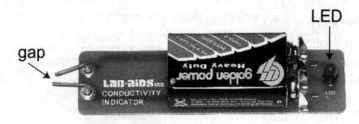

Fig. 136 Conductivity indicator

How to Use the Conductivity Indicator

1. Use a fresh 9 volt battery, not rechargeable variety. Keep it in a separate bag. It will last a long time.

2. Handle the tester with great care. Everything depends on the gap at the tips of the wires.

3. Buy distilled water, more than one kind. You need to find a variety that shows <u>no</u> conductivity.

4. Attach battery to tester. Fit one side of battery first. Then swing battery into the other side of connector. This prevents accidental damage.

5. The tester light should not be on. If it is, separate the tips of the wires with a piece of paper. Bend them apart very gently till no light comes on when the paper is removed.

6. Turn off all room lights. It should be dark.

7. Open water jug, stick tester into distilled water, not above the wires. Light should not go on.

8. If the light goes on it is not suitable water. Try a different distilled water. When you have a distilled water that does not turn on the light you are ready to start.

9. Pour distilled water into the containers you want to test for metal seepage. Allow a suitable time, like 2, 12 or 24 hr.

10. Rinse the device before each test, in the distilled water, giving it a shake to dry it. Do not use anything to dry it except a very <u>soft tissue</u>. Use a <u>very soft touch</u>. If you do not dry it

before you lay it down it could short later and turn the light on by itself. That would drain the battery.

11. Now dip the device in each water container, not above the wires. Keep it in about 20 seconds, moving it around. Cup your hands around it to make it darker so you can see better. There should be no light, not even the faintest glimmer. That is a good container. Even the faintest glow is too much; discard the container.

12. After each test, wash the electrodes in the distilled water as in #10.

13. Well water, chlorinated water and rainwater all have considerable conductivity. Only distilled water <u>may</u> not.

14. This does not test for malonic acid or solvents or dyes. It is not as sensitive as a Syncrometer®. It does not detect the weaker metals such as germanium or thallium very well. A conductivity meter is better in some ways.

The Centrifuge Way

The method: Purchase an inexpensive table centrifuge, with centrifuge tubes for holding liquids and a small brush (similar to a bottle brush) for cleaning them. Caps are not needed. Make a 7-day water sample. You need not wait for oil and grease to rise with this method. The centrifuge speeds it up.

Pour water to fill 2 centrifuge tubes nearly to the top. Label them and arrange them across from each other in the centrifuge, leaving the other holes empty. Or use other holes

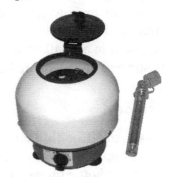

Fig. 137 Centrifuge and tube

to test other kinds of water, including clean water. Arrange them all symmetrically. This keeps the centrifuge from wobbling. After centrifuging at least 30 minutes at the highest

583

speed it is capable of, set the tubes upright in a drinking glass to store till you can test for grease at your convenience.

Then choose one of these test methods:

1. Dip a piece of oil detection paper into the surface. Set it aside to "develop" any oily color.

2. Dip your conductivity indicator into the surface and note light intensity or other kind of evidence of the conductivity. Compare this with the conductivity of this same water that has not been centrifuged.

3. Wait till an oil film appears at the surface. It may take the form of grease "particles" instead of a flat film at the surface. It may come in patches or swirls. It could take a week.

NOTE: If you dipped paper into the surface the oil would have been removed or disturbed so the other two methods will no longer be useful.

How to Make Saliva Test Samples

Homeographic Saliva Sample

Being able to capture the frequency pattern of a saliva sample in pure water is important to be able to transport it safely and to be able to store it for an indefinite time. You can capture it in a small bottle of water (Method 1) or in a zippered plastic bag of water (Method 2). You will need:

Method 1

- a small bottle that fits snugly in your hand so there is maximum surface contact between hand and bottle. A ½ oz. amber bottle of glass or plastic, with non-metal cap, is fine.
- paper, such as kitchen towel, unfragranced, uncolored. Cut or tear a 2" x 2" piece (5 cm x 5 cm).
- water from cold faucet
- zippered plastic bags

A sample of the water and paper should be made as "controls." Dip a small piece of paper in the water; shake to remove drips and place in separate zippered bag. Label it CONTROL.

Stuff the small square of paper in your mouth and chew till wet but not dripping. Spit it into a zippered plastic bag without touching it with your hands.

Add 4 tsp. (20 ml) water to the saliva sample; no exact measurement is needed. Zip shut. Squish the paper wad, in the bag, with your fingers a few times to mix saliva and water. Set aside. (If you used too big a piece of paper there will not be enough water to do this successfully.)

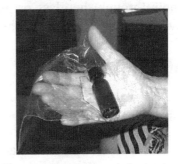

Chewed paper wad is in bag under bottle.

Fig. 138 Homeographic saliva sample

Next, prepare the water sample that will receive the frequency pattern.

Put 2 tsp. water in the ½ oz. bottle. This leaves room for shaking. Close.

Holding the bag in your hand, place the bottle of water on top of it (the bag). The bottle should be positioned above the paper wad. Grip both tightly. If you used too big a bag this will not be possible. Shake 130 times vigorously (20 shakes per 5 seconds; practice this beforehand). Label the bottle "Saliva #3, Manual."

Explanation: Saliva, as you produce it, is given the number "1". After adding water, it is called #2; its electronic properties are changed. The copy of #2 is called #3; if copied by hand it is called "Manual". If it is copied on copy maker, it is called "electronic".

Protect your copy of saliva from direct sunlight and magnetic fields. That is why the amber color and plastic lid were chosen. Wrap the bottle in layers of packaging material, or "bubble wrap" to keep it safe from magnets while traveling. No refrigeration needed.

Further copies made from your #3 bottle are numbered #4, #5, etc. They are not identical.

Evidently, your body is supplying the high frequency energy needed to "carry" (modulate) the pattern from the saliva sample through the glass or plastic into the water. The action may be similar to homeographic copy-making (see page 112).

Method 2

You will need only the paper, water and zippered plastic bags. First we will make the saliva sample; then we will copy it into some clean water in a second bag.

Cut or tear a piece of paper towel without fragrance or a printed pattern. The size should be about 2 or 3 inches square. Stick it all in your mouth and chew it till it is quite damp. Spit it into a zippered plastic bag of sandwich size, about 6 inches square (not bigger) without touching it with fingers. This is called a #1 sample because it has had nothing added. Next, add about 1 tbsp. water, without measuring; there should be about twice as much water as paper wad. Squish the paper wad several times to release the saliva. Such water is labeled saliva #2 because only water has been added. Close the bag securely. Set aside.

Put about 1 tbsp. of water into a second zippered bag.

We will copy the frequency pattern of the saliva sample into this water sample.

Check each bag for leaks, expelling some air so the bags will lie flat on each other.

Place the saliva bag in your strongest hand so the corner with the sample is in your palm. Place the water sample on top of it, also in your palm. Fold the empty portions of the bags inward so you are holding all of it in your hand. If you chose large bags this will not be possible. Gripping it tightly, shake it 150 times as fast as you can. Aim for 4 shakes per second. You may take rests. You may switch hands without starting the count over. It is better to change hands to rest than to slow down.

Even if the bags loosened and got misaligned, and a few drops escaped, the frequency will probably transfer. If water escaped, close the bags again very tightly. Rinse them under the faucet and dry each side carefully. Throw away the bag with saliva sample. For shipping, place the newly made water sample in a second zippered bag and both of these in a plastic bottle (used vitamin bottle).

During shipment all the seals will open!

You may also pour your water sample into a small bottle for shipping. The bottle should have no rubber stopper, nor metal lid. Label it Saliva #3.

Both #1 and #2 saliva samples can be tested directly, but, of course, a #3 is no longer considered a biological fluid. It is safe and can be shipped without special precautions.

How to Stop your Pitcher Filter from Seeping

Take out the filter unit. Bring tap water to a near-boil and pour it into the pitcher. Fill the pitcher to the top. Cover and let stand for ½ hour. If the plastic is very flexible, you should do this twice, because there may be a lot of DAP in it. (DAP is a serious carcinogen.)

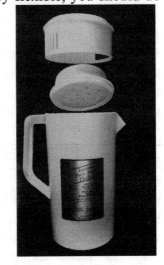

Next we will stop the metal seepage from the filter unit. If you are not very handy, draw it first, so you can put it back together correctly.

Take it apart. Pour the charcoal into a steel saucepan and set aside. Put the fiber or other cushioning into its own saucepan and set aside. Place the plastic parts into a third saucepan. Cover them with tap water. Bring to a near-boil. When steaming, turn

Fig. 139 Water pitcher with filter

587

heat off. Cover and let stand for ½ hour. Drain and rinse twice with tap water.

Cover the fiber with near-boiling water. Let stand 5 minutes and drain. Repeat 2 more times. Rinse with tap water.

Cover the charcoal with a huge excess of <u>tap water</u> (nearly a quart). Bring to a boil and boil 5 minutes. Drain carefully so charcoal stays in pan. Add a bit more <u>tap</u> water and drain a second time. If you used distilled water you will recontaminate the charcoal. Spoon the charcoal back onto its padding and reassemble the filter unit. Pour your distilled water into the filter pitcher. DO NOT FILL IT SO FULL IT TOUCHES THE FILTER. Leave 1 inch (2½ cm) of space. Pour through the filter into a non-seeping glass or a zippered bag. Test with conductivity indicator.

You could, of course, test each part separately before reassembling it. Clean your charcoal by boiling it 5 minutes every 2 weeks. Other parts do not need reheating.

Trouble Shooting the Filter

You can't assume the filter is doing its job even if you put it all together correctly. Test the water by Syncrometer® for ruthenium, strontium, aluminum, beryllium, rubidium, and rhodium, even if the conductivity indicator detects nothing. You may make the tester more sensitive by making the gap smaller. Be sure to rinse and dry very gently after each test now to avoid accidental "shorting". Keep the test water covered to reduce carbon dioxide absorption from the air, which raises conductivity.

If the water shows you some conductivity, don't drink it. Study your filter. The fit of the filter unit may be so loose that the distilled water is bypassing the filter. In this case, put a tan rubber band around the base to tighten the fit. Boil the rubber band a minute first. Then rinse 3 more times in steaming hot water. Choose #65 rubber bands. If this fixes the problem you may do final testing of your filtered water. Test by Syncrometer® for malonic acid, DAP, thallium (which is not very conductive), and traces of strontium, beryllium, aluminum, ruthenium, and rubidium. The ruthenium comes from the charcoal itself and from the distilled water, even if properly disinfected. That is why the boiling is done in tap water.

Double Filtering

It may be easier and certainly more reliable to filter your water twice. Even ultra traces of strontium or ruthenium are harmful to advanced cancer patients or lung disease patients (see page 225).

Making a 1-Glass Filter

It is convenient to travel with a small filter that cleans your water a glass at a time. You can make a 1-glass filter out of 4 HDPE♲ plastic glasses.

You will need:
- 4 tall plastic glasses
- activated charcoal, NSF
- fiber padding
- drill or ice pick

Make a dozen, or so, pinholes in the bottom of two plastic glasses. A drill bit of $^1/_{32}$ or an ice pick to pierce holes are suitable size.

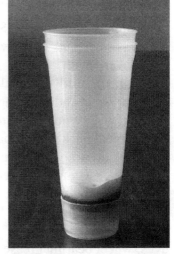

This invention is a gift to you from JOSE, the inventor.

Fig. 140 1-glass "JOSE" filter

Cut a circle of padding material taken from a filter pitcher. Peel off a very thin layer of padding for this purpose. Place it inside the glass to cover the holes. Add 2 or 3 tbsp. boiled (5 minutes) charcoal. Add another layer of padding cut slightly larger to fit snugly over the charcoal.

Place the second glass inside the first one, also pierced with holes. This is your filter.

Cut a third glass to act as a holder for your new filter. First fit your new filter into the third glass to see where the fit would be snug. Draw a line 1 or 2 inches above the snug point. Remove filter and cut the third glass at the line. This gives you a small holder so you can travel with your 1-glass filter. The 4th glass is for drinking. Use a large zippered bag, in addition, to prevent spillage accidents. When the flow is satisfactory and the water tests zero in conductivity, take it all apart and harden each part in near-boiling water for ½ hour.

How to Clean Activated Charcoal

Dump new or used NSF-grade charcoal, wet or dry, into a stainless steel pan. There will be 3 or 4 tbsp.

Cover with about 3 cups tap water (NSF-bleach disinfected). Boil charcoal 5 minutes. Drain. Add another ½ cup tap water and drain again. (If you accidentally rinse with distilled water you will reload the filter with ruthenium.) Spoon the charcoal back into its padding.

This does not clear laundry bleach from activated carbon. To clean PCBs and benzene from laundry bleached charcoal, pour carbon into stainless steel pan. Cover with 5 to 10 times as much tap water. Boil 5 minutes at rolling boil. Pour off. Repeat twice. This does not clear the hypochlorite, asbestos, dyes, wheel bearing grease or motor oil from charcoal.

Filter Padding

Save the fiber padding from old filters to use in homemade ones. They are easily cleaned, just under the hot faucet. When padding is not available, a piece of nylon hose tested for laundry bleach works well, too. Boil the whole hose 5 minutes first and rinse under faucet. When dry cut a 5 or 6 inch length, tying a knot at one end. Spoon in the clean charcoal and tie other end. This can be made to lay flat in the pitcher filter, 1 cup filter, or HDPE♲ gallon filter (here it is tucked into the funnel).

SOURCES

This list was accurate as this book went to press. Only the vitamin sources listed here were found to be pollution-free, and only the herb sources listed here were found to be potent, although there may be other good sources that have not been tested. The author has no financial interest in, influence on, or other connection with any company listed, except for having family members in the Self Health Resource Center.

Note to readers outside the United States of America:

Sources listed are typically companies within the United States because they are the ones I am most familiar with. You may be tempted to try a more convenient manufacturer in your own country and hope for the best. I must advise against this! In my experience, an uninformed manufacturer most likely has a polluted product! Your health is worth the extra effort to obtain the products that make you well. One bad product can keep you from reaching that goal. This chapter will be updated as I become aware of acceptable sources outside the United States. Best of all is to learn to test products yourself.

When contacting these *Sources*, ask first for their **retail department**. They may wish to direct you to a nearby distributor. Be patient.

When ordering chemicals for internal use, always ask for the food grade variety.

Item	Source
Activated carbon	See charcoal
Amber glass or polyethylene bottles, ½ ounce	Drugstore, Continental Glass & Plastic, Inc. (large quantities)
Amino acid mixture, liquid for IV use and other IV liquids in glass bottles	Abbott Laboratories; Mexican pharmacies
Amino acids, dry	Spectrum Chemical Co.; Seltzer Chemicals, Inc.
Anatomy set	See microscope slides
Arrowroot starch, #P170	San Francisco Herb & Natural Food Co.
Aspartic acid	Spectrum Chemical Co.
Baking soda (sodium bicarbonate)	Spectrum Chemical Co.
Beeswax	Brushy Bee
Betaine hydrochloride	Seltzer Chemicals, Inc.
Black cherry concentrate	Bernard Jensen Products; health food store
Black Walnut Hull tincture	See Green Black Walnut Hull
Bleach, USP	See dental bleach
Bottle-copies	See homeographic copies
Bottles	See HDPE bottles
Borax	Grocery store
Boric acid	Spectrum Chemical Co.; health food store; pharmacy; animal feed store
Cactus, Prickly Pear, tablets (Nopales)	Plantas M. Anahuac, C.A. de C.V.
Canning jars	Ball / Kerr Mason jars, ½ cup
Cascara sagrada	San Francisco Herb & Natural Food Co.
Charcoal	Self Health Resource Center
Chlorination supplies	Pool and spa store; garden supply store; Ecolab; Spectrum Chemical Co.; Edwards-Councilor Co. Inc.
Cholecalciferol	See vitamin D_3
Citric acid	Univar; health food store
Cloves	San Francisco Herb & Natural Food Co. (ASK for fresh); Starwest Botanicals, Inc.
Coenzyme Q10	Seltzer Chemicals Inc.; Spectrum Chemical Co.
Coffee mill	Lehman's
Colloidal silver maker	CTS Originals; SOTA Instruments, Inc.

Item	Source
Compass	Camping store; science store
Conductivity indicator	Dr. Clark Store; Lab-Aids, Inc.
Dental Bleach	Self Health Resource Center
Dental chemicals	I have not found dental chemical supply companies to be reliably pure. Order your dental chemicals from regular chemical companies like Spectrum Chemical Co.
Dental help in Europe	Naturheilverein
Dental impression compounds	Patterson's Dental Supply, Inc.; Bosworth Company; GC America, Inc.; Waterpik Technologies, Inc.
Dental probe	Make your own
Digestive enzyme mixture	Self Health Resource Center
Electronic parts	A Radio Shack near you; Mouser
Empty gelatin capsules size 00	Capsugel; health food store
Enema equipment	Dr. Clark Store; Medical Devices International; "Fleet" bottle is available at pharmacies; drugstores
Epoxy coating for copper pipes	American Pipelining; Cura Flo
Essential oils	San Francisco Herb & Natural Food Co.; Starwest Botanicals, Inc.
Eucalyptus leaf, organic	San Francisco Herb & Natural Food Co.
Fat emulsion for IV use	Abbott Laboratories; Mexican pharmacies
Filters, pure charcoal	Pure Water Products (pitchers); Seagull Distribution Co. (faucet, shower, whole house)
Folic acid	Spectrum Chemical Co.
Food mill	See coffee mill
Germanium 132	Henry's Marketplace; Provitaminas; health food store
Germanium, organic	Hydrangea, coconut or other nuts
Ginger capsules	San Francisco Herb & Natural Food Co. (bulk)
Glutathione	Seltzer Chemicals, Inc.
Goat milk	Zip International Group
Goldenrod tincture	Blessed Herbs; Self Health Resource Center
Grains	Bob's Red Mill
Grain alcohol (ethyl	Liquor store; Everclear, search for the ¾

Item	Source
alcohol)	liter or 1 liter size.
Gravel root (herb)	San Francisco Herb & Natural Food Co.; Starwest Botanicals, Inc.
Green Black Walnut Hull freeze-dried capsules	New Action Products; Consumer Health Organization
Green Black Walnut Hull tincture	New Action Products
Hats, broad-brimmed	Nacho Hats
Henna hair dye, black, red	Karabetian Imp. Exp., Inc.
Herbs, in bulk	San Francisco Herb & Natural Food Co.
HCl	See hydrochloric acid
HDPE (only) bottles	Spectrum Chemical Co. (lids of different plastic need to be hardened)
Homeographic copies	Century Nutrition of Mexico
Hydrangea (herb)	San Francisco Herb & Natural Food Co.
Hydrochloric acid, USP	Spectrum Chemical Co. You must dilute the 10% solution purchased (#HY105) to a 5% solution by adding an equal volume of water. For internal use, must be made by pharmacist.
Hydrogen peroxide 35% (food grade)	Univar
Inspection mirror	Automotive store
Insulation	Bonded Logic, Inc.
Iodine	Spectrum Chemical Co.
Lactase enzymes	Mother Nature Advanced Enzyme System (Rainbow Light)
Lipase-pancreatin enzyme mixture	See individual ingredients
L-glutamic acid powder (this is not glutamine.)	Spectrum Chemical Co.
Lipase	Spectrum Chemical Co
L-lysine powder	Spectrum Chemical Co.
Lugol's iodine	Spectrum Chemical Co.; or farm animal supply store (for disinfection and slide staining, not internal use). For internal use must be made from scratch by pharmacist.
Magnesium oxide	Spectrum Chemical Co.
Magnopatch	Cut a 1-inch square from a magnetic sheet available at any craft store. Glue on one-third inch round magnet in the

Item	Source
	center, south side up. Round bottom magnet .312 x .125 available from The Cutting Edge.
Maple syrup	US Foods
Marshmallow root (herb)	San Francisco Herb & Natural Food Co.; Starwest Botanicals, Inc.
Microscope slides	Carolina Biological Supply Co.; Ward's Natural Science, Inc.; Southern Biological Supply Co.
Niacinamide	Spectrum Chemical Co.
Oil detection test paper	The Science Source
Olive leaf powder	San Francisco Herb & Natural Food Co.
Oregano oil	Starwest Botanicals, Inc.; North American Herb & Spice Co.
Oregano oil tooth powder	Wholesome International
Organ samples preserved on microscope slides	See microscope slides
Ornithine	Spectrum Chemical Co.; Seltzer Chemicals, Inc.
Ortho-phospho-tyrosine	Use homeographic copies
Oscillococcinum, homeopathic flu medicine	Boiron Borneman; health food store
Ozonator	Superior Health Products
P24 antigen sample	Use homeographic copies
Parasites, bacteria, viruses preserved on microscope slides	See microscope slides
Pancreatin	Spectrum Chemical Co
Pau D'Arco	Starwest Botanicals, Inc.
Peppermint oil	Starwest Botanicals, Inc.
Peroxy	See hydrogen peroxide
pH strips	Pharmacies, drugstore
Pipettes (HDPE♲)	Spectrum; Univar
Plastic-coated water pipes	See epoxy coating
Plastic eyedropper	Drugstore
Plastic lids for Ball's canning jars	Alltrista Corporation
Polyethylene dropper bottles	Spectrum
Potassium chloride	Spectrum Chemical Co.
Potassium iodide	Spectrum Chemical Co.

Item	Source
Pump, water lubricated	F.E. Myers
Salt (sodium chloride)	Spectrum Chemical Co.
Salt (sodium-potassium)	Self Health Resource Center
Seltzer maker	Fante's; KegMan
Slides	See microscope slides
Soap, homemade	See *Recipes*
Sodium alginate	Spectrum Chemical Co.; health food store
Sodium hypochlorite, NSF	See chlorination supplies
Sonicator	Any ultrasonic jewelry cleaner
Stainless steel cookware	Chefmate; restaurant supply stores, department stores
Stainless steel platters	Tableware International Inc.
Strainer, stainless steel	San Francisco Herb & Natural Food Co.; Self Health Resource Center
Sucrose	Spectrum Chemical Co. (#SU103, Crystal, N.F.)
Syncrometer® video	New Century Press
Tapioca pearls	Bob's Red Mill
Tea ball, stainless steel	San Francisco Herb & Natural Food Co.; Self Health Resource Center
Tubes, shielding	Use 1" electrical conduit. Available at hardware stores.
Uva Ursi, herb	San Francisco Herb & Natural Food Co.
Vegecaps	Capsugel
Vermiculite insulation	See insulation
Virtual copies	See homeographic copies
Vitamin A (acetate)	Spectrum Chemical Co.
Vitamin B_1	Spectrum Chemical Co.
Vitamin B_{12}	Spectrum Chemical Co.
Vitamin B_2	Spectrum Chemical Co.; Seltzer Chemicals, Inc.
Vitamin B_6	Spectrum Chemical Co.; Seltzer Chemicals, Inc.
Vitamin C (ascorbic acid), synthetic	Roche Vitamins, Inc. (all other sources tested had either toxic selenium, yttrium, or thulium pollution!)
Vitamin C, organic	Rose hips are naturally high in vitamin C - San Francisco Herb & Natural Food Co.
Vitamin D_3	Spectrum Chemical Co.
Vitamin E	Bronson Laboratories

Item	Source
Watercress, fresh	Grocery store
Watercress seeds (*Nasturtium officinale*)	Garden store
Watercress, tablets (Berro)	Plantas M. Anahuac, C.A. de C.V.
Water filter pitchers	See filters
Water-lubricated pump	See pump
Wormwood capsules, mixture	New Action Products
Wormwood seed	R.H. Shumway
Yeast	Industria Mexicana de Alimentos S.A. de C.V.
Yunnan Paiyao	Health food store; Internet
Zapper kit	Make your own
Zinc oxide	Spectrum Chemical Co.

Abbott Laboratories
100 Abbott Park Rd.
Abbott Park, IL 60064
(847) 937-6100
www.abbott.com

Alltrista Corporation
PO Box 2729
Muncie, IN 47307-0729
(765) 281-5000
www.alltrista.com

American Pipelining
PO Box 5045
El Dorado Hills, CA 95762
(916) 933-4199
www.americanpipelining.com

Ball/Kerr Mason Jars
www.homecanning.com

Brushy Mountain Bee Farm
(800) 233-7929
www.beeequipment.com

Bernard Jensen Products
535 Stevens Ave.
Solana Beach, CA 92075
(800) 755-4027

Blessed Herbs
109 Barre Plaines Rd.
Oakham, MA 01068
(508) 882-3839
(800)489-4372
www.blessedherbs.com

Bob's Red Mill
5209 SE International Way
Milwaukie, OR 97222
(800) 349-2173
Fax (503) 653-1339
www.bobsredmill.com

Boiron Borneman
6 Campus Blvd.
Newtown Square, PA 19073
(800) 258-8823
(610) 325-7464

Bonded Logic, Inc.
411 East Ray Rd.
Chandler, AZ 85225
(480) 812-9114
www.bondedlogic.com

Bosworth Company
7227 N. Hamlin Ave.
Skokie, IL 60076
(800) 323-4352
www.bosworth.com

Bronson Labs
350 South 400 West, Ste. 102
Lindon, UT 84042
(800) 235-3200 retail
(800) 610-4848 wholesale
www.bronsonlabs.com

Capsugel
PO Box 640091
Pittsburgh, PA 15264-0091
(888) 783-6361
(864) 223-2270
www.capsugel.com

Carolina Biological Supply Co.
PO Box 6010
Burlington, NC 27216-6010
(800) 334-5551
(336) 584-0381
www.carolina.com

Century Nutrition of Mexico
S. de R.L. de C.V. Mexico
Fax 52-664-683-4454

Chefmate®
www.chefmate.tripod.com
www.target.com

Consumer Health Organization of Canada
1220 Sheppard Ave. E, Ste. 412
Toronto, Ontario M2K 2S5
(416) 490-0986

Continental Glass & Plastic, Inc.
841 West Cermak Road
Chicago, IL 60608-4582
(312) 666-2050
www.cgppkg.com

CTS Originals
PO Box 64
Lemon Grove, CA 91946
Fax (619) 644-8635

Cura Flo
1265 North Manassero Street, Ste. 305
Anaheim, CA 92807
(800) 620-5325
Fax (714) 970-2105
www.curaflo.com

Dr. Clark Store
(866) 372-5275
(619) 795-0568
Fax (619) 795-0569
www.drclarkstore.com

Ecolab
(651) 293-2233
www.ecolab.com

Edwards-Councilor Co., Inc.
1427 Baker Road
Virginia Beach, VA 23455
(757) 460-2401
(800) 444-8227
Fax (757) 464-6551
www.sanitize.com

Fante's
1006 S. 9th St.
Philadelphia, PA 19147-4798
(800) 443-2683
www.fantes.com

F.E. Myers
1101 Myers Parkway
Ashland, OH 44805
www.globalspec.com

GC America, Inc.
3737 W. 127th St.
Alsip, IL 60803
www.gcamerica.com

Henry's Marketplace
www.wildoats.com

**Industria Mexicana de
Alimentos S.A. de C.V.**
Km. 70.5 Carretera Federal
Mexico – Puebla, San Martin,
Texmelucan, Puebla
52 (5) 541 9602
Fax 52 (5) 541 9675

Karabetian Import
2021 San Fernando Rd.
Los Angeles, CA 90065
(323) 224-8991

KegMan
(800) 292-6633
 www.kegman.net

Lab-Aids, Inc.
17 Colt Court
Ronkonkoma, NY 11779
(800) 381-8003
Fax (631) 737-1286
www.lab-aids.com

Lehman's
(888) 438-5346
www.lehmans.com

Medical Devices International
3849 Swanson Ct.
Gurnee, IL 60031
(579) 336-6611
www.cprmicroshield.com

Mother Nature
322 7th Avenue, 3rd Floor
New York, NY 10001
(800) 439-5506
Fax (212) 279-4290
www.mothernature.com

Mouser
1000 North Main St.
Mansfield, TX 76063-1514
(800) 346-6873
www.mouser.com

Nacho Hats
Jose Velasquez
1722 N. L Street
Lake Worth, FL 33460
(561) 683-5128

**Naturheilverein "Hilfe zur
Selbsthilfe"**
e.V. Postfach 1238
D-65302 Bad Schwalbach
Germany
49-06128-41097

New Action Products (USA)
PO Box 540
Orchard Park, NY 14127
(800) 455-6459 (USA only)
(716) 662-8000
 New Action Products
(CANADA)
PO Box 141
Grimsby, Ontario
(800) 541-3799
(716) 873-3738
www.newactionproducts.com

New Century Press
(Book Publisher)
1055 Bay Blvd., Ste. C
Chula Vista, CA 91911
(800) 519-2465
www.newcenturypress.com

North American Herb & Spice Co.
PO Box 4885
Buffalo Grove, IL 60089
(800) 243-5242

Patterson Dental Supply, Inc.
1031 Mendota Heights Rd.
Saint Paul, MN 55120
(651) 686-1600
(800) 328-5536
www.pattersondental.com

Plantas M. Anahuac, S.A. de C.V.
Oriente 255 no 57 col. Agricola
Oriental CP 08500 Mexico D.F.
52-557-63-75-20
Anahuac (U.S. office)
7522 Scout Ave.
Bell Gardens, CA 90201
562-927-6414

Provitaminas
PO Box 351991
Los Angeles, CA 90035
(800) 510-6444
(310) 845-9350
Fax (310) 559-2112
www.provitaminas.com

Pure Water Products
10332 Park View Ave.
Westminster, CA 92683
(800) 478-7987

R.H. Shumway
PO Box 1
Graniteville, SC 29829
(803) 663-9771

Roche Vitamins, Inc.
340 Kingsland St.
Nutley, NJ 07110-1199
(800) 892-6510 (no retail sales)

San Francisco Herb & Natural Food Co.
47444 Kato Road
Fremont, CA 94538
(800) 227-2830 wholesale
(510) 770-1215 retail
www.herbspicetea.com

Seagull Distribution Co.
3670 Clairemont Dr.
San Diego, CA 92117
(858) 270-7532

Self Heath Resource Center
1055 Bay Blvd. Suite A
Chula Vista, CA 91911
(800) 873-1663

Seltzer Chemicals, Inc.
5927 Geiger Ct.
Carlsbad, CA 92008-7305
(800) 735-8137
(760) 438-0089
Fax (760) 438-0336
www.nutritionaloutlook.com

SOTA Instruments, Inc.
PO Box 1269
Revelstoke, BC
Canada V0E 2S0
(800) 224-0242
Fax (250) 814-0047

Southern Biological Supply Co.
PO Box 368
McKenzie, TN 38201
(800) 748-8735
(901) 352-3337

Spectrum Chemical Co.
14422 South San Pedro Street
Gardena, CA 90248
(800) 791-3210
(310) 516-8000
www.spectrumchemical.com

Starwest Botanicals, Inc.
11253 Trade Center Dr.
Rancho Cordova, CA 95742
(800) 273-4372
(916) 638-8100
www.starwestherb.com

Superior Health Products, LLC
13549 Ventura Blvd.
Sherman Oaks, CA 91403
(800) 700-1543
(818) 986-9456
www.superiorhealthproducts.com

Tableware International Inc.
770 12th Ave
San Diego, CA 92101
(619) 236-0210
Fax (619) 236-0130
Tableware@pacbell.net

The Cutting Edge
Befit Enterprises LTD
PO Box 5034
Southampton, NY 11969
(631) 287-3813

The Science Source
PO Box 727
Waldoboro, ME 04572
(207) 832-6344
info@thesciencesource.com
"What's in the Water 1500 Kit"

Univar (wholesale only)
2100 Hafley Avenue
National City, CA 91950
(800) 888-4897
(619) 262-0711

US Foods
www.usfoodservice.com

Ward's Natural Science, Inc.
5100 West Henrietta Road
Rochester, NY 14692
(800) 962-2660
(716) 359-2502
www.wardsci.com

Waterpik Technologies, Inc.
1730 E. Prospect Rd.
Ft. Collins, CO 80553
(970) 484-1352
www.waterpik.com

Wholesome International
P.O. Box 2475
Rancho Santa Fe, CA 92067
Fax (619) 284-9000
www.wholesomeintl.com

Zip International Group
2723 W. 15th St.
Brooklyn, NY 11224
(718) 372-1113
www.ekmol.ru

Food and Product Dyes

Numbers after dash are Color Index (CI); Square brackets are CAS numbers

4-amino-3-nitrotoluene (S) —37110

Chlorotoluidines, liquid (S)

(DAB) 4-dimethyl aminoazobenzene 4-isothiocyanate dye (S) [7612-98-8], D-872

(DAB) p-dimethylaminoazobenzene [60-11-7], CI 11020, Sigma #D-6760 causes elevated alkaline phosphatase enzyme in blood tests.

Fast Blue BB Base (S) —37175

Fast Blue RR Base (S) —37155, [6268-05-9], EEC No 228-441-6, F-0375

Fast Garnet GBC Base (S) —11160 causes death of T4 helpers; dye is found on most fish, fresh or canned and poultry.

Fast Green FCF (S) —42053 blocks BUN and creatinine making enzymes, increases rate of mitosis.

Fast Red 1 TR Salt Practical Grade (S) —37150

Fast Red AL salt (S) —37275

Fast Red RC Salt (S) —37120

Fast Red TR Base (S) —37085

Fast Red Violet LB Salt (S) —may be 32348-81-5 causes lymph blockage and effusions, inhibits maleic anhydride detoxification

Fast Scarlet TR Base (S) —37080

Fast Violet B Base (S) —37165

Nitrotoluidines, mono (S)

Sudan Black B Practical Grade (S) —26150, [4197-25-5], Sigma #S-2380 causes elevated lactic dehydrogenase enzyme in blood tests.

Sudan I—12055

Sudan II (SP) (S) —12140

Sudan III (SP) (S) —26100

Sudan IV (S) —26105, Spectrum #SU120, [85-83-6], Sigma #S-8756

Sudan Orange G (S) —11920

Tartrazine (acid yellow 23, FD + C #5) (SP)

Testing Laboratories

(For testing heavy metals, including lanthanides, in carbon filters.)
Alchemy Environmental Laboratories, Inc.
315 New York Road
Plattsburgh, NY 12903
(518) 563-1720
www.aelabs.com

(For testing heavy metals, except lanthanides, in carbon filters.)
Braun Intertec Corp.
11001 Hampshire Ave. S.
Bloomington, MN 55483
(952) 995-2000
www.braunintertec.com

Phoenix Environmental Laboratories, Inc.
587 East Middle Turnpike
PO Box 370
Manchester, CT 06040
(860) 645-1102
Fax (860) 645-0823
www.phoenixlabs.com

(For testing benzene, heavy metals, including lanthanides, in carbon filters.)
SRC Analytical Laboratories
422 Downey Road
Saskatoon, Sask. S7N 4N1 Canada
(306) 933-6932
www.src.sk.ca

B

chow, 461, 463, 472, 473
chromium III, 12, 274, 279, 287, 301, 392, 393
chromosome breakage, 66
chromosome ends, 166
citric acid, 42, 43, 229, 271, 288, 295, 429, 527, 528, 530, 531, 535, 536, 537, 541, 542, 543, 566, 575, 576
clone, 128
Clonorchis sinensis, 57, 103, 178
clostridium bacteria, 574
clotting problem, 351, 354, 355, 357
clotting time, 351
coconut, 40, 528, 551, 593
collagenase, 59
colloidal silver, 332, 339
colostomy, 386, 387
coma, 365, 366, 379, 467
comfrey root, 371
common cold, 52, 89, 172, 304
compass, 150, 196, 227, 229, 247, 344, 502, 503, 525
complement C_3, 24, 25, 27, 276, 290, 406, 462
conductance channels, 230, 475
conductivity, 86, 114, 115, 148, 226, 238, 240, 241, 253, 260, 286, 364, 442, 443, 469, 526, 535, 552, 554, 556, 558, 578, 581, 582, 583, 584, 588, 590
constipation, 169, 177, 362, 558
coriander, 41, 81, 82, 128, 531, 548, 549, 550
corn, 36, 41, 44, 103, 163, 170, 172, 224, 237, 242, 262, 281, 284, 287, 289,

292, 296, 297, 299, 323, 325, 539, 577
cortisone, 192, 265, 393, 433
cosmetics, 199, 240, 320, 373, 434, 511
cosmic dust, 147, 148, 149, 153, 155
coughing, 157, 168, 170, 172, 177, 447, 546
coumarin, 46, 48, 162, 178, 181, 185, 187, 282, 284, 289, 290, 320, 323, 354, 356, 358, 539
Coxsackie viruses, 52, 65
criminal behavior, 349
crowns, 221, 333
cyst, 136, 137, 138, 419, 434
cystic fibrosis, 317
cytochrome C, 277, 285, 292, 299
cytochrome enzymes, 228
Cytomegalovirus (CMV), 172, 224

D

dandruff, 576
d-carnitine, 189, 242, 284, 290, 291, 292, 299, 309, 383, 391
dead teeth, 333
dementia, 347
dental bleach, 592
dental mirror, 341
dental plastic, 349
dentist phobia, 330
detoxifying ability, 15, 130, 233, 371
detox-illness, 74, 76, 89, 90, 98, 99, 101, 109, 113, 130, 169, 176, 177, 199, 236, 238, 246, 266, 461, 473, 547, 549, 550
d-forms, 65, 66, 185, 307

diabetes, 32, 33, 55, 58, 140, 397, 515, 516
diallyl sulfide, 61, 103, 187, 201, 422, 423
diamagnetic, 152, 459, 505
differentiate, 136
digestive enzymes, 22, 29, 53, 61, 89, 102, 160, 162, 164, 201, 217, 222, 244, 245, 262, 277, 297, 298, 299, 304, 373, 383, 385, 416, 431, 447, 461, 468, 537
digestive organs, 29, 99, 436
Dirofilaria, 52, 74, 103, 143, 162, 178, 266, 276, 282, 284, 292, 299, 308, 391, 412
distilled-filtered water, 113, 239, 297, 324, 450
diuretics, 372
D-mannitol, 36, 187, 357, 538, 539, 542
DNA, vi, ix, 4, 5, 21, 68, 88, 135, 141, 144, 145, 155, 163, 164, 165, 183, 223, 228, 230, 234, 276, 283, 284, 292, 299, 307, 309, 389, 393, 455, 458, 459
DNA polymerase, 88, 165, 276, 284, 292, 299
domains, 150
Dr. Benjamin Arechiga, 334
Dr. Hal Huggins, 334
Dr. Robert Gardner, 419
drainage tube, 367
duplexes, 26, 27, 34, 62, 136, 433, 455, 457

E

earrings, 119, 226, 321
Echinoporyphium recurvatum, 54, 81, 82, 103, 391

Echinostoma revolutum, 54, 81, 82
ecological allergists, 398
ecological allergy, 31
edema, 177, 212, 375, 376
EDTA, vi, 68, 186, 383, 385, 408
EDTA chelation, 186, 383
effusates, 212, 371, 376
effusions, 67, 177, 212, 232, 367, 368, 372, 399, 413, 414, 547, 603
elder leaf, 42
electrical energy, 523
electronic language, 113
ellagic acid, 536
emphysema, 232, 262
enamel, 213, 278, 425, 552
enamel cookware, 213
enema, 194, 196, 248, 263, 269, 270, 295, 296, 298, 405, 408, 411, 415, 426, 448, 449, 450, 465, 469, 555, 558, 559, 560, 561
eosinophilia, 30
eosinophils, 201, 571
epidemiology, 6, 7, 8
epidermal growth factor, 164, 170, 437
epinephrine, 364, 365, 436
Epstein Barre Virus (EBV), 172, 225
erythroblastosis, 164
Escherichia coli, 168, 275
estradiol, 49, 265, 519
estriole, 265, 519
estrogen, 265, 329, 349, 432, 433
estrogens, 262, 265, 519
estrone, 49, 265, 433, 519
Eucalyptus, 89, 90, 128, 245, 246, 264, 291, 295, 297, 298, 304, 431, 532, 593
European laundry bleach, 15, 400, 412, 425

609

613

Penicillium fungus, 222, 275, 289, 365
peppermint oil, 548
peritoneal, 52
peritoneal fluid, 52
peroxidase, 140, 267
PGE2, 59, 60, 63, 66, 67, 174, 178, 182, 184, 192, 237, 265, 267, 277, 280, 282, 285, 288, 292, 299, 305, 308, 309, 355, 356, 382, 430, 438, 459, 460, 461, 462, 534
pH strips, 249, 595
phagocytosis, 68, 144
phenol, 38, 186, 188, 268, 352, 357, 492, 521, 524
phenolic allergies, 398
phenylisothiocyanate, 36, 184, 186
phloridzin, 32, 33, 34, 37, 38, 40, 49, 50, 57, 69, 126, 127, 187, 188, 242, 243, 276, 283, 284, 290, 297, 305, 313, 377, 399, 404, 420, 427, 433, 461, 542
phosphatidyl serine (PS), 68, 167, 277
phthalates, 237, 325, 572
pineal gland, 187, 366, 373, 374, 409
pipettes, 264, 443
pituitary cells, 24, 41, 44, 49, 69, 133, 136, 276, 283, 284, 288, 290, 305, 418, 427, 455, 456, 457, 533
placenta, 5, 60, 135, 136, 307, 397, 428
plague, 382, 508, 511
plastic fillings, 341, 344
plastic ingredients, 327, 349, 408, 416
platelets, 23, 121, 187, 201, 222, 279, 340

polarity, 150, 202, 228, 267, 294, 345, 393, 503, 504, 505, 525
polio vaccine, 140
polyethylene dropper bottles, 443, 448, 450
polymerization, 525
pomegranate, 46, 82
porcelain, 347
potassium chloride, 538
potatoes, 31, 46, 61, 62, 103, 164, 242, 243, 284, 286, 289, 290, 291, 292, 299, 301, 369, 459, 460, 522, 527
pre enemas, 448
pregnancy hormone, 5
primary host, 51
primary tumor, 28, 29, 30, 139, 186, 188, 189, 190, 381
primitive societies, 52, 61
prion protein, 65, 174, 275, 280, 468, 477, 534
prions, 52, 75, 81, 82, 89, 159, 168, 174, 175, 176, 200, 220, 224, 245, 265, 266, 279, 302, 327, 328, 365, 427, 448, 521, 534, 547, 552
Progenitor, 171
prolactin, 137
prostaglandin, 59, 277
protective drops, 122
pseudometastases, 184, 189
Pseudomonas aeruginosa, 74, 157, 171, 225
PT, 351, 416
PTT, 351
pump house, 16, 221, 250
pump station, 250
pure salt, 336, 338, 339, 538, 543, 544
pyruvic aldehyde, 145, 165, 241, 261

392, 393, 396, 502, 504, 525

southerly zone, 65, 524

soy products, 33, 47, 242, 430, 533

soybeans, 47, 430, 534

special enemas, 65, 176, 177, 385, 415

square wave, 83, 105, 485

SRC, 75, 141, 143, 163, 164, 179, 183, 275, 281, 284, 289, 296, 395, 424, 426, 427, 428, 464, 604

stainless steel saucepans, 526

stainless steel strainers, 336

Staphylococcus aureus, 74, 169, 226, 275, 394, 426, 463

starvation, 76, 130, 142, 143, 175, 177, 450

stem cell factor, 67, 68, 71, 134, 135, 138, 152, 155, 183, 191, 192, 208, 220, 230, 232, 276, 418, 423, 434, 438, 456

stem cells, 135, 136, 230

stray south fields, 525

Streptococcus, 74, 125, 157, 170, 177, 224, 226, 275, 279, 281, 282, 343, 359, 361, 364, 394, 426, 438, 463

Streptococcus G, 74, 170, 226, 275, 282, 426, 463

Streptococcus pneumoniae, 125, 157, 170, 224, 226, 275, 281, 359, 364, 394, 426, 463

sucrose, 539

Sudan Black, vi, 11, 117, 121, 212, 278, 289, 313, 315, 366, 367, 384, 466, 603

suppositories, 577

SV 40 virus, 55, 138, 140, 182, 183, 200, 263, 268, 283, 328, 329, 381, 394, 404, 415, 428, 437, 455, 457, 458, 459, 462, 463, 533

sweats, 66, 168, 170, 225

T

take-out bottle, 112, 118, 120, 122, 127, 374, 451

talc, 325

tangerine, 45, 530

tapioca, 47, 531

tattoos, 320, 330, 342, 343

taurine, 294, 325, 354, 447

telomerase, 164, 166, 167, 178, 179, 277, 284, 285, 293, 300, 423

telomerase inhibitor, 164, 167, 178, 179, 277, 284, 285, 293, 423

telomerase inhibitor II, 178, 179, 277, 284, 285, 293, 423

tetra cobalt dodecacarbonyl, 149, 153

thiourea, 88, 127, 144, 145, 155, 165, 193, 284, 459

thrombin, 354

thrombocytosis, 30

thulium, 12, 192, 195, 220, 241, 254, 274, 280, 287, 294, 379, 392, 454, 554, 596

thyroid, 65, 66, 68, 185, 188, 216, 245, 248, 265, 315, 378, 403, 429, 433, 519

Thyroid Stimulating Hormone, 132

Thyrotropin Releasing Hormone, 133

tin, 12, 84, 150, 228, 229, 343, 505

tin cans, 150
Tobacco smoke, 323
tolerance, 130
tomato, 48, 286, 301, 369,
    399, 419, 522, 543
tomatoes, 48, 286, 301, 399,
    522, 543
Tooth Truth, 343
tooth zappication, 375
tooth zappicator, 329, 343,
    344, 345
toothpaste, 199, 259, 319,
    343
toxic amines, 165
toxicity effects, 67, 371
toxicity-illness, 176, 511
transcription factor, 163
TRH, 133
tricalcium phosphate, 97, 98,
    123, 178, 249, 264, 272,
    276, 277, 278, 283, 291,
    298
triiron dodecacarbonyl, 149,
    153
triplet, 27, 28, 29, 62, 69, 133,
    455, 457, 458
trophoblast, 5
tropism, 49, 50, 61, 175, 267,
    356, 430
tropisms, 49, 50, 81, 82
trypsin, 264, 310, 383
tryptophane, 36, 187, 365,
    366, 374, 537
TSH, 40, 132
turmeric, 48, 82, 143, 160,
    162, 163, 245, 248, 263,
    269, 295, 296, 298, 299,
    373, 404, 405, 411, 415,
    426, 429, 447, 449, 465,
    542, 549, 550, 555, 557,
    558
twinge, 308, 431
Tylenol, 363

U

ubiquitin, 178, 217, 277, 285,
    292, 299
ultra trace minerals, 154, 155
ultrasound, 136, 237, 371,
    434
umbelliferone, 49, 143, 173,
    184, 186, 187, 282, 290,
    292, 304, 378, 382, 395,
    396, 397
unfragranced products, 324
unnatural metals, 223, 267,
    392, 393
uranium, 13, 92, 119, 214,
    221, 251, 252, 261, 274,
    279, 286, 294, 301, 522
urea, 168, 218, 313, 402
urea synthesis cycle, 168, 218
urease, 217, 218, 223, 319
urethane, 329, 341, 408, 418,
    420, 572
urine test, 87, 404, 409
Uva Ursi, 561, 562, 563, 596

V

vascular set, 97, 98, 295
vasopressin, 40, 137
vein valves, 3, 163, 188, 284
veins, 27, 84, 87, 92, 95, 96,
    163, 188, 201, 266, 284,
    336
vet, 441, 442, 448, 453, 467,
    469, 472, 474
vinegar, 175, 186, 187, 322,
    324, 552, 572, 576
viral integrase, 207
vitamin B_2, 78, 213, 244, 294,
    354, 362, 383, 384, 429,
    431, 447, 466, 538

vitamin B$_6$, 561, 562
vitamin D$_3$, 248, 249, 264, 272, 283, 298, 315, 342, 429, 592
vitamin K, 355, 356
voltage, 83, 84, 85, 86, 91, 112, 113, 117, 134, 452, 475, 476, 479, 485, 487, 491, 492, 501, 523, 524

W

Walter C. Rawls, 393
watch, 25, 200, 226, 270, 320, 579
water pick, 336, 338, 339, 340
water regulations, 16, 472
watercress, 48, 82
water-holding, 375
weapons, 104, 111, 201
weeping, 90, 304
weight loss, 65, 127, 177, 379
well water, 17, 255, 256, 285, 286, 288, 388
white iodine, 332, 556
white thyme, 81, 82

wintergreen, 160, 265, 356, 548
wormwood, 55, 79, 81, 82, 128, 143, 163, 246, 291, 298, 411, 416, 418, 422, 448, 469, 472, 548, 550, 551

X

x-rays, xvi, 132, 329, 342, 343, 396, 403

Y

yeast buds, 159, 160, 161, 263, 268

Z

zappicator, 154, 195, 226, 244, 248, 261, 262, 341, 343, 344, 345, 414, 445, 492, 493, 503, 504, 505, 524, 525
zearalenone, 179, 221, 284, 352

Acknowledgements

It was the microscope slide of Fasciolopsis buski, made by Frank Jerome, D.D.S that turned out to have the parasite responsible for causing malignancy in cancer. The generous loan of his parasite slide collection, around 1990, made this discovery possible. Now four more slides that were in his collection will take part in finding the true beginning of all tumors. Thank you, again, Dr. Jerome!

As a student he had mounted and stained the entire adult Fasciolopsis buski fluke. It was not shipped in from China or India. It was obtained from the local abattoir on a day when hog slaughtering was done and the same day as his parasitology class. All flukes needed to be very fresh and alive in order to be mountable on a glass slide. It would need to be pressed flat while alive; otherwise it would be too hard to make into a thin specimen. Only a very thin specimen, perfectly expanded to show all details and beautifully stained would garner an "A" grade in this class. Pigs yielded handfuls of these slithery parasites, besides Ascaris worms, which filled buckets. Other animals could yield a few flukes, but not as many as pigs or a wild deer or moose that was accidentally killed on a highway.

Other flukes, especially lung flukes (Paragonimus) were plentiful, too. Pancreatic flukes (Eurytrema) were easy to pick out, as, of course the ever present Fasciola hepatica.

Later, when dissecting the frog, some of these same parasites were encountered again in smaller versions. They were not too strict about their host.

In 1999, the collaboration with Erika Hüther, M.D., of Germany made possible our discovery of mercury, thallium and phenylalanine in every malignant melanoma in combination with the expected parasites. Later, we discovered the tumor nucleus and its role in all tumor formation. Her contributions are deeply appreciated.

Thanks are due the entire staff of Century Nutrition of Mexico, whose personal dedication to the salvage of advanced cancer patients was inspirational; I am deeply indebted.

I gratefully acknowledge the help of my son, Geoffrey A. Clark, as provider of toxin-free food, environmentally safe lodging, and later as computer editor of this book. This project could not have been done without him.

The help of my sister, Edna Bernstein, was also indispensable, as literature researcher.

Gratitude is due our oral surgeon, C.D. Benjamin Arechiga, C.M.F. Without his expertise and innovation; none of our terminally ill cancer patients could have recovered. I also thank our innovative denture maker, Dr. Virgilio Oscar Solario.

Thanks are due my financial supporters, as well as Tim Bolen and those attorneys who protected me from the legal onslaughts of vested interests who would incarcerate me for publishing these findings.

And finally, Mexico itself is to be commended on its research-friendly climate. I am truly grateful to this forward-looking country that made this venture possible.

Notes

Notes

Notes